T0215195

Professional Identity in the Caring Professions

Professional identity is a central topic in all courses of professional training and educators must decide what kind of identity they hope their students will develop as well as think about how they can recruit for, facilitate and assess this development.

This unique book explores professional identity in a group of caring professions, looking at definition, assessment, and teaching and learning. *Professional Identity in the Caring Professions* includes overviews of professional identity in nursing, medicine, social work, teaching, and lecturing, along with a further chapter on identity in emergent professions in healthcare. Additional chapters look at innovative approaches to selection, competency development, professional values, leadership potential and reflection as a key element in professional and interprofessional identity. The book ends with guidance for curriculum development in professional education and training, and the assessment of professional identity.

This international collection is essential reading for those who plan, deliver and evaluate programs of professional training, as well as scholars and advanced students researching identity in the caring professions, including medicine, nursing, allied health, social work and teaching.

Roger Ellis is Emeritus Professor at the University of Ulster and the University of Chester, UK. He edited *Professional Competence and Quality Assurance in the Caring Professions* in 1988, of which this book is in many ways the successor. Both represent his long-standing interest in professional identity where he has published widely. His academic managerial career has been mainly in the education of caring professions pre and post registration, for which work he received the Order of the British Empire. He has taught and managed in five universities and enjoyed a synergy between his teaching, leadership and research in promoting student learning, professional identity development and research and evaluation capability. He is the Director of the Social and Health Evaluation Unit International, which has completed a number of programme evaluations in social and healthcare. His main current research interests include identity in the caring professions, programme evaluation, personal development and learning disability, and value-based recruitment.

Elaine Hogard is the Director of Assessment and Program Evaluation and Professor of Program Evaluation at the Northern Ontario School of Medicine. She has served for the past 10 years on the Northern Ontario School of Medicine's curriculum committee that focuses upon professionalism and medical ethics. She has a long-standing interest in professional identity and its evaluation and measurement and has numerous publications in the field. One of her current research areas includes value-based recruitment for medical education and she is developing a unique psychometric instrument for this purpose: Medi-Match. Her abiding interest in professionalism and identity goes back to original graduate work. It was particularly stimulated by her first large-scale program evaluation which was of an emergent hybrid professional identity. This interest in professionalism and identity led to her working primarily in professional faculties and schools throughout her academic career across Canada, the US, the UK and Ireland. She has supervised a number of PhD scholars who were concerned with professional identity.

Routledge Key Themes in Health and Society

https://www.routledge.com/Routledge-Key-Themes-in-Health-and-Society/book-series/RKTHS

Available titles include:

The Story of Nursing in British Mental Hospitals
Echoes from the corridors
Niall McCrae and Peter Nolan

Living with Mental Disorder
Insights from qualitative research
Jacqueline Corcoran

A New Ethic of 'Older'
Subjectivity, Surgery and Self-stylization
Bridget Garnham

Social Theory and Nursing
Edited by Martin Lipscomb

Older Citizens and End-of-Life Care
Social work practice strategies for adults in later life
Malcolm Payne

Digital Technologies and Generational Identity
ICT Usage Across the Life Course
Sakari Taipale, Terhi-Anna Wilksa and Chris Gilleard

Partiality and Justice in Nursing Care
Marita Nordhaug

Loss, Dying and Bereavement in the Criminal Justice System
Edited by Sue Read, Sotirios Santatzoglou and Anthony Wrigley

Professional Identity in the Caring Professions
Meaning, Measurement and Mastery
Edited by Roger Ellis and Elaine Hogard

Professional Identity in the Caring Professions

Meaning, Measurement and Mastery

Edited by Roger Ellis and Elaine Hogard

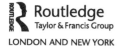
Routledge
Taylor & Francis Group

LONDON AND NEW YORK

First published 2021
by Routledge
2 Park Square, Milton Park, Abingdon, Oxon OX14 4RN

and by Routledge
52 Vanderbilt Avenue, New York, NY 10017

Routledge is an imprint of the Taylor & Francis Group, an informa business

British Library Cataloguing-in-Publication Data
A catalogue record for this book is available from the British Library

Library of Congress Cataloging-in-Publication Data
Names: Ellis, Roger, 1937- editor. | Hogard, Elaine, editor.
Title: Professional identity in the caring professions : meaning,
measurement and mastery / edited by Roger Ellis and Elaine Hogard.
Description: Abingdon, Oxon ; New York, NY : Routledge, 2021. | Series:
Routledge key themes in health and society | Includes bibliographical
references and index. |
Identifiers: LCCN 2020038717 (print) | LCCN 2020038718 (ebook) | ISBN
9780367458263 (hardback) | ISBN 9781003025610 (ebook)
Subjects: LCSH: Medical personnel. | Social workers. | Teachers. |
Professional employees. | Human services personnel--Professional ethics.
| Group identity.
Classification: LCC R690 .P7624 2021 (print) | LCC R690 (ebook) | DDC
610.73/7--dc23
LC record available at https://lccn.loc.gov/2020038717
LC ebook record available at https://lccn.loc.gov/2020038718

ISBN: 978-0-367-45826-3 (hbk)
ISBN: 978-1-003-02561-0 (ebk)

Typeset in Goudy
by KnowledgeWorks Global Ltd.

Contents

Figures

Tables

Boxes

Contributors

Adrian Furnham is currently an Adjunct Professor of Management at the Norwegian School of Management. Previously a lecturer in Psychology at Pembroke College, Oxford, he was Professor of Psychology at University College London from 1992 to 2018. Adrian has lectured widely abroad and held scholarships and visiting professorships at, among others, the University of New South Wales, the University of the West Indies, the University of Hong Kong, and the University of KwaZulu-Natal. He has also been a Visiting Professor of Management at Henley Management College. He has written over 1300 scientific papers and 89 books.

Balázs Ákos Vass, MA in Social Work, is a Social Worker Practitioner. He has gained experiences in the criminal justice system and in child protection and family support services. He has been involved in a number of research projects on social worker identity since 2004. He conducted a sociodemographic study on the career orientation of applicants to a social work study programme at the University of Szeged. As a student at the University of Pécs, he started a longitudinal study on the career profile of social workers.

Astrid Frotjold is a Senior Lecturer in Acute Care Nursing at the Susan Wakil School of Nursing and Midwifery, University of Sydney. She also holds the position of Academic Lead for Simulation and Health Technology. She is a registered nurse with a strong educational background and extensive experience as an academic at several universities in Australia.

Frotjold's research background focuses on clinical simulation, interprofessional learning, digital health and clinical practice. She currently coleads a number of research projects in the areas of interprofessional education, digital health technologies, and the use of artificial intelligence in wound care.

Audrey Roulston qualified as a Social Worker in 1996 and worked predominantly in adult services, specialising in palliative and end-of-life care for 14 years. Since moving into academia at Queen's University Belfast in 2010, she has conducted a number of small-scale research studies on palliative and bereavement care and published research with social work students around placement satisfaction, readiness to practice, professional identity, failing placement, resilience, and well-being. She is currently conducting research around value-based recruitment and how the COVID-19 pandemic impacted on the values, resilience, and developing professional identity of student social workers.

Calum T. McHale is a Health Psychologist and Research Fellow in the School of Medicine at the University of St Andrews, Scotland. While completing his PhD at the University of St Andrews, Calum conducted multi-method research to investigate weight-related communication in primary health-care consultations. Calum's research interests include healthcare communication, psychological intervention development and delivery, and medical research ethics. Calum is a Chartered member of the British Psychological Society, and he currently sits on the School of Medicine Ethics Committee at the University of St Andrews and on the research committee of the International Association for Communication in Healthcare (EACH).

Carl Schneider is a Senior Lecturer in Pharmacy Practice at The University of Sydney School of Pharmacy, Faculty of Medicine and Health at The University of Sydney, Australia. Carl has worked as an academic in pharmacy practice over the past decade in both Australia at The University of Sydney and previously in the United Kingdom at Aston University. In addition to his role as an academic, Carl is a registered pharmacist and registered nurse and has practiced as a clinical pharmacist in Australia and the United Kingdom in both hospital and community practice settings. Under the research theme of patient safety, Carl is an active researcher in health services and health education with a national and emerging international profile in these fields.

Carol Hall is a Nurse and Academic whose role includes enabling high-quality international education for nursing and health-care professions. Carol has extensive experience in the design, delivery and quality assurance of nursing education within the United Kingdom and more widely, through roles in curriculum development and validation and accreditation.

Carol is Professor of Nursing and currently Director of Undergraduate Education within the School of Health Sciences at the University of Nottingham. She was awarded PFHEA by the Higher Education Academy in November 2014.

Christopher Roberts is an Associate Professor in Medical Education at Sydney Medical School. He has held a number of senior positions within Sydney Medical School, within the wider University of Sydney, and before that in the United Kingdom. He is part of the leadership team for the design and implementation of a new MD curriculum. He is a past chair of the Sydney medical and dental admissions committee, through which he led the implementation of the multiple-mini-interview in 2008. He has been an active clinical teacher for over 30 years and has much experience at undergraduate and postgraduate levels, including large-scale interprofessional learning. He has received teaching wards at the faculty, university, and Australian national level. He is a member of the Royal College of Australian General Practitioners.

Christopher Wilkins is a Professor of Education and has been an Initial Teacher Education Tutor at the University of Leicester for the past 20 years, including 5 years as a programme leader and 8 years as director of teacher education. His experience of four Ofsted inspections during this time has contributed to a research interest in the accountability culture of teacher education and in particular the ways in which high-stakes accountability systems impact both on professional development cultures in schools and universities and in the nature of the educational experience they provide. Chris also has significant international experience of supporting teacher education reform, particularly in Eastern Europe and the Middle East and North Africa region.

Colin McNeill is a Research Psychologist working for Identity Exploration Ltd in Northern Ireland. He has 18 years' research experience as a social psychologist specialising in the description and analysis of personal and group identity using Weinreich's research procedure "Identity Structure Analysis" (ISA). He studied under Professor Weinreich. His research interests include development and change in personal identity and intergroup relations, with a focus on personal values used to construe aspects of self and others in situ. He lectured on the use of ISA in research at the University of Ulster during the 1990s and since 2002 has used identity analysis to address and explore social and cultural issues in the workplace and the community.

Damian Day is the Head of Education at the General Pharmaceutical Council, the regulator for pharmacy in Great Britain. He is responsible for national regulatory education policy development in pharmacy, the quality assurance of pharmacy education, and for the pharmacist national examination, the Registration Assessment. He has worked for the Quality Assurance Agency in a number of roles, has worked for the General Medical Council as an accreditor, and in a number of QA roles in Saudi Arabia, Lithuania, and elsewhere.

A graduate of the University of Durham and Royal College of Music, he is a musicologist by background and worked as an academic for 15 years before moving into regulation.

George Brown is a Retired Professor from the University of Nottingham. In his early career, he developed video-training for student, teachers and academics. In the 1970s, he established Staff Development at the University of Nottingham. As National Coordinator of Academic Staff Development for the CVCP in the 1980s, he contributed to Staff Development in the United Kingdom. He was awarded an honorary doctorate in odontology for his contributions to dental education in Europe. He has published several articles and texts in Higher and Medical Education.

Joanne E. Cecil is a Lecturer in Behavioural Science in the School of Medicine at the University of St Andrews. Her research interests include eating behaviour and obesity; health-care communication; well-being; and health behaviours. Her research investigates the bio-phsychological controls of appetite, eating behaviour, and obesity in children and adults and follows an interdisciplinary approach, straddling physiological, genetic, and psychological domains. She combines her obesity expertise with teaching interests in clinical communication, where she investigates health-care communication within the context of patient overweight and obesity in primary care. Her research on well-being investigates health behaviours and how they contribute to stress, resiliency and burnout in medical students and doctors.

Jacqueline Bloomfield is an Associate Professor and Director-International in the Faculty of Nursing and Midwifery (Sydney Nursing School) at the University of Sydney. This role encompasses the directorship of degree programs in Singapore and the development and implementation of international educational and research activity for the faculty. Jacqueline teaches in both Sydney and Singapore and her teaching focuses on cancer, clinical skills, evidence-based practice, and research methods. Jacqueline's research background and interests focus on two major areas: supportive care for patients with cancer; and nursing and interprofessional education. She is particularly interested in how nurses can be educated and supported to care for patients in the cancer and palliative care setting.

Joel Lanphear's career spans 45 years as a medical educator and administrator in medical schools in the United States, Canada, and abroad. In addition to developing four new medical schools, he was responsible for leading the successful accreditation process in the US and Canadian schools. He has served in a broad range of administrative roles in medical schools ranging from Acting Dean, Vice President, Provost, Associate Dean for Medical Education, Senior Associate Campus Dean, and Executive Associate Dean. Lamphear retired from the Northern Ontario School of Medicine as Professor of Medical Education and was named the school's first Emeritus Professor in 2013. He continues to publish and pursues an active role in medical education activities involving social accountability, curriculum development, and quality assurance.

Julie Gustavs works as a Manager, Education Development and Research at the Australian Medical Council (AMC), the standards setting body for the continuum of medical education in Australia. She is the lead educationalist at the AMC responsible for ensuring that accreditation and assessment practices are underpinned by sound educational principles and methods. Julie is committed to codesign methods and the adoption of holistic approaches to educational design and implementation. Her work experience is underpinned by sound research and academic qualifications. She has published book chapters and journal articles on her research interests, which include education, organisation studies, and medical education and has presented at both national and international conferences.

Marie C. Matte is the Associate Dean, Compliance, Assessment, and Evaluation at Central Michigan University College of Medicine (CMED). She has more than 25 years of experience in higher education as an academic administrator.

She has extensive and comprehensive experience in health science programme development, curriculum development, student assessment, programme evaluation, and programme delivery/implementation. For over 20 years, Marie has served as an accreditation survey team member, and survey team chair for the Canadian Medical Association (CMA). She is also a member of the Liaison Committee on Medical Education (LCME) accreditation survey team group, where she holds the position identified as educator.

Marta B. Erdos, PhD, is an Associate Professor in Mental Health and Clinical Social Work at the Department of Social and Community Studies, Faculty of Humanities, University of Pécs. Her main area of research interest is programme evaluation. She is leader and founder of Social Innovation Evaluation Research Centre, which was established in Hungary in 2008 and is now affiliated with Social and Health Evaluation Unit International. Before starting her career as a lecturer and researcher in 2000, she used to work as a crisis counsellor. She has studied contexts and conditions for identity transformations in the frameworks of discursive psychology.

Norma Reid Birley is a Mathematician, Statistician, and Social Scientist, with a specialism in research methodology. At Ulster University, she established one of the first multidisciplinary health research centres in the United Kingdom, the Centre for Applied Health Studies, which drew on expertise across the sciences, social sciences, and humanities. Her interest in the Delphi technique was triggered by this interdisciplinary collaboration. She held Senior Academic posts at Ulster and Coventry University and then was a Deputy/Pro-Vice-Chancellor at Coventry and Plymouth Universities. She then became the first woman Vice-Chancellor of the University of the Witwatersrand, in South Africa, one of Africa's premier universities. She continues to write and engages with pleasure with Ulster University, of which she is an Associate Professor, and of which her late husband was the Founding Vice-Chancellor—and also with her other alma mater, Sussex University.

Rebeka Javor is an Assistant Lecturer in General and Social Psychology at the Department of Community and Social Studies, Faculty of Humanities, University of Pécs. In 2020, she defended her Ph.D. dissertation in Cognitive Psychology—Psycholinguistics at the Psychology Doctoral School, Cognitive and Evolutionary Psychology Doctoral Programme, University of Pécs. She analysed positive effects of bilingualism on cognitive and social skills. As a practitioner, she worked for the Association of Hungarian Talent Support, where she was responsible for talent development and support, career guidance, talent counselling, personality development, and talent identification. She also worked as a mentor for international students at the University of Pécs.

Sarah Edmunds is a Senior Lecturer in Exercise Psychology in the Department of Sport and Exercise Sciences at the University of Chichester. After completing her Ph.D. at Liverpool John Moores University, she worked as a Lecturer in the Department of Sport and Exercise Science at St Mary's University

College, and then as a Research Fellow in the Department of Psychology at the University of Westminster, before joining the University of Chichester in 2013. Her research interests are in exercise motivation and behaviour change, and the pedagogy of teaching and learning.

Stuart Lane is an Associate Professor at the Sydney Medical School. He graduated from the Medical School at the University of Newcastle-upon-Tyne, United Kingdom. He commenced his appointment with Sydney Medical School in 2007, along with his clinical role as a Senior Staff Specialist in Intensive Care Medicine at Nepean Hospital. He is currently Coordinator of Clinical Studies and Chair of the Personal and Professional Development (PPD) teaching theme for the Sydney Medical Program. His primary research interest is phenomenological analysis of human experience. He has implemented the first Intensive Care Unit (ICU) follow-up clinic in NSW, developing knowledge and theory to optimise patient experience and management, while they are in the ICU and beyond.

Theanne Walters is the Deputy Chief Executive Officer of the Australian Medical Council. Theanne has 25 years' experience in accreditation of medical programmes, and national and international collaborations on standards setting and accreditation. Theanne contributes to international evaluations of medical programmes and accreditation systems via the World Federation for Medical Education and the Western Pacific Association for Medical Education. Theanne is a Senior Adviser for the World Federation for Medical Education. In Australia, Theanne is Deputy Chair of the Health Professions Accreditation Collaborative Forum, a coalition of the independent accreditation councils for the regulated health professions.

Tomi Gomory is an Associate Professor at the College of Social Work, Florida State University (FSU) and has worked at FSU since 1998. His primary research interests are homelessness, mental health, evaluation of practice, philosophy of science, and social work education. Before beginning his academic career, he spent 10 years working as a social worker, including as a clinician, director of the first adult homeless shelter in Brooklyn and a stint as the San Francisco project director of the Robert Wood Johnson and HUD coordinated federal Homeless Families Model Project. Currently, he has developed a non-coercive, psychosocial educational model of helping called Solving Problems in Everyday Living (SPIEL) and also has developed a routine brief (five item) student educational feedback scale (BSEFS) currently being piloted at FSU utilized to improve the quality of the classroom student experience and enhance teacher skills.

1 Introduction

Professional identity: issues and approaches

Roger Ellis and Elaine Hogard

This chapter is intended as an introduction to the other 20 chapters in the book, linking them to the book's title and its themes. The book's title was of course intended to be clearly indicative of its content; however, its apparent clarity flatters to deceive. Identity, profession and caring are all quite difficult to pin down. What makes a particular activity worthy of the title profession? How do we describe identity at the interface of an individual and a profession? Which professions can be described as caring and which excluded?

One simple definition is that a profession is a paid occupation that involves a prolonged formal training. Even simpler is the idea that a profession is a job with good remuneration together with social responsibilities. All true. However, there is more to it than that.

Flexner (1910)[1] identified six characteristics of a profession and its professionals, and he is still widely quoted. The six characteristics he believed are: (1) 'professions involve essentially intellectual operations with large individual responsibility', (2) 'they derive their raw material from science and learning', (3) 'this material they work up to a practical and definite end', (4) 'they possess an educationally communicable technique' (their own language), (5) 'they tend to self-organisation' and (6) 'they are becoming increasingly altruistic in motivation'. This is alright so far as it goes, and it has certainly stood the test of time. However, it is mainly cognitive and intellectual in orientation. A professional is defined primarily by 'intellectual operations' and these operations must be based on science and learning to which the profession has contributed giving it responsibility for its own knowledge and a communicable language in which it is expressed. However, this intellectual- and research-based material must be worked up to a practical and definite end. Here we begin to see the practical behaviours and competencies which are the professional's manifest stock in trade. Professionals have to do things not just think about them. Professionals must also have 'large individual responsibility' and tend to 'self-organisation'. So, autonomy is an important aspect of being a professional. Professionals must also become 'increasingly altruistic' that is dedicated to the good of others. This is a window into the ethical values which are the third important element of professionalism.

We would suggest, therefore, that the three main features of a profession are knowledge, competency and values. A professional is defined by what they know, what they can do and the values that underpin this. Training curricula reflect this with classroom teaching and learning covering an appropriate knowledge base and activities in the university and work placements developing a set of complex skills and competencies. By the end of the programme, students must have demonstrated knowledge and competencies through the assessment programme. In this structure, values are a significant Cinderella. While their importance is recognised, there are problems when it comes to their teaching, learning and assessment. These problems first appear when students are selected for a programme when it is thought important that students have the right values for the profession. This leads to attempts at so-called values-based recruitment.

Adding the word identity to profession brings these issues into a sharper focus and at the same time makes them more complex. Identity is open to a number of definitions depending on the theoretical perspective adopted. One theorist (Weinreich and Saunderson 2013)[2] suggests identity might be conceived as the totality of values, attitudes, memories, convictions, aspirations and reflections that are unique to an individual. However, professional implies some selection or reorientation from such a list relevant to the individual's role as a member of a recognised profession which adheres to generally recognised standards and involves an extended training and preparation.

For this book, the recognised professions would be ones considered to be 'caring'. Does that help our focus? – conventionally – yes. Caring is certainly used commonly to describe social and health professions such as medicine nursing, and social work that are involved with looking after people who are ill or who need help in coping with their lives. Teaching has probably sneaked into the category although it is largely provided for pupils who are neither ill nor having problems coping, although some certainly will. The category is by no means watertight. Other professions might reasonably claim they are there to help people, including law, the church and even accountancy and estate agency. Caring also has several connotations one indicating not only that the professional cares for people with health or social needs but also indicating that the professional cares about what they are doing and that they discharge their duties with care.

Perhaps this analysis is unnecessary when we have defined caring ostensively through the choice of medicine, nursing, social work and teaching. However, the label certainly influences what needs to be known, what skills are employed and particularly what values should underpin action.

Professional identity has both internal and external aspects. On the one hand, it is the way the individual sees themselves; on the other, it is the way they are seen. A comprehensive view of professional identity includes all the knowledge that a professional is expected to have and all the things they are able to do to help their patients and clients. The professional curriculum reflects this with components dedicated to knowledge and competence. However, underpinning what is done and what is known is a set of values which determine ethical standards for practice. Developing a professional identity including the right values is both fundamental to the curriculum but also the most challenging for teaching, learning and assessment.

Both professional identity and values are slippery concepts. Neither are directly observable but have to be inferred from observable behaviour. Rather than being objective entities that can be recorded and quantified, they are hypothetical constructs open to different interpretations. Notwithstanding these problems, we will aim in this book to offer some practical findings, advice and suggestions – regarding meaning, measurement and mastery through the curriculum.

The kind of knowledge we have of professional identity tends to be implicit rather explicit. This can come to a head in professional training when supervisors feel that a student is falling short of the professionalism required but find it difficult to say exactly why. They are making a judgement which might be both valid and reliably shared with other supervisors but difficult to objectify in the way an assessment scheme requires.

Meaning, measurement and mastery were chosen to highlight the three themes of the book that is clarifying the meanings attached to professional identity, addressing the problems of measuring it and informing the challenges faced by curricula which aim to develop it. If meaning is problematic, measurement is consequently and inherently more difficult. Mastery depends on clarity in both. So, the three themes are interdependent. In the absence of some form of measurement (of which more anon), meaning will remain imprecise and the curriculum and mastery no more than an aspiration.

We are using 'measurement' as both a general and a would-be precise term. Generally, I would suggest that measurement begins with reliable and objective recognition. Recognition then has to be captured in description. Objective and reliable description may lead to quantification and then true measurement.

So, we might claim to be able to recognise whether or not a practitioner has developed an appropriate professional identity. Recognising is one thing and describing the cues that underpin recognition is another. If the indicators of identity can be described objectively (that is making them apparent to others) and reliably identified, then the next step might be to apply some kind of numerical value to them.

We would argue that some form of measurement is essential for two reasons. First, in addressing professional identity, it makes what can be intangible and implicit more objective and grounded. Second, measurement is essential to assess the outcomes of professional training where we ask – have the students developed an appropriate professional identity, how do we know and how do we validly and reliably assess it.

Returning to meaning, the terms profession, professional, professional identity and professionalism are, as pointed out by Stuart Lane in Chapter 2, used widely in the caring professions but often interchangeably. Definition and empirical grounding are essential to clarify this potentially confusing melange. All the chapters in the book are intended to contribute to this clarification. In particular, there are chapters concerning medicine, nursing, social work, school teaching and university lecturing which consider what professional identity means in that profession.

We were keen that each of these chapters should express individual views from an authority in the profession concerned rather than responding to specific editorial questions. It is interesting to see how each chapter approaches professional identity and how it is conceived and described. How does it balance private and public identity and individual and collective identity? How has identity developed historically and how does it develop in each individual? What social and political factors contribute to the identity? This description and analysis explore our concern with meaning. Additionally, each chapter addresses the problems of measuring and assessing professional identity and finally how identity can be mastered, developed, encouraged, taught and assessed in the curriculum.

So, each of these contributors was asked to address meaning, measurement and mastery for their chosen profession. Chapters include Stuart Lane's chapter on PI in Medicine, Carol Hall's on PI in Nursing, Chris Wilkins' on PI in School Teaching, Audrey Roulston's on PI in Social Work and George Brown's on PI in Higher Education Lecturing. This is by no means an exhaustive list of possible professions, but arguably a representative sample of caring professions. We hoped that each chapter would be not only interesting for its own profession but also raising issues and ideas of relevance to other caring professions. We believe issues of and approaches to meaning, measurement and mastery transfer readily across professions.

Complementing these central chapters are explorations of aspects or contexts for professional identity. Competence is one important aspect of identity. Adrian Furnham explores competence in Medicine as an aspect of PI and Julie Gustavs and Theanne Walters look at the development of competency-based approaches to the accreditation of medical programmes. Marta Erdos and Tomi Gomery compare and contrast PI in Social Work in the United States and Hungary. Stuart Lane identifies the importance of reflection in professional identity. New emergent professional identities are considered by Damian Day, and Stuart Lane and his colleagues look at interprofessional identities.

The second major theme, measurement is covered by three methodological chapters. Roger Ellis and Elaine Hogard look at psychometric approaches to measurement or rather one in particular, Weinreich's ISA/Ipseus, which they apply in a nurse identity instrument and which they anticipate for a medical instrument. Medi-Match Measurement figures also in three other chapters: Marta Erdos and colleagues describe an instrument to explore social work identities in Hungary, Colin McNeill reports on an instrument to measure leadership potential in nursing and Graham Passmore an instrument to explore identity crisis in school teaching.

After psychometrics, two other approaches are described. Elaine Hogard and Roger Ellis consider four key consultative methods and Elaine and Norma Reid Birley look in greater depth at one consultative method, the Delphi technique.

The third approach considered is naturalistic observation and this is addressed by Jo Cecil and Calum Mc Hale.

Not only do these chapters consider the three major approaches methodologically but also they all report on empirical studies carried out by the authors and each includes a substantial case study. We believe these studies together with studies reported in other chapters by Marta Erdos, Graham Passmore and Colin McNeill make up a unique set of research studies involving the measurement and elucidation of professional identity and ranging across nursing, school teaching, social work and medicine.

In this book, we will take a comprehensive view of professional identity suggesting that it has three main components: knowledge, competence and values, that is what the professional knows, what they can do and what they believe. Developing and measuring knowledge and latterly competence are well established in the teaching–learning and assessment procedures of the professional curriculum. When it comes to the values which are the core of professional identity, there are difficulties both in developing and assessing them. The problem of assessing and measuring values surfaces first when students are selected for a program.

As indicated previously, a number of chapters in the book address the measurement of professional identity and values and several describe studies which employ a particular method to measure identity: Identity Structure Analysis and its linked psychometric measure Ipseus. Other chapters concerned with the measurement of PI include ones on observational methods, consultative methods and the Delphi technique. As it has turned out, then measurement and methods of investigation have proved a major emphasis in the book. This reflects our present state of knowledge of professional identity and the need for further studies to provide the firm basis of empirical material required.

The third theme of the book is mastery that is the development of a professional identity through the curriculum. Clarifying meanings and measuring identity and values should all contribute to the curriculum. Contributors were asked to suggest ways in which their chapter might contribute particularly, and their guidance and their views are brought together into a new curriculum model in the final chapter on professional identity and the curriculum. One chapter by Joel Lanphear and Marie Matt addresses the first stage in curriculum, selection and how selection processes can be geared to assessing factors that harmonise with the school's mission. This chapter relates to the outline of Medi-Match in Ellis and Hogard's psychometric chapter where the developments of instruments for selection are described.

After mentioning each of the chapters in the context of the book's design, we will now conclude with a fuller abstract of each chapter.

1. Introduction: professional identity: issues and approaches

This chapter will outline the issues and challenges implied by the title of the book. These include problems of definition and operationalisation of professional identity, problems of measurement and assessment of professional identity, and problems in teaching and learning professional identity. The chapter will consider the ways in which the book addresses these issues and introduces each chapter.

2. Professional identity in medicine

The terms profession, professional, professional identity and professionalism are quoted many times in medicine and are often used interchangeably. This can lead to confusion as to what the concepts really are, and we therefore need to be careful what we mean when we quote them, and, more importantly, what we understand about how they relate to our personal clinical practice. Medical students and doctors are constantly being told in lectures, tutorials and workshops, that they need to demonstrate professionalism in their future careers, so what is vital in their professional development is that they understand not only how everybody else defines professionalism, but most importantly what it means to them, that they have got it right and they keep getting it right throughout their careers.

To achieve this, clinicians need to be aware of concepts that will allow them to develop and truly understand professionalism and professional identity, along with role modelling the types of behaviour that are expected of them. Some of the most pertinent and beneficial to harness the development of one's beliefs and attitudes towards professionalism and professional identity are intellectual humility, growth mindset, belonginess and situational awareness. These concepts are integral to how students and doctors develop. Having a greater understanding and a desire to want to understand and utilise them can only improve your practice, clinical decision-making, lifelong learning and working relationships, and therefore the care you provide to patients and ultimately the way you live your life.

3. Professional identity in nursing

The identity of nursing as a profession is comparatively young and during the last 100 years of its development, in particular, has experienced challenges not usually associated with those professions that are more established. Nonetheless, the nature of professions more widely is now facing challenges in a rapidly changing world, nursing as a profession is increasingly recognised as fundamental in supporting future health and well-being across the globe. The World Health Organisation will recognise 2020 as the year of the nurse, and it is timely, therefore, to reflect on the status and professional identity of the nurse today.

This chapter will consider the defining nature of nursing as a profession and examine historical issues faced by nurses across the world in relation to the perceptions and images of nurses as professionals.

Using the best evidence, the chapter explores the contemporary global nursing and the complexity of professional identity across some very different sociological contexts. It will consider the importance of nurses as leaders and explore the contemporary trend of ensuring preparing young leadership identities for nursing through education and exemplary practice as one means for providing for a strong future profession.

The chapter will propose future directions in relation to assuring a well-led profession that can optimise professional practice for the future benefit and well-being of health communities.

4. Professional identity in social work

This chapter provides a historical overview of professional identity within the context of social work, what we mean by professional identity, how we measure it and how we teach it to students. Through exploring definitions of professional social work identity and findings from empirical research involving social workers and students, we identify challenges for educators, based on competing social work discourses and multiple identities of practitioner, researcher and educator. Findings from empirical research, conducted by the author in Northern Ireland, highlight the learning activities that student social workers found most useful in terms of developing readiness for practice competence and professional social work identity. This research offers insights into the differing perspectives of students based on the placement setting and stage of training, as well as the perceived usefulness of specific learning activities. This chapter concludes with some evidence-informed advice to curriculum developers.

5. "Social workers" professional identity in its social context: A comparative analysis

This chapter is a comparative analysis of social workers' professional identity in the United States and Hungary. Beginning in the UK toward the latter part of the second half of the 19th century, social work by now has become a global profession The question may arise whether the multiplicities of roles and methods of the profession, reflecting the possible complexities of the various cultures and societies, could yield a universal definition on social work – or are there viable variations of the social work profession? The International Federation of Social Workers (IFSW) defines core constituents and basic values that are at the heart of the profession, but the different social contexts and differing problems demand varied the application of the principles and practices, establishing the plausibility of a comparative analysis.

For the social worker, one's self-identity is often that of an instrument of helping. The profession works with 'difficult' or 'underprivileged' populations, promotes 'social justice' and has a special, systemic perspective on human problems with a focus on the person-in-the-environment. The authors discuss the similarities and differences in social workers' professional identities in two countries, the United States and Hungary, with regard to historical and contextual factors shaping these identities. At the rebirth of the profession after several decades of dictatorship in Hungary, there was a hopeful intention in the political atmosphere that social work might make progress in amending possible distortions of the regime change on the social system a mission impossible for a practically newborn profession and its impact a drop in the bucket on the systematic inertia. In the United States, the birth of social work was facilitated by strong social movements, especially religiously inspired beneficence, the rapidly emerging professional struggles for control over 'the personal problems jurisdiction') and alignment with the medical model of helping (social work being the hand-maiden of psychiatry).

In both countries, there are ongoing debates concerning possible roles of the 'social justice project' and the 'professionalisation project' in the development of social work). Both projects have a great influence on the identity of the social worker. Key features of professionalisation – such as its role as a social control government agent, prestige, influence, monopolies of certain activities, working conditions and professional autonomy – have been shaped by the profession's history and the current contexts and challenges of social work in the two countries. The social justice project is not concerned about formal rules and institutions but about the core values and basic mission of social work. The contents of the two projects serve as the basic dimensions for a comparative analysis.

6. Professional identity in teaching

This chapter explores two key strands of conceptualising teacher identity – first, through the fundamental values that shape teachers' world view and influence how they create a self-image of themselves as a teacher and, second, through the 'modes of professionalism' that have been used to relate teachers' thinking about their work in relation to regulatory policy contexts. The chapter focuses in particular on the role of initial teacher education (ITE) in England has played in shaping professional values. It discusses the ways in which successive governments have sought to influence these values through the demands it makes on ITE providers in respect of both the core content of their programmes and the Ofsted inspection framework used to 'police' provision. However, although the specific policy context this chapter is the English ITE system, the wider discussion of concepts of teacher identity and teacher professionalism draws on international perspectives.

7. Changes of academic identities in UK universities

This chapter provides a brief, accessible introduction to the changes in the identities of universities and their academic staff in the United Kingdom (UK). These are heads of universities, their senior officers, heads of departments and lecturers. However, identity is an elusive, polymorphous concept so at the outset of this chapter we provide our conception of identity. Put simply, we regard identity as concerned with how we see ourselves and others see us. Changes in the identity are described, wherever possible, in terms of demographic characteristics, changes in roles and tasks and changes in perceptions of identities and self-perceptions. These changes include changes in identities within subjects and the influence of changes in academic staff training. All of these have changed for academic staff in universities as the identities and functions of universities have changed.

This chapter examines the changes in identity of academic staff, including vice chancellors, senior staff, heads of departments and lecturers. The term 'identity' in this chapter refers to how people see themselves and how other people see them. These changes in identity of staff are influenced by the changes in the universities, particularly since World War I. These in their turn have been affected by changes in governmental policy from promoting collegial approaches to their firm insistence on neoliberal economic policies. This insistence has led to the removal of many organisations, tighter control over research and teaching, learning and assessment and the introduction of hefty student fees. Other changes which influence academic identities are the relationships between employers and academics, subject identities and academic staff training and development. The chapter ends with an overview and a discussion of further possible avenues of research on academic identity. These include limitations of both collegiality and neoliberalism and the effects on student recruitment of schooling and other community services.

8. Evolving professional identities in healthcare: the case of associate professions

The United Kingdom (UK) healthcare workforce is changing rapidly and as traditional roles are reshaped, new ones are being introduced to redistribute the delivery of healthcare in more flexible and responsive ways. In England, primary care delivery is being built around local primary care networks in which the anchor profession remains the general practitioner (GP, or family doctor), but the standard configuration of a GP practice with a single professional group is being replaced with networks in which GPs work alongside practice nurses, practice pharmacists, physiotherapists, paramedics and others. Newer professions are joining the healthcare workforce as well-physician associates, pharmacy technicians and nurse associates, for example. Similar realignments are taking place across the National Health Services (NHSs) in the other countries of the UK.

A conventional view of the new professions is a vertical one: that while they are professions in their own right, they draw heavily on longer established, cognate roles – doctors (linked to physician associates), pharmacists (linked to pharmacy technicians) and nurses (linked to nurse assistants) and that the older roles are their parents. That is true to an extent, but this chapter suggests an alternative, horizontal rather than vertical, approach. In the Office for National Statistics' (ONS) occupational classifications, doctors, pharmacists and nurses are classed as 'professionals', with a shared set of characteristics. Pharmacy technicians, on the other hand, are 'associate professionals', with a different set of characteristics, which they share with the very new professions of physician associates and nurse assistants (as well as paramedics, dispensing opticians and others). That relationship is horizontal not vertical.

The chapter suggests that the precedent for introducing these roles is now well established but may reshape the healthcare workforce in ways that are not yet fully understood. It uses pharmacy technicians and their working relationship with pharmacists and other healthcare professionals as a case study.

9. Professional identity and competence to practise in medicine

This chapter will attempt to assess the way in which the medical profession and patients define, determine, regulate and evaluate competence as a key part of the professional identity of doctors. The concept of competence is both multidimensional and remains ambiguous, which makes any analysis of this issue problematic. Furthermore, it has numerous synonyms such as sufficiency, capacity and adequacy, none of which quite tap the subtlety of the actual concept of com-petence as applied in professional quality assurance. Moreover, the concept gets expanded to cover new areas such as the current interest in cultural competence. As a consequence, much has been written about a 'competency-based medical curriculum'. Many professionals attempt to instil, by formal and informal social-isation and education, a certain degree or level of competence in a large number of specific, profession-related skills. These skills are usually assessed by a formal examination. The central question is which skills, and how best to instil and measure them.

There are essentially three ways of teaching/training people: classroom/ward teaching using traditional teaching methods, active learning through practice and assignments and personal coaching. We are now also seeing the emergence of e-learning and teaching. Most doctors are trained by all four methods. One ques-tion for those in medical education is how to use different methods to achieve maximum competence at minimum cost to the taxpayer. This question is at the heart of the issue of professional identity in medicine for academics, politicians and members of the general public.

10. The future starts now – the identity and competence of doctors and the impact of accreditation

Identity and competency are central tenets of a doctor's practice and key hallmarks of the medical profession. In this chapter, we explore evidence from the literature and undertake qualitative research to identify the stories and per-spectives of a range of doctors, the multi-professional team and their patients. We draw on the works of the French philosophers Michel Foucault and Bruno Latour to trace the impacts of knowledge/power on changing doctor identities and perceptions of competence, and the impact of non-human as well as human agency on changes to past, present and future conceptions of doctor identity and competence).

We focus specifically on the impact of the 21st-century medical education devel-opment, which recognises the importance of professional qualities, non-technical roles as well as clinical expertise on doctor identity and conceptions of compe-tence. We do, however, see further disruption and opportunities on the horizon with technology enhancement rendered through machine learning and artificial intelligence (AI). We conclude this chapter with observations on proposed future directions for medical education innovation and accreditation strategies to better prepare doctors to navigate anticipated change and disruption to their ways of being and competence.

11. The measurement of leadership qualities as an aspect of nursing identity

This chapter focuses on leadership, an aspect of professional identity in nursing and a study using an ISA/Match instrument to measure this.

There are many challenges facing the nursing profession and a need for lead-ership for meeting them – leadership to build quality work environments, imple-ment new models of care and bring health and well-being to an exhausted and stretched nursing workforce. Leadership in its rich variety of types is needed to enhance nurse satisfaction, recruitment, retention and healthy work environments, particularly in this current and worsening nursing shortage.

Identification and development of student leadership capacity and efficacy is critical to this process. To this end, the chapter describes the new Nurse Match Leadership (NML) psychometric instrument and its use in assessing the personal nursing values and leadership qualities of students at a school of nursing.

Recent theoretical and empirical developments in the leadership literature are receiving attention. This chapter will demonstrate how the NML test and software can provide better quantitative and qualitative research data on leadership in nursing than is currently available and better inform schools of nursing about the leadership talent in their annual student intakes. The model of leadership used will be authentic leadership, but the developmental processes behind NML test design permit the appraisal of transformational and relational leadership and other types of leadership, required in the management of capital, cash and resources.

12. Are we admitting the right students?: Seeking the "best fit" with institutional values and professional identity development and professionalism in US medical school admission processes

The development of professional identity for any student in the health professions involves the process of learning about oneself, the content and processes of patient care and the milieu in which one will practice.

The context of medical practice in the United States has changed as a result of a number of influences. Amongst them are the increasing cost of healthcare, lack of primary care physicians in less populated areas, lack of minority students and practitioners, increased preventable health problems related to diet and lifestyle, the need to develop team approaches to healthcare and the positive and negative impact of social media, to name a few.

Some medical students and institutions have developed new courses, new curricula and modified their mission statements in an effort to address the changing environment. Other medical schools, particularly those whose mission statements and curricula are focussed specifically on addressing the issues listed previously, are asking 'are we admitting the right students?' Is there a way to change our admissions and selection processes to identify and measure the candidates most likely to fit the mission of the school and to maximise the development of their professional identity? This chapter describes how some North American medical schools have addressed these issues.

Topics covered in the chapter will include the following:

1   Historical approach to admissions: the old men behind the desk interview
2   AAMC project for admissions
3   Early McMaster work on the OSCE-based MMI
4   CMU admission approaches – results to date
5   Online written approaches
6   Change in MCAT

13. Identity structure analysis as a means to explore social worker professional identity

Key concepts in this chapter are social work, professional identity, resilience, wounded healer, interpretive phenomenological analysis and Identity Structure Analysis.

There are diverse traditions on social work as a profession in the different countries. In Hungary, state-socialist ruling regime claimed that the system was an ideal context for human development and was free from exploitation. Consequently, problems that are the usual targets of social or mental health interventions were not even present in contemporary public discourse before the transition of the social system in 1989. Critical-reflective voices that are normally at the centre of social professional practice were silenced. After 1989, initial responses to problems facilitated the development of two closely related professions: social policy, a more prestigious area with its close contact to government initiations, and social work to help clients via direct interactions. The latter, however, has long been the subject of misunderstandings and misinterpretations concerning its main mission and competency areas.

In the current chapter, authors focus on social workers' identity development processes. How does one become a professional social worker? What are the core professional values, attitudes and visions of a social worker? How are these identity constituents shaped in the direct practice of the profession, and by the volatile and anomic setting of the Hungarian society? In what ways, do social workers serve as role models for their clients? Results of a content analysis on professional documents and practitioner interviews suggest that certain personal skills and attitudes, namely empathy, self-reflective skills and resilience, are of central importance in becoming a competent social worker in a number of different work environments. How do social workers acquire these skills? How does this learning process relate to the development of their professional identity?

Strength-based methods in social work empower clients to cope with stresses in life and maintain hope even in seemingly hopeless situations. In order to apply these methods, social workers must develop certain skills and attitudes via experiential learning. This may begin in a formal learning environment, but the majority of the helpers are also 'wounded healers'. A preceding trauma in their lives motivates them in their career choice and leads them to enter formal training. The trauma can (and in a helper's role, must) be solved in profound and constructive life-transformation processes. Formal training adds underpinning theories to social workers' own stories of redemption, facilitating congruent and empathetic responses to clients, as well as further development of self-reflective skills and a motivation to continuously practice the care of self.

The study involves a more specific exploration on the wounded healer concept as a core constituent of SW identity, concentrating on the role of professionals' own traumatic experiences and resilience in the formation of their professional identities. Interviews with practitioners are analysed, employing interpretive phenomenological analysis (IPA), a hermeneutic method for in-depth analysis of individual experiences and meaning-making on a sensitive issue. Qualitative methods, in addition to yielding insight into the area, also serve as an input for an ISA/Ipseus specification for the in-depth study of the formation of social worker identity to further explore the dynamics of professional values, identifications and conflicted areas.

14. Reflective practice and professional identity

Reflection and reflexivity ensure and enable the optimal development of a person's learning and understanding of their professional identity, and reflective practice is the cornerstone of maintaining this development throughout your career. Good communication, including non-verbal aspects such as tone of voice and facial expressions, along with the giving and receiving of honest feedback, and the ability and desire to immerse in metacognition are vital to establishing the development of effective reflective practice. Reflective practice involves an action-based set of ethical skills and is a skill which can be focussed and polished.

The competency matrix is a learning development theory that is referred to frequently in healthcare learning, especially in the context of simulated learning environment. It describes the inability to recognise one's limitations relating to the learning a new skill, behaviour, ability or technique. While popular in the healthcare environment, there are some significant flaws in the theory based around the omission of ongoing lifelong reflective practice and the profound effect that human rationalisation can have on a clinician's perception of their abilities and professional identity. Therefore, reflective practice needs to be an ongoing process throughout a practitioner's career, always present in the background and even the forefront of their thinking. Patients are the ultimate beneficiary of their learning and development, which is why it is paramount that clinicians start to ensure it develops optimally as early as possible in their career. This requires reflecting with the right people at the right time in the right manner, including themselves.

15. Crisis in teacher identity: ISA guided mentorship and teacher turnover

The chapter uses Weinreich's (2003) Identity Structure Analysis (ISA) to explicate the nature of the teacher identity in crisis. It explores how through a combination approach, ISA and mentoring, can help develop and enhance professional identity by providing insights into issues, conflicts and concerns that trainee teachers can work through with the help of a mentor. The chapter builds on previous work that considered how the combined approach can help trainee teachers develop their professional identity during their training. In its consideration of a combined ISA and mentoring approach to identity crisis, the chapter also explores the psychology of stress and how knowledge of professional identity can be applied to mediate the negative effects of high stress in the workplace. This is also discussed in terms of professional development programmes and mentoring schemes which aim to increase the retention of qualified teachers, currently experiencing a crisis within the United Kingdom, suggesting that the use of ISA can provide more structure and impact.

16. Interprofessional education and interprofessional identity

Interprofessional education has been described as occurring 'when students from two or more professions learn about, from, and with each other to enable effective collaboration and improve health outcome'. Interprofessional education has been mandated internationally across health curricula, and the development of interprofessional competency–based education has been identified as a priority in many tertiary institutions. Historically, interprofessional education within health curricula has been opportunistic with little consideration given to the formation of professional identity.

Professional identity is developed throughout a person's life and career, and this identity has three distinct elements; in being members of groups (social identity), having certain roles (role identities) or being the unique biological entities that they are (personal identities). With increasing exposure and utilisation of interprofessional education amongst healthcare students, all three aspects of their identity formation are altered. Subsequently, their professional identity can be well formed and even rigidly set, long before they graduate from their respective degrees into the healthcare environment, affecting their sense of belonging and the ability to simultaneously identifying themselves with both their own profession, and that of the interprofessional community. Therefore, the need to develop a suitable professional identity and professionalism, in relation to one's colleagues as well as themselves, is essential for ensuring optimal patient care from practitioners working as part of a healthcare team.

17. Psychometric measurement of professional identity through values in nursing and medicine

After reviewing approaches to measuring professional identity, this chapter introduces a novel psychometric method for measuring professional identity through professional values. This method combines an established methodology for identity measurement, ISA/Ipseus, with the Ideal Match method which relates actual to ideal profiles. The instrument measures the values held by respondents and compares these with an ideal pattern for a professional. This approach is based on Identity Structure Analysis and its tool Ipseus, and the approach is described in detail. The chapter then describes Nurse Match: the development, use and evaluation of an instrument for value-based recruitment in student selection and tutorial guidance in nursing. The evaluation of the instrument is summarised. Finally, the chapter considers the potential and first steps for developing a similar instrument in medicine.

18. Explicating professional identity through consultative methods

This chapter considers how professional identity, particularly key attributes and values, can be explicated through consultation with professionals. Four consultative methods are described: reconstitutive ethnography, critical incident technique, expert systems approach and the Delphi method. A case study of the clinical facilitator in nurse education is presented. This study of a hybrid identity combining nursing and educational professional identities was based on consultation with practitioners combining the four methods outlined in the chapter.

19. The potential contribution of the Delphi technique to the study of professional identity

This chapter introduces the Delphi technique as an important consultative method and justifies its use in relation to the study of professional identity. The technique is explained in detail; options within it are considered and guidance is given for its use. Finally, the Delphi technique is exemplified through a case study of its use in nurse education.

20. Observing identity: measuring professional identity empirically in the healthcare professions

Shared values are a defining characteristic of professional identity. Within the healthcare professions, such values include compassion, respect and dignity for patients as well as a belief in equity of care and patient-centred practices. The implications that professional identity has for effective patient care have made professional identity a core component in medical education and continual professional development. Aspects of professional identity are complex, abstract and can be challenging to assess; however, the influence that professional identity has on an individual's practice can be observed and measured.

In this chapter, we propose that values and attitudes associated with professional identity in the healthcare profession can be meaningfully studied through the analysis of communication and behavioural practices, observed directly from healthcare professionals' interactions with patients during clinical consultations. This chapter will provide a narrative review of research that has employed direct observation of communication and behaviour to assess professional identity. It will also present a detailed case study of how direct observation methodologies, i.e. video observation, can be used to identify and quantify communications and behaviours associated with professional identity within a primary healthcare setting.

Observational methodologies are key to studying and understanding the characteristics that make up professional identity. We suggest that direct observation of communication and behaviour during clinical interactions can enhance the development and assessment of professional identify during clinical training, support the maintenance of professional identity within the healthcare services and provide the best practice in healthcare settings.

21. Conclusion: professional identity and the curriculum

In conclusion, this chapter reviews the material in the rest of the book and identifies guidance for those who plan, deliver and validate professional curricula.

Particular foci are on selection, curriculum content, teaching and learning assessment and careers guidance when the focus is on the development of a professional identity. The chapter introduces a new model, of a Curriculum for Professional Identity Development (CuPID), for making professional identity development the central focus of the curriculum.

We hope that readers find the chapters of interest not only for their own profession but also for the cross professional fertilisation of ideas which was an important aspiration for the book.

Notes

1. Flexner, A. (1910). Medical Education in the United States and Canada: A Report to the Carnegie Foundation for the Advancement of Teaching. New York, NY, USA: The Carnegie Foundation for the Advancement of Teaching.
2. Weinreich, P., & Saunderson, W. (Eds.) (2013). *Analysing Identity: Cross-Cultural Context, Societal and Clinical Contexts*. Psychology Press.

2 Professional identity in medicine

Stuart Lane and Christopher Roberts

The terms profession, professional, professional identity and professionalism are referred to numerous times in medicine and often used interchangeably. This can lead to confusion as to what the concepts really are, and therefore clarity is needed as to what we mean when we quote them, and more importantly what we understand about how they relate to clinical practice, from both a personal and a generic perspective. Medical students and junior doctors are constantly being told in lectures, tutorials and workshops that they need to demonstrate professionalism in their future careers, so what is vital in their professional development is that they understand not only how everybody else defines professionalism but most importantly what it means to them that they have got it right, and that there is a need to constantly re-conceptualise it throughout their careers so that they keep getting it right.

The American philosopher Mortimer J. Adler defined a professional as 'a man or woman who does skilled work to achieve a useful social goal. In other words, the essential characteristic of a profession is the dedication of its members to the service they perform'.[1] So if professionals belong to a profession, what does it take to be part of one? In the early 20th century, EP Scarlett defined what he believed were the seven pillars of a profession; technical skill and craftsmanship, renewed by continuing education; a sense of social responsibility; a knowledge of history; a knowledge of literature and the arts; personal integrity; faith in the meaning and value of life; the grace of humility.[2] This 'list' of attributes, as to what defines a person or a concept has become common within modern society, and just as humans have a 'tick-box' of what they may desire in a future friend, partner or colleague, healthcare organisations have 'tick-boxes' as to what they expect of their members. For example, the Accreditation Council for Graduate Medical Education defined professionalism in another seven-point list that defined the core competencies of a doctor as respect, compassion, integrity; responsiveness to needs; altruism; accountability; commitment to excellence; sound ethics; sensitivity to culture, age, gender and disabilities.[3] We can see that professionalism is an expected attribute to be a member of the medical profession, but it also seems to align with old-fashioned values considered to be core properties of a profession, and the people who define these pillars are not just the profession themselves, but society as well. The profession has a contract with society that society grants them self-determination and awards them an elevated status, in return for civic responsibility, community leadership and professionalism.

So, what is the connection between professional identity and professionalism? Burke states that 'Identities are the meanings that individuals hold for themselves, what it means to be who they are. These identities have bases in being members of groups (social identity), having certain roles (role identities) or being the unique biological entities that they are (personal identities)'.[4] This is important for medical students as they develop their identity during their time at medical school, and also junior doctors as they develop through their early careers, and what is often forgotten is that it also refers to senior clinicians as they navigate their established careers. Tajfel and Turner proposed that people tend to categorise themselves into one or more in-groups, deriving their identity from the group and forming boundaries with other groups.[5] This group identification promotes self-esteem within the group and leads to greater commitment to the group, even if the group's status is low. They believed that the three major components of social identity are[6]: (1) categorisation: putting others or ourselves into categories, labelling the person as a way of defining the person; (2) identification: the way in which we define our self-image through association with a group, in-groups being the ones with which we identify and out-groups those who we do not; (3) comparison: we compare our own groups to others and create favourable biases towards our own. This process is very strong within people's cognition and internal beliefs and leads to stereotyping. If doctors are stereotyped as being caring, altruistic individuals by one person, they may now be stereotyped in another person's minds as greedy and arrogant. Ultimately once these stereotypes are formed, they can become rigid.

Coulehan distinguishes three types of professional identity in medicine[6]: (1) technical identity: the doctor abandons traditional values, becoming cynical about duty and integrity and narrowing the sphere of responsibility to the technical arena; (2) non-reflective identity: the doctor espouses and consciously adheres to traditional medical values while subconsciously basing behaviour, or some of it on opposing values, thus being self-deluded and detached; (3) compassionate and responsive identity: the doctor overcomes conflicts between tacit and explicit socialisation, internalises the virtues and values professed and manifests these in behaviour. What is worrying is that Coulehan demonstrated that a large percentage of medical graduates can be classed as having a non-reflective professional identity, maintaining that this outcome is most likely where there are conflicting values in the learning environment. This identity is taken with the students into the clinical environment and with poor role modelling can quickly become reinforced and established. His work further demonstrated that the inability to reflect appropriately was demonstrated by the participants when there were deficiencies in their clinical reasoning, which further highlights the need for good role modelling and mentorship.

This role modelling and mentorship has to begin from when medical students commence medical school; however, there are inherent problems with this, as identity formation has been occurring in every individual since the day they are born, and by the time medical students eagerly arrive to commence their training, they have already have an identity to 'who they are' and 'what they wish to become'.[7] Every person's journey to arrive at this point has been different, as will their journey throughout medical school and their medical career; therefore, educators and educational interventions which aim to explicitly support professional identity formation within medical education need to ensure that medical students, interns, residents and all levels of doctors come to 'think, act and feel like a physician'.[7] This also applies to senior doctors, who need to maintain the ability to self-promote this mindset. Creuss and Creuss explain this further in Figure 2.1, and as previously described by Burke, socialisation has a significant part to play in this process.

The diagram demonstrates that individuals enter the process of socialisation with partially developed identities and emerge with both personal and professional identities (upper portion). The process of socialisation in medicine results in an individual moving from legitimate peripheral participation in a community of practice to full participation, primarily through social interaction (lower portion).

To be more descriptive and prescriptive, what is it that we are aiming for when we state the doctors should 'think, act and feel like a physician'. Greater context is given by Wald with a suggestion that the professional identity formation process involves 'deepening one's commitment to the values and dispositions of the profession into habits of mind and heart, and is fundamentally ethical (including an ethic of caring) with development of a set of internal standards or

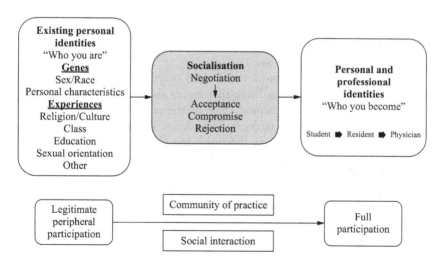

Figure 2.1 A schematic representation of professional identity formation and socialisation of medical students and residents: a guide for medical educators.

Source: Cruess R, Cruess S, Boudreau J, et al. Academic Medicine. 2015 (permission for use granted by Wolters Kluwer).

an "internal compass" regulating the professional's work'.[8] Wald reinforces the notion of continuous lifelong learning of the development of professional identity, by describing it as a transformative journey in which one integrates knowledge, skills, values and behaviours of a competent humanistic physician with one's own unique identity and core values. It is further described as a continuous process which fosters personal and professional growth through mentorship, self-reflection and experiences that affirm best practices, traditions and ethics of the medical profession, and that professional identity formation is the foundation for all medical student education.[8]

Taking a closer look at this journey through medical school and junior doctor education, there must be a focus on how the development of professional identity can be measured, assessed and learned. With the age-old adage of 'assessment driving learning', one of the arguments put forward is that it is not about the actual content of the assessments, but rather the way in which assessments are conducted. Jarvis-Selinger et al. take this approach and make the point that the heavy reliance on specific assessments within medical curricula has missed the interconnectedness of how physician roles shape future physicians, which prevents the development of professional identity. They argue that rather than assessments focusing on 'the work of a physician', they should focus on 'being a physician'.[9] This can be achieved by conceptualising the assessment medical students as the assessment of 'being a doctor' as replicating their future clinical practice, which can also apply to junior doctors going through the early stages of the postgraduate career. Rather than the traditional high-volume high-stakes end-of-year summative assessments, of system of multiple, lesser-volume, low-to-medium stakes assessments, encompassing rich-narrative feedback, such as the method of programmatic assessment as suggested by Schuwirth and Van der Vleuten, could develop the utilisation of expert subjective opinion for the benefit that it can truly be.[10]

Programmatic assessment is a summation of assessments rather than a summative assessment, with each assessment giving rich narrative feedback to the student on where they can improve rather than awarding a binary pass–fail decision. It is the rich narrative feedback that makes the decision for an assessee's progression requirement for learning clear, as the program of assessment gives multiple expert opinions from multiple assessments. This translates to a progression decision that is not only very defensible but also very constructive for the assessee and will ultimately produce the lifelong reflective learners we aspire to produce. This aligns with the idea of 'being a doctor' as the student must complete these multiple small-stakes assessments while continuing to learn within their clinical working environment. This changes the idea of 'assessment for learning' to 'assessment as learning', which once again resonates with their future clinical practice. A further aspect of programmatic assessment is the need for students to triage their learning, and prioritise their assessment completion and submissions, as per their future clinical practice. Furthermore, failure to complete these low-stakes assessments can lead to a failure of progression for students, reinforcing the message that all assessments and learning situations are important, not just the large end-of-year summative assessments. Teaching professionalism in this manner must once again align with future CPD (continuing professional development) requirements, where guidance and expectations would be outlined by professional accreditation bodies and organisations.[11] Therefore, professionalism should be framed and taught explicitly to ensure that medical students and junior doctors understand the nature of professionalism and of their professional obligations. This argument was put forward by Cruess, who also states that it would appear desirable to be explicit about the nature of professional identity formation, making students aware of the concept of professional identity, its links to professionalism, the role of socialisation and the characteristics of the good physician.[11] The goals are to engage learners as active participants in the process of identity formation and to encourage them to trace their own progress through the journey.[11]

However, there are inherent difficulties in teaching medical students to develop a professional identity and to act with the professionalism of a doctor, because in the minds of many, including themselves, they are not yet fulfilling this role. This tension has been vividly described by Sharpless et al., where student illuminate their efforts at 'pretending' during their 'medical education'.[12] In this first example quote, the student makes it clear how the expectations of them do not align with the learning they have received. The student stated:

> Being a first-year medical student gives me latitude to admit ways in which I am an imposter. I am taught clinical skills but have not yet learned how the information I gather fits into diagnosis or treatment, or even what is relevant. When I prod standardized patients, I am often admonished to push harder, to 'use a firmer touch.' To some degree, I fear hurting these patient actors—after all, I will not heal their 'imposter' illnesses, so any discomfort seems unwarranted.

In this example, the student explains how they do not feel they have the right to perform as requested, as they are not yet in the role where they would demonstrate this practice; however, despite feeling like an imposter there is a desire to be part of the profession as demonstrated by this second quote:

> First and second year of medical school, it seems our goal is pretense. We role-play with standardized patients, we dress up, and we fumble with our ophthalmoscopes. We wear our white coats, but we consciously do not yet inhabit the role they signify. As a second year, I feel more comfortable doing an interview and physical exam, but I am only just learning how to use this information to provide care. I am most aware of my pretenses when I inadvertently fool the hospital staff into thinking I have a role on the medical team that I do not yet know enough to inhabit—when I am asked to write orders or call consults. But I admit I enjoy my imposter role: I am thrilled to look competent enough to be mistaken for part of the medical team and can enjoy my successful pretenses because the stakes and my responsibilities are still minimal.

The student describes the same feelings as the previous student, not feeling competent to perform the procedures as their current knowledge is not aligned to their level of performance; however, the final few lines show the desire to be seen as and be accepted as part of their future profession. This shows the power of role modelling, since with poor supervision and mentorship, new doctors may internalise beliefs that certain unvirtuous behaviours are virtuous, since that is 'the way things are in medicine', that is to say it is the cultural norm. However, another major factor in the development of a person's professional identity is the influence of another concept, the notion of belongingness. Belongingness is the human emotional need to be an accepted member of a group. Whether it is family, friends, co-workers or a sports team, humans have an inherent desire to belong and be an important part of something greater than themselves. This implies a relationship that is greater than simple acquaintance or familiarity. The need to belong is the need to give and receive affection from others.[13] Without belonging, a person cannot identify oneself as clearly, thus having difficulties communicating with and relating to one's surroundings. This implies that belongingness is related to identity. However, there is a danger with belongingness in that the desire to belong can lead to conformity, which can lead to the lack of self-regulation, both personally and within the group. From somebody's personal perspective, they may view themselves as better as or more worthy than others because they may have stereotyped their group of which they are a member. Ultimately, once these stereotypes are formed, they can become rigid. This reinforces the need for junior doctors to continually reflect with their peers and other colleagues in the right manner as they develop their professional practice. And this is what brings us back to the notion of professionalism.

When you look at the definitions of medical professionalism, there are numerous differing statements. For example, the University of Ottawa states that professionalism embodies the relationship between medicine and society as it forms the basis of patient–physician trust. It attempts to make tangible certain attitudes, behaviours and characteristics that are desirable among the medical profession.[14] The medical protection society in the United Kingdom devotes a large amount of narrative to discussion of the concept but does not come forward and give a definition.[15] The Australian Medical Association (AMA) makes a statement on it 'While the expression medical professionalism is used in different ways, for the purposes of this position statement we are using it to refer to the values and skills that the profession and society expects of doctors,[16] encapsulating both the individual doctor–patient relationship and the wider social "contract" between the profession and society; however, it remains very vague as a concept'.

The previous discussion and statements suggest that professional identity is constructed at the level of the individual, whereas professionalism is constructed by the community and medical profession. These community and society ideals are articulated in professional codes, institutional frameworks and formal medical curricula, which may or may not be a reality. However, professional identity is a reality that might not correspond to the ideal, for reasons that can be either valid or non-valid. It is based on one's beliefs about what it means to be professional, and a doctor's beliefs may differ from those of the community or other health professionals. It therefore follows that a responsive and reflective professional identity is more likely to develop where there is alignment between the understandings and expectations of others, self-identity and personal values, the social identity of the professional group, and the cultural milieu of the working environment. Since identity implies values and goals, it will also determine motivation; thus, it has important educational implications for self-regulated learning. This means that professionalism must be defined by the individual, and that they must ensure that their personal beliefs and concepts of what professionalism means resonates with the organisations and society in which they operate.

What this discussion of belongingness and identity highlights is that there are many external social and environmental factors that can influence the behaviour and development of doctors throughout their careers. Ensuring that one develops an appropriate identity, defines professionalism to themselves in the correct manner and necessitates critical reflection. This reflection can occur at either a superficial, moderate or deep level,[17] and it is this deeper level of reflection that makes it critical. Superficial reflection is purely descriptive, and while it might refer to existing knowledge, it does not critique it. With moderate reflection, often called dialogic reflection, the person takes a step back and starts to explore thoughts, feeling, assumptions and gaps in knowledge. The reflector makes sense of what has been learnt from the experience and what future action might need to take place. Deep or critical reflection leads to a change due to the experience. To achieve this, the learner needs to be aware of the relevance of multiple perspectives from contexts beyond the chosen incident – and how the learning from the chosen incident will impact on other situations.

So, what is it that allows this appropriate reflection to occur and allows the development of an appropriate professional identity? We shall now explore some further concepts which are integral in the development of beliefs and attitudes, and ultimately professional identity: intellectual humility, growth mindset and situational awareness. These concepts also relate to clinical decision-making, lifelong learning and the development of working relationships.

Intellectual humility has been described as 'Having a consciousness of the limits of one's knowledge, including a sensitivity to circumstances in which one's native egocentrism is likely to function self-deceptively, sensitivity to bias, prejudice and limitations of one's viewpoint. Intellectual humility depends on recognising that one should not claim more than one knows. It does not imply spinelessness or submissiveness. It implies the lack of intellectual pretentiousness, boastfulness, or conceit, combined with insight into the logical foundations, or lack of such foundations, of one's beliefs'.[18] Put simply it means that people have 'knowledge of ignorance'. When considering intellectual humility from a learning perspective, it could be described as a balance between the extremes of intellectual arrogance, overconfidence in one's own opinions and intellectual powers and undue timidity in one's intellectual life or even intellectual cowardice.[19] This allows us as individuals to remedy headstrong decisions and reconsider incorrect interpretations and ultimately allows interacting more constructively with one another. In the clinical environment, it allows us to revisit diagnoses when things 'do not quite fit', thus avoiding cognitive biases such as attribution, affective and confirmation bias.

The concept of intellectual humility can also be seen to be mirrored within the context of ethical decision-making, and once again clinical practice. If we consider the '4 pillars of medical ethics': autonomy, beneficence, non-maleficence and social justice, non-maleficence or 'first do no harm', the latter is often the most poorly understood. How can a doctor do harm, how can they act in a way that does not provide good? Many beneficial procedures that doctors perform and therapies that they provide inherently have associated risk; however, the context of whether this risk is justified is whether the potential benefits outweigh the risks. The context where the risk outweighs the benefit is either when the procedure has no therapeutic benefit, or when the person providing the procedure is neither qualified nor skilled to perform it. This is where intellectual humility comes into play, in that a doctor must recognise that the task in front of them is beyond their level of expertise, and there are the time and resources for it to be provided by another doctor. The doctor recognises the limitations of their skills and ultimately provides good by not doing harm.

Experimentation is a vital part of learning, since when learners experiment, they are more likely to make mistakes, and learning from making mistakes is vital for the development of mastery and for developing cognitive resilience.[20] These are the principles developed from the work of Dr. Carol Dweck who outlines the connection between experimentation and the development of cognitive resilience in her theory of 'Growth Mindset'. Dweck describes how individuals can be placed on a continuum according to their implicit views of where ability comes from. Some individuals believe that their success is based on innate ability, and these people are said to demonstrate a 'fixed' theory of intelligence. Other individuals believe that their success is based on hard work, learning, training and doggedness and are said to demonstrate a 'growth' theory of intelligence. Individuals may not necessarily have an awareness of their own mindset; however, it can still be discerned on the basis of their behaviour, especially in their reaction to failure. Fixed-mindset individuals are terrified of failure, as they see it is a negative statement on their basic abilities, while growth mindset individuals do not have a fear of failure to the same degree, as they realise their performance can be improved and from failure they can learn.[21] These two mindsets play an important role in all aspects of a person's life, not just their professional practice. Dweck argues that the development of a growth mindset will allow a person to live a less stressful and more successful life.

When considering Dweck's theory, doctors who possess a fixed mindset believe that their basic abilities are just fixed traits, and they only have a certain limited amount which can be both reached and exhausted. Their goal in the learning environment is farmed around the perceptions of others rather than what is beneficial to themselves, their goal is to look intelligent all the time. With a growth mindset, students understand that their abilities can be developed through effort, good teaching and persistence. This is important because individuals with a 'growth' mindset are more likely to continue working hard despite setbacks, and an individual's theory of intelligence can be affected by subtle environmental cues. For example, learners given praise such as 'good job, you're very smart' are much more likely to develop a fixed mindset, whereas if given compliments like 'good job, you worked very hard' they are likely to develop a growth mindset.[21] In other words, it is possible to encourage students and doctors, for example, to persist despite failure by encouraging them to think about learning in a certain way. Therefore, once again the role of the role modelling and mentorship in this learning process is critical, since even with the correct environment of psychological safety, and the correct emotional arousal, the students still require the correct feedback to develop their growth mindset.

A growth mindset aligns closely with recognised educational learning theories, especially the circumplex theory of human emotion and learning as described by Lisa Barrett. The circumplex model of human emotion[22] suggests that if something is learned in a greater state of arousal, irrespective of whether the state of arousal is in a negative or positive manner, then the information is better retained. This knowledge is referred to as activated rather than inert knowledge. Circumplex theory also suggests that learning in highly activated states, which is recalled when similar states are invoked, that positive emotion and mastery under stress can be anchored, is harder to erase. Figure 2.2 shows the graph of positive and negative human emotions with levels of activation and deactivation.

According to circumplex theory, people learn better if they are situated at the upper portions of the graph during learning. However, this state of arousal can be either unpleasant or pleasant, as seen in the diagram by the terms nervous and tense versus alert and excited. From the perspective of a growth mindset, people are more likely to feel nervous and tense when they are out of their comfort zone, and this will be usually when they are challenging themselves often

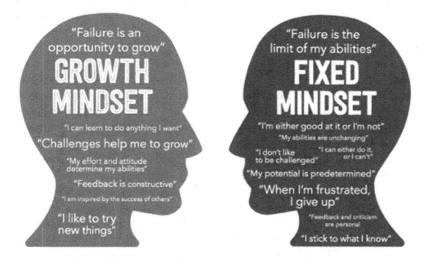

Figure 2.2 The circumplex model of human emotional learning.

with something they have not experienced regularly, which will be an ongoing experience for all doctors throughout their medical career. Challenging one's self implicitly carries the risk of failure, and therefore challenges can only be embarked upon when you possess the ability to accept the potential for failure: in essence when you possess a growth mindset.

The third aspect we will consider is situational awareness and emotional intelligence (EI). EI, often measured as an EI quotient, describes a concept that involves the ability, capacity, skill or a self-perceived ability, to identify, assess and manage the emotions of one's self, of others and of groups.[23] EI allows clinicians to gain greater rapport with patients that enables them to extract more valuable data, to make more informed clinical decisions. Situational awareness is defined as 'the perception of elements in the environment within a volume of time and space, the comprehension of their meaning, and the projection of their status in the near future'.[24] People with good situational awareness have a good 'feel' for situations and people, and events that play out due to variables the subject can control.

There are three levels of situational awareness: perception, comprehension and projection. Perception is about achieving the status, attributes and dynamic elements in the environment. This involves the processes of monitoring, cue detection and simple recognition, which leads to an awareness of multiple situational elements and their current states. Comprehension involves a synthesis of the disjointed elements of perception through processes of pattern recognition, interpretation and evaluation. This requires integrating this information to understand how it will impact upon the individual's goals and objectives. This includes developing a comprehensive picture of the world, or that portion of the world concerned to the individual. Projection is the highest level of situational awareness and involves the ability to project the future actions of these elements in the environment. This level is achieved through the knowledge of the status and dynamics of the elements and comprehension of the situation and then extrapolating this information forwards in time to determine how it will affect future states of the operational environment.

Individuals vary in their ability to acquire situational awareness thus providing the same systems for learning and training will not ensure that there is similar situational awareness across different individuals. Situational awareness also involves a temporal and a spatial component since time is an important concept in all three levels. The individual's actions, task characteristics and the surrounding environment dictate the change in tempo of a situation, and as new inputs enter the system, the individual incorporates them into this mental representation, making changes as necessary in plans and actions in order to achieve desired goals. As mentioned earlier, a doctor with good situational awareness will extract more useful information form patients due to greater rapport; however, this generation of rapport can be replicated across all relationships in the healthcare environment, making your working environment more pleasant, and fostering a better working culture. This is because the possession of good situational awareness usually translates to a perception of empathy.

Empathy has been defined as 'the feeling that you understand and share another person's experiences and emotions: the ability to share someone else's feelings'.[25] However, there is disagreement about what true empathy is, and its role in healthcare, especially among physicians. Another definition is 'A predominantly cognitive (as opposed to affective or emotional) attribute that involves an understanding (as opposed to feeling) of patients' experiences, concerns, and perspectives combined with a capacity to communicate this understanding: an intention to help by preventing and alleviating pain and suffering is an additional feature of empathy in the context of patient care'.[26] The latter definition expands on the first definition by discussing the importance of cognition in empathy, rather than a purely emotional response. Halpern expands this further by suggesting that 'empathy is an experiential way of grasping another's emotional states, it is a perceptual activity that operates alongside logical inquiry'.[27] Empathy can be practiced and can be improved, and the three ways in which you can achieve this are improve your ability to see another person's perspective – this requires listening and time, improve your ability to articulate how others are feeling – this requires listening and time, connect emotionally with other people – this requires listening and time.[28] The lesson is therefore very straightforward, if a doctor wishes to become more empathic and improve their working relationships, they need to give their colleagues time and listen to their stories. This will ultimately benefit them, since clinicians who possess greater empathy suffer less from burnout.[27]

Bringing all these concepts together, can they all be encapsulated by one overriding concept? During my own research, into interns who were faced with giving open disclosure communication, the interns not only encapsulated what the essence of professionalism was, but also it personally resonated with me and made me consider it in my own practice, and if I am to write about the development of the correct professional identity and professionalism, and state that doctors should know what it mean to them, then I should lead by example and know what it means to me. Professionalism as defined by myself to myself is based on 'three rights': (1) I know what the patient has a right to; (2) I know what the right thing to do is, and I will do it; (3) I know the right manner to do it in. This conveniently for me encompasses the legal, ethical, moral aspects of my clinical practice, and I believe it is summarised by the concept of integrity: integrity for me is what defines professionalism. To translate this into a clinical concept, consider the delivery of open disclosure. I know the patient has a right to an apology, I am aware of need rationale and need to apologise and I want to apologise. To ensure that I hopefully continue to practice in this way, I reflect with the right people, at the right time, in the right manner, meaning I do not seek out those who will always agree with me, and I ask them for an opinion before I state my beliefs, while I am ready to listen to their suggestions.

As doctors navigate their medical careers, they have to continually amass new knowledge, as well as learn new techniques and procedures; however, understanding themselves and those around them to a greater depth is the best piece of armamentarium they can acquire as they begin to forge their medical careers.

Understanding concepts such as intellectual humility, growth mindset, situational awareness is concept beyond the basic curricula; however, they are essential to ensure that a doctor's career is successful and fulfilling as possible and need to become part of mainstream curricula. Finally, and most importantly, having a greater understanding of these concepts does not count for anything unless the doctors have desire to want to understand and utilise them, improving their practice and the care you provide to patients, and ultimately the way they live their lives.

References

1. Manning PR, DeBakey L. 2003. *Medicine: Preserving the Passion in the 21st Century.* London: Springer Publishing.
2. Scarlett EP. 1967. The Medical Jackdaw. Patrick Lewis Papers 1949–1987.
3. Accreditation Council for Graduate Medical Education (ACGME). 2001.
4. Burke P. 2004. Identities and Social Structure: The 2003 Cooley-Mead Award Address. *Social Psychology Quarterly* 67 (1):5–15.
5. Tajfel H, Turner J. 1986. *The Social Identity Theory of Intergroup Behaviour.* New York, NY: Psychology Press.
6. Coulehan J, Williams P. 2003. Conflicting Professional Values in Medical Education. *Cambridge Quarterly of Healthcare Ethics* 12 (01):7–20.
7. Cruess RL, Cruess SR, Boudreau J, et al. 2015. A Schematic Representation of the Professional Identity Formation and Socialization of Medical Students and Residents. A Guide for Medical Educators. *Academic Medicine* 90 (6):718–725.
8. Wald HS. 2015. Professional Identity (Trans)Formation in Medical Education. Reflection, Relationship, Resilience. *Academic Medicine* 90 (6):701–70.
9. Jarvis-Selinger S, Pratt DD, Regehr G. 2012. Competency Is Not Enough. Integrating Identity Formation into the Medical Education Curriculum. *Academic Medicine* 87 (9):1185–1190.
10. Van der Vleuten C, Schuwirth L, Driessen E, et al. 2012. A Model for Programmatic Assessment Fit for Purpose. *Medical Teacher* 34 (3):205–214.
11. Cruess RL, Cruess SR, Boudreau JD, et al. 2014. Reframing Medical Education to Support Professional Identity Formation. *Academic Medicine* 89 (11):1446–1451.
12. Sharpless J, Baldwin N, Cook R, et al. 2015. The Becoming. Students' Reflections on the Process of Professional Identity Formation in Medical Education. *Academic Medicine* 90 (6):713–717.
13. Fiske ST. 2004. *Social Beings: A Core Motives Approach to Social Psychology.* London: Wiley.
14. http://www.med.uottawa.ca/students/md/professionalism/eng/what_is_professionalism.html
15. http://www.medicalprotection.org/uk/advice-booklets/professionalism-an-mps-guide/chapter-1-medical-professionalism-what-do-we-mean
16. https://ama.com.au/position-statement/medical-professionalism-2010-revised-2015
17. Reflective Practice in Health Sciences. Types of Reflection. 2010. http://latrobe.libguides.com/content.php?pid=177292&sid=1498201
18. http://www.criticalthinking.org/pages/valuable-intellectual-traits/528
19. https://www.templeton.org/what-we-fund/grants/the-philosophy-and-theology-of-intellectual-humility
20. Paige K. 2012. The Four Principles: Can They Be Measure and Do They Predict Ethical Decision-Making. *BMC Medical Ethics* 13 (2012):10.

21. Dweck CS. 2012. *Mindset: How You Can Fulfil Your Potential*. London: Constable & Robinson Limited.
22. Barrett L. 1999. The Structure of Current Affect: Controversies and Emerging Consensus. *Current Directions in Psychological Science* 8 (1):10–14.
23. Ioannidou F, Konstantikaki V. 2008. Empathy, and Emotional Intelligence: What Is It Really About? *International Journal of Caring Sciences* 1 (3):118–123.
24. Endsley M. 1995. Toward a Theory of Situation Awareness in Dynamic Systems. *Human Factors* 37 (1):32–64.
25. Bellet PS, Maloney MJ. 1991. The Importance of Empathy As an Interviewing Skill in Medicine. *JAMA* 226 (13):1831–1832.
26. Hojat M, Vergare M, Maxwell K, Brainard GC, Herrine SK, Isenberg JA. 2009. The Devil Is in the Third Year: A Longitudinal Study of Erosion of Empathy in Medical School. *Academic Medicine* 84 (9):1182–1191.
27. Halpern J. 2003. What Is Clinical Empathy? *Journal of General Internal Medicine* 18 (8):670–674.
28. https://www.psychologytoday.com/au/blog/making-change/201411/want-better-relationships-learn-be-more-empathic

3 Professional identity in nursing

Carol Hall

Introduction

The professional identity of nursing is comparatively young when compared with other professional groups (eg medicine) and this is significant. It is important to note that during the last 100 years of development in particular, nursing has thus faced challenges to the very nature of professional identity and how any claim to such a definition might be justified. This chapter will consider collective definitions of nursing as a professional organisation and examine historical contexts in relation to the changing perceptions and public images of nurses over time. Changing world contexts relating to the way in which professional identity may be viewed is also important and impacts upon professional status. The chapter also considers contemporary global nursing and the complexity of professional identity across different sociological contexts. The role of personal identity of the individual in determining professional identity is also critical and will be considered to illuminate ways that professional identity is described, conceptualised and operationalised in relation to nursing. Evidence about how professional identity has been measured and applied will be using best empirical evidence from key studies, notably those by Aiken et al (2014) in relation to the impact of registered nurses on patient outcomes and also the Tuning Educational Structures in Europe (Tuning Study) (2011) and its contribution in defining educational characteristics of the profession of nursing. Finally, the chapter will look forward in exploring ways in which professional identity can be taught to nursing students today and learnt by those becoming professionals. The importance of nurses as leaders is a fundamental component in concluding this discussion and will explore the contemporary trend of ensuring preparing young leadership identities for nursing through education and exemplary practice as one means for providing for a strong future profession.

The World Health Organisation (2020) identified 2020 as the International Year of the Nurse with the intention of further raising the profile of nursing across the world. It is thus a timely and relevant opportunity for this chapter to reflect on the professional identity of the nurse today.

Setting the scene – early identities

Modern nursing popularly identifies Florence Nightingale as a key historical instigator in defining nursing. Nightingale's books and writings (especially 'Notes on Nursing – What it is and What it is not' (1865) held a global appeal. Her observations moved a considerable way towards establishing the singularity of the nurses' role that could be considered more than an unprepared assistant to the fast emerging hospital-based medical profession of the time, particularly in Western Europe and the United States. Nightingale identified how nurses could use their voices to create change and enable better patient care in a way that went beyond the pure remit of medical treatment of patients. She embraced the need for nurses to promote well-being and a safe environment for the maintenance of homoeostasis and the provision of holistic patient care, and recognised the need for some nurses (although not all) to engage with and to understand best evidence in order for effective care to be assured. Nightingale's view on professionalism was strongly focussed upon the vocational nature of the work of nursing and the responsibilities of the individual nurse for their own quality of nursing provided. Today, personal identity is recognised as one component of an extremely complex concept of professionalism in nursing, yet it is important.

Nightingale (2020) was adamant that nursing was a vocation that required moral integrity of the individual to provide quality care to patients directly. She was neither overly interested in the development of professional regulation, nor in the notion that nurses should be accountable to any external professional body. She did not consider that nurses should necessarily be afforded rights as an autonomous profession. Indeed, she actively campaigned against this until the end of her life in 1910, on the grounds that professional regulation was no certain arbiter of quality (Royal College of Nursing (RCN), 2019). This stance was challenged by others in nursing at the time who saw benefits in the development of the profession from a more collective viewpoint. In particular, in the United Kingdom, Bedford-Fenwick and Swift identified that collective recognition of nursing status could enable regulation and thus the removal of 'slackers' in the system who called themselves nurses and brought the identity of nursing into disrepute (Royal College of Nursing (RCN), 2019). This they identified, could be best served by a collective definition including the presence of the Royal College of Nursing (established in 1916) and the identification of standard requirements for the assurance of all 'registered' nurses including a declaration of professional 'good standing' that continues to be included within requirements to this day (Nursing and Midwifery Council, 2019). Regulation commenced for general nursing in the United Kingdom in 1919, and today some form of registration is instituted in many countries worldwide as a means of public protection (removal from the register to prevent unsafe nurses from practicing and to reduce the risk of misdemeanour is certainly considered an important feature in making patients feel safe and trust nurses to deliver effective care). Registration has also been integrated as a requirement within sectoral directives at European level for nursing (EU/36/2005 amendment EU/55/2013) with some benefit including sectoral recognition enabling mobility of regulated professionals across Europe and the presences of a monitoring system to address individual concerns regarding nurses mobile across the European Union (Internal Marketing Information System, IMI).

The notion of a collective professionalism thus had long support and some credence in terms of operationalising systems for regulating and monitoring the nursing profession. However, Nightingale's point that regulation is not a certain arbiter of quality has also been demonstrated within public inquiries, even recently. Regulation does not result in an automatic professional identity for nursing either, as this is much more nuanced and layered with the impact of other influences. There is validity within arguments for both individual and collective approaches in the assurance of professional integrity within nursing and both of these elements must be considered when considering the conceptual nature of professional identity today.

The concept of professional identity in nursing

The achievement of particular generic criteria for professions has long been accepted as a means to determine the validity of those aspiring to claim, and doubtless this is evidenced throughout this text. Indeed, one classification of criteria relating to what makes a profession was illuminated originally in relation to social workers by Flexner in 1915 as:

- Essentially intellectual operations with large individual responsibility
- Derive raw material from science and learning
- Knowledge that is communicable
- Tendency for self-organisation/regulation
- Altruistic in motivation

(Flexner cited by Morris McGrath 2008)

Flexner's characteristics plus variations added by others (eg Parsons, 1939; Greenwood, 1957; Etzioni, 1969) have formed the basis for debate around collective professional status widely since this date and this has also included many aspects relevant to nursing. However, such criteria are dynamic and socially contextualised and are subject to critical challenge. Consequently, defining the constructs of the profession specifically has been controversial. In nursing, specific challenges in establishing a clear-cut definition of the profession have related both to the capacity of others to ascribe professional status (or not) through interpretation of professional criteria, and by nursing in being able to effectively determine adequate evidence for such criteria. Cogan (1955), a US Academic, acknowledged such challenges in embarking upon a path to professional identity, warning that on accepting the desire to recognise any definition of a profession one must also acknowledge the complexity of its very nature. Cogan concluded 'The man who addresses himself to the problem of defining a profession should be able to say with equanimity: "It is better to light a little lantern than to curse the darkness"'. (Cogan, 1955, p105).

While it is beyond this chapter to enter deeper consideration around the philosophical utility of professional identity and regulation in nursing (this is addressed in work by Johnson et al (1995) and Saks (2010, 2012)), it is important to note that efforts to measure the integrity of the profession against externally recognised characteristics have been a pre-occupation since the development of the Royal College of Nursing in 1916. This continued, with a peak of anxiety during the 1970–1980s that reached across the globe and became incorporated with the concerns of other disciplines, in terms of defining the professions more widely (eg White, 1984; Matthews, 2012).

Longstanding and evident public debates have questioned the nature of nursing and whether it can be truly identified as profession due to the multidimensional identification of nursing knowledge and practice as both an art and a science, as well as including work that is strongly vocational as well as intellectual in nature. In 1919, defining a specific knowledge base for nursing was a challenge for those nurses undertaking the claim for nursing registration in 1919, largely because of the complex relationship between caring and science where the focus at the time was strongly upon the requirement for a professional body offering stringent regulation and quality assurance (Royal College of Nursing (RCN), 2019). As the requirement of regulation was achieved in the United Kingdom, debates around nurses pay, conditions, autonomy and recognition continued within a deep sociological context emerging around the development of health service provision and the subsequent changing nature and need for nursing within the NHS. The exploration of the full history of nursing over this period is useful to appreciate the timeline of events fully but is beyond the remit of this chapter. For those interested, Abel-Smith (1961) and Baly (2002) offer seminal comprehensive historical UK reviews in significant detail, whilst Davies (1980), Maggs (1996) and Rafferty (1996) complement and enrich the interpretations made with updated commentaries. A US timeline similar to the one produced by Baly is offered by Matthews (2012) and outlines key events in US nursing history.

Development of nursing education

Throughout the 20th century, there was pressure upon the profession to assure that the need for nurses to understand and create evidence in their practice was to be supported, (Hockey, 1985). However, ongoing acknowledgement of the need for UK nursing to move towards greater academic learning (eg Wood Report, 1947; Briggs Report, 1972) failed to be heeded by successive governments. Only in 1990 with the implementation of Project 2000 (United Kingdom Central Council for Nursing, 1986) did the move to higher education begin, as nursing qualifications were moved to Diploma level, finally reaching degree in 2015. By this time, the NMC was under pressure from the European Higher Education Area, who had begun to use the Tuning project (Gonzalez and Wagenaar, 2008) to identify the characteristics of a first cycle degree. In this work, nursing was considered as a specific case and the detailed mapping contributed significantly to the realisation the requirements of nursing more than fitted within the criteria and level for bachelor's-degree-level study. While this may seem recent compared with older academic studies, it is not unique, and is a move that continues globally (eg see Willetts and Clarke, 2013 for Australian context).

Developments in nursing education were complemented by peaks and troughs fuelled by political influences of subsequent governments. In the United Kingdom, this was particularly important, as the NHS has always been an important political pawn. In the 1980s, the need for affirmation as a profession came to a head as the level of preregistration education was increasing for nurses and moving from certificate-level education towards nursing diploma and subsequently to degree and needed to silence those concerns that challenged professional identity (White, 1984). In her seminal paper 'Altruism is not enough', White (1984) considered barriers to the advancement of the nursing profession at the time as political, and this remains globally important today as professionalisation is moving across the world's countries at different speeds. Indeed, it was not always external scrutineers who caused damage to nursing's professional integrity, as nurses themselves have also been complicit at times. Threats perceived by the advancements of nursing to diploma and degree programmes led to UK nurses questioning whether educated nurses were 'too posh to wash' (BBC News, 2004). Although submitted as a provocative resolution intending to make a point at RCN Congress about concerns over education in nursing being disproportionate to practice, the nurse proposers created a catchphrase used by the media to challenge the need for nursing and education progression for many years.

In 2010, a further challenge related to the ethical code of practice of a body of professionals was illuminated through the publication of the first Independent Inquiry (Francis Report, 2010) into care given by nurses at the Mid-Staffordshire NHS Foundation Trust. As Traynor and Buus (2016) identified, this inquiry had a notable effect on the professional identity of nursing due to the espoused view of Francis that pre-registration nursing education did not fully prepare students for the world of the NHS. A flurry of activity forced the production of new nursing curriculum focussed upon caring and the publication of the 6 C's (Care, Compassion, Commitment, Courage, Competence and Commitment) Commissioning Board Chief Nursing Officer and DH Chief Nursing Adviser, 2012 and the NHS Constitution and Values. The image of highly educated nurses who needed to be reminded of these values challenged professional autonomy and caused some to suggest that nursing in the United Kingdom should be refocused onto vocational roots and political sentiment at the time reiterated this desire (Andrew, 2012). The Cavendish Review (2013) focussed upon training of Health Care Assistants but identified the need for those entering nursing to experience caring practice. All of these reports served to define the focus upon the scope of nursing knowledge at registration and the requirements of registered nurses as professionals. For further contemporary consideration regarding nursing roles and the perceptions of nurses in respect of their development of professional identity in context, Traynor (1999), Traynor and Buus (2016) led the profession in offering evidence around internal policy perspectives.

The Willis report, 'Raising the Bar' commissioned as an independent review by Health Education England (2015) recognised the critical need for nurses to enhance their academic status to be effective as registered and accountable professionals in the United Kingdom, with recognition for the need for advanced practice taking nursing knowledge closer than before to roles previously occupied by medical practitioners. Post-registered nurses in the UK prescribing could undertake further study to prescribe medication and treatments and had been doing so since the Nurse Prescribing Act (Medicines Control Agency (MCA), 2002), but impending demographic change suggested the need for development of advanced roles such as those of 'clinical nurse specialist' and the 'advanced nurse practitioner'. While the Nursing and Midwifery Council have been slow to acknowledge this need, substantial work in defining standards in the UK is now accredited to the RCN (Royal College of Nursing, 2018). These roles are not unique to the United Kingdom, but have a strong international following (particularly in the US) and are pivotal in the determination of unique identity of the registered nurse and the preparation of others to support them.

One global profession – many faces – the challenges in developing a global professional identity the development of professional nursing identity across the world

Across the world, the influence of Nightingale was profound, and it is important to recognise her undoubted impact as a global leader of her time. Many countries developed nursing schools in accordance with her guidance and in her name that remain to this day. Nightingales lasting legacy (identifiable by the regular patronage to Florence's birthday on the World International Nurses Day), celebrated every year on the date of her birth and the International Year of the Nurse in 2020, is so recognised as the bicentennial of her birth in 1820. However, while the influence of Nightingale was evident and much sought after by countries attempting to define nursing, her work identified nurses in training schools that prepared nurses as supportive partners linked tightly to the medical professions, rather than as autonomous and independent practitioners in their own right. Since this establishment in early 20th century, development of nursing as an international profession has taken different routes. In some countries, this has been as the result of different educational backdrops (eg The US Model of nursing care delivery, identified nursing quite differently, including a different education model leading to a degree, where nurses were considered more liberal and highly educated than the rather obedient, conscientious and compassionate carers encouraged by Nightingale), and in others, development has related strongly to other existing professions. In some central European countries, where the Nightingale tradition of nursing was not followed, there was no development of nursing schools by nurses and 'nursing' was derived as clear role of medical assistant (Keighley, 2012). Nursing education in these setting was historically limited and subordinated, led by medical practitioners and the development of nursing has been impacted more by external influences. Still other countries developed according to the Nightingale influence (including development of nursing schools), but then were restricted from further developments through national political circumstances that limited development or refused to recognise nursing status.

The impact of the media and public image

Much has been made of the public image of nursing and correctly so, indeed public image regarding any professional entity offers a key thread within the contextual fabric in which a profession might thrive or wither. However, the way in which media has portrayed the nurse has cultivated different images through time that nursing must challenge. It is not a function of this chapter to dwell on historical stereotypes, but to point them out and consider growth away from them. In this context, the summary by Ten Hoeve et al (2013) is simply a useful way to illuminate these issues as faced within a western context. Ten Hoeve (2013) reviewed 18 papers relating to the ways that nurses have been portrayed in the media and found that the impact of early stereotypes of the nurse as 'angels of mercy', 'the doctor's handmaiden', 'battleaxe' and 'sexy nurse' are still perpetuated by the media despite latter recognition by others as nurses with a more 'careerist' image (Kalisch and Kalisch, 1983, cited by Ten Hoeve, 2013). This is changing as public recognition of nursing is beginning to include a more careerist stance and the profession itself rejects physical embodiments of previous times. Nonetheless, changing public perception is challenging and takes time. Images of nursing in particular have been shown to develop in childhood, and these are retained and latently supported by media. An excellent example of the lasting impact of stereotyping can be seen in the following example:

> Despite considerable work currently being undertaken by the NHS Horizons Team and Nursing Now England during 2018/19 to reframe the portrayal of nurses in the UK (including the changing of media perceptions of uniform by school children including presentation of contemporary mini uniforms to schools which include Scrubs tops and trousers) the Guinness World GWR faced criticism when a nurse dressed in her own contemporary uniform was not considered to have succeeded in achieving a world record for the fastest marathon in a nurses uniform because the clothing worn did not conform to their requirements which stipulated that a nurse's uniform must include a blue or white dress, a white pinafore apron and a traditional white nurse's cap.
>
> (Otte, 2019)

GWR were forced into changing the rules and awarding the record, but the illustration of the potential impact of media is an important factor in regularising latent stereotypes within collective professional and that despite efforts to change, Ten Hoeve et al (2013) conclusion that the media does not yet meet the professional image of nursing remains supported. In considering stereotypes though, there is an important issue of professional cultural identity that must be respected and should be noted with extreme care when defining nursing. The above scenario is British and framed by UK expectations. In other settings, nurses may wear uniforms of the nature described without issue. However, within the United Kingdom, there is a conflict between the concepts of the nurse within a contemporary UK context that includes a very different type of clothing (notably in this case 'scrubs') identified by GWR as being more associated with medical staff. A bigger issue, related to this scenario, though must relate to the lack of diversity within the images of nursing portrayed by the media. Despite image of multi-ethnic backgrounds increasing in the popular media, the idea that nursing as a profession is diverse remains a work in progress.

Further challenges associated with public image of the collective identity of nursing as a profession may relate to a public views that nurses are caring and that caring is equated to vocational rather than professional, and technical rather than academic due to the perceived ability of caring to be inherent rather than learnt. This point is raised by Andrew (2012) (in her consideration 'Professionalism – Are we there yet'? When she also pertinently questions if nursing, and its roots in professional practice rather than academia is being set up to fail by the competing requirements of academy teaching and research and practice.

Finally, professional culture is an aspect of identity that is critical to the development of nursing across the world. Cross-cutting elements (including gender, status, politics, religion and professional expectations both within and outside of nursing) form key cultural perspectives about the acceptability and status of the profession of nursing to populations and also to nurses themselves. In the next section though, it is important to return to Nightingales consideration of individual responsibility as discussed in the introduction to this chapter.

Nightingale identified that individuals in nursing have a role to play in the development of the profession and that collective regulation was no arbiter of quality. While this was opposed at the time and regulation has become fundamental across the world, it is important to consider the role of individuals in determining professional identity and in enhancing and developing professional practice.

Measuring the effectiveness of professional identities

Attempts to determine the efficacy of roles within nursing have been acknowledged as beneficial in respect of assuring the quality of a workforce for care and to counter arguments regarding the need for registered nurses to be educated within higher education and to the minimum of degree level. Most recently, in the RN4CAST Consortium, Aiken et al (2014) led the world in significant work in this area across the world through comparative studies that have empirically explored the relationship between patient outcomes and the number of registered nurses and degree qualification. These studies have affirmed the need for a highly qualified workforce to enhance care and reduce patient mortality.

Individual professional identity

While collective status has offered the mainstay over many years in defining the professional identity of nursing (and has served some purpose in regulating and elevating the status of a profession), the above discussion shows that this is contextual and can be damaged as a country changes its politics or scrutiny reveals discrediting weaknesses. Further, despite initial standpoints of those requiring professional registration and a collective identity, this ideology is more nuanced in practice where nursing is reliant upon more than simply the characteristics that define it. From a sociological perspective, the work of Giddens (1991) identified the importance of self in establishing professional identity, noting that explaining or enabling professional identity simply on the basis of characterising a profession is not a feasible position. Although controversial in many ways to experts of sociology and philosophy, (of which I am neither) Gidden's work on structuration explained sociological relationships between professions as social organisations and individual agency of professionals and professional behaviours. He countered that such a consideration is always necessary, as individual perceptions, positions and personal esteem can strongly influence the way in which the professional views themselves and are viewed by others. This stance is compelling in respect of nursing because the way that nursing is seen as profession also depends upon who is looking, and may have capacity to influence any outcome (as we saw in the Francis inquiry example before). Andrew (2012) in asking 'Professional identity in nursing - are we there yet?' embraced the challenge faced by a merging view of professional identity of the individual and of the organisation. Andrew also looked at the impact of professional change upon perceptions of professional identity, identifying in particular the impact of nurse educators of changes in professional identity relating to movement from health-based nursing schools into university department. Social identity theory (SIT) (Willetts and Clarke, 2013) may have also utility in considering nursing identity since it embraces the capacity to consider a range of social identities including those that are key to determining professional roles and also the impact of cross-cutting individual roles that are unique but impactful. SIT enables the perception of nursing to be explored from individual perspectives in a way that is contextualised to their situation. For nursing, which has struggled with attracting individuals to the profession and which has a wide base for recruitment, understanding how people value nursing as a profession and see themselves within it is clearly important. An example of work undertaken to attempt to relate to cross-cutting identities includes the impact of generational identity upon the work of nursing. This work attempted to consider both personal identities and the relationship to organisational needs and identity in an attempt to recruit and retain nurses within the NHS.

Johnson et al (2012) took the notion of self-concept and professional identity in nursing further by focussing upon the role of the individual in creating their own critically important professional identity. While this may be criticised for not including the contextual organisational elements, Johnson et al (2012) posit that the professional identity of the individual is influential and that groups of individuals with strong and well-articulated professional identities are needed in order to move the whole institution of nursing forward as a profession. For nursing education, these points made by Johnson et al (2012) are critically important as they identify professional identity as a career-long element of an individual's contribution and notes that professional identity is likely to change throughout this span. Threats to professional identity at an individual level must be addressed by education and also by the profession if the development of nursing's professional identity is to be a coherent and positive articulation strongly visible to others outside of nursing. As a modern theory, this holds considerable weight and it is easy to see how this is being adopted as a more credible stance in assuring the future of nursing. Major global initiatives such as 'Nursing Now' aimed towards raising the awareness and profile of nursing globally have focussed their efforts on the development of leaders for nursing – identifying the potential impact of nurses in the development of the world's health and in supporting the Global Sustainable Development Goals. The Nightingale Challenge (Nursing Now, 2019) focusses effort upon global communities committing to enhancing leadership development of young registered nurses and the aim of achieving 20,000 new young leaders in nursing in 2020.

Implications of professional identity for teaching learning and curriculum

Professional identity is critical for nursing and educators play a key part in the way in which this continues to be developed across the world. Professional identity and the way in which nursing is accorded within any countries legislative status significantly influence how and where nursing education might take place. In some countries (eg Germany, Austria, Luxembourg), full progression towards degree-level education has been limited through the legal identification of nursing as being vocationally led. While this is changing, there are still many challenges to the further enhancement of the profession. For nurse educators, this has also meant that they have had conflicting expectations. Countries (eg United Kingdom, Ireland) entering higher education for the first time need to meet requirements for academic status as well as retaining credible professional identities. Andrew (2012) identifies that being expert clinical professionals and educators as well as having a credible research and academic base can be stressful and lead to stress and low esteem. In other countries, a move towards higher or advanced-level education may be limited due to their countries legal position. In Portugal, the development of PhD's in nursing has been can only be awarded by universities and the subject of nursing can only be taught by nurse teachers employed within nursing schools (not in universities). Since the subject expert must supervise PhD studies, innovative collaborations between universities and partnering nursing schools have had to be employed to enable the development of PhD's for nursing in Portugal and the situation remains a complex one. Yet there have also been advantages, the development of higher education across some countries of the world has meant a movement of nurses to gain PhD's and develop research capacity. Educators in particular, have been supported by governments in order to develop capacity. Many post-registered nursing students attend UK universities from across the world to learn about advanced nursing practice and to research their own health care systems. They bring new ideas and a new sense of global professional identity while they achieve their degrees. With the right support in the future, these nurses also offer the benefit of new professional identities across the world.

For nurse educators the opportunity to participate in global accreditation of programmes for nursing is an immense privilege and one that affords opportunities for considering the content of study programmes that can enhance leadership and professional identity at an early career stage. Individual encouragement and inclusion of students in important global development, whether in education or research or in practice, fosters recognition of the critical importance of early professional identity. Nurse academics play a significant role in recruitment of students and in enhancing their developing perceptions of nursing. Johnson et al (2012) address these points well in terms of how personal professional identity develops and may be challenged throughout a nursing career, but it is educators and practitioners who can support developing roles consider how new nurses experience their careers as well as envisage this for the profession of nursing.

Note bene – the role of leadership

Finally, it is prudent to consider the role of leadership in developing future professional identity for nursing. Nursing leadership has traditionally been hierarchical and positional, with nurses earning promotion and credibility throughout their careers. In concluding this chapter, it is proposed that this system is insufficient to assure future nursing and maximise the contribution of all. There is increasing recognition of the need for a more devolved leadership and contribution supported by key initiatives such for quality (eg the US-led Magnet Status for hospitals) and employing techniques that value the contributions of all, such as the business model of appreciative inquiry (Cooperider and Whitney, 2005). To prepare nurses for a future that is more collaborative will however require considerable investment; educators, practitioners and clinical managers must work together to support education and practice to enable the achievement of such expectations and manage existing prejudices. Junior leadership programmes such as 150 Leaders (UK Council of Deans for Health) and the European Junior leadership academy, combined with new opportunities for nursing including the contemporary application of reverse mentoring, enable possibility for future thinking that may develop individual and collective nursing identities in new ways.

References

Abel-Smith B (1961) History of the Nursing Profession. London: Heinemann.
Aiken LH, Sloane DM, Bruyneel L, et al (2014) Nurse staffing and education and hospital mortality in nine European countries: a retrospective observational study. Lancet 383, 1824–1830.

Andrew N (2012) Professional identity in nursing: are we there yet? Nurse Education Today 32(8), 846–849.

Baly MF (2002) Nursing and Social Change (3rd Edition). London: Routledge.

BBC News (2004) Nurses cannot be too posh to wash. 10 May. http://news.bbc.co.uk/ accessed 6/6/2020.

Cavendish C (2013) The Cavendish review: an independent review into healthcare assistants and support workers in the NHS and social care settings. https://assets.publishing. service.gov.uk/government/uploads/system/uploads/attachment_data/file/236212/ Cavendish_Review.pdf accessed 12/10/20.

Cogan ML (1955) The problem of defining a profession. The Annals of the American Academy of Political and Social Science 297 (1), 105–111.

Commissioning Board Chief Nursing Officer and DH Chief Nursing Adviser (4 December 2012) Compassion in Practice: Nursing, Midwifery and Care Staff Our Vision and Strategy. London: NHS Commissioning Board/Department of Health.

Cooperider D, Whitney D (2005) Appreciative Inquiry: A Positive Revolution in Change. San Francisco, CA: Berrett-Koehler Publishers.

Davies C (1980) Rewriting Nursing History. London: Croom Helm.

Etzioni A (1969). The Semi-Professions and Their Organization: Teachers, Nurses, Social Workers. New York: Free Press.

Giddens A (1991) Modernity and Self-Identity: Self and Society in the Late Modern Age. Stanford: Stanford University Press.

Gonzalez J, Wagenaar R (2008) Universities Contribution to the Bologna Process the Tuning Project (2nd Edition). Bilbao, Spain: University of Deusto.

Greenwood E (1957) Attributes of a Profession. Social Work 2 (3), 45–55.

Health Education England (2015) Raising the Bar Shape of Caring: A Review of the Future Education and Training of Registered Nurses and Care Assistants Chair Lord Willis London HEE https://www.hee.nhs.uk/ accessed 12/10/20.

Hockey L (1985) Nursing Research: Mistakes and Misconceptions. Churchill, Edinburgh: Livingstone.

Johnson M, Cowin L, Wilson I, Young H (2012) Professional identity and nursing: contemporary theoretical developments and future research challenges. International Nursing Review 59, 562–569.

Johnson T, Larkin G, Saks M (Eds.) (1995) Health Professions and the State in Europe. London: Routledge.

Keighley T (2012) Accession to the European Union 2001–2010: a reflection on some of the ethical issues for nursing. Nursing Ethics 19(1), 160–166.

Maggs, C (1996) A history of nursing: a history of caring? Journal of Advanced Nursing 23, 630–635.

Matthews J (2012) Role of Professional Organizations in Advocating for the Nursing Profession OJIN. The Online Journal of Issues in Nursing 17(1), 3.

McGrath MP (2008) Reinterpreting Abraham Flexner's Speech, "Is Social Work a Profession?": its meaning and influence on the field's early professional development. Social Service Review 82(1), 29–60.

Medicines Control Agency (2002) Proposals for Supplementary Prescribing by Nurses and Pharmacists and Proposed Amendments to the Prescription Only Medicines (Human Use) Order 1997. MLX 284. London: Medicines Control Agency.

Nightingale F (2020) Notes on Nursing: What It is, and What it is Not 160th Anniversary Edition. London UK: Wolters Kluwer.

Nursing and Midwifery Council (2019) Guidance on Good health and Character. London NMC January. https://www.nmc.org.uk/ accessed 06/06/2020.

Otte J (2019) Nurse in Trousers told her London Marathon Record would not count. *The Guardian*. Saturday 5th May. https://www.theguardian.com/ accessed 6/6/20.

Parsons T (1939) The professions and social structure. Social Forces 17, 457–67.

Rafferty A (1996) The Politics of Nursing Knowledge. London: Routledge.

Report of the Committee on Nursing (1972) Chairman: Professor Asa Briggs, CMND. 5115, London: HMSO.

Report of the Mid Staffordshire NHS Foundation Trust Public Inquiry (2013) Chair Robert Francis QC. CMD HC 947. London: TSO/HMSO.

Report of the Working Party on Recruitment and Training of Nurses (1947) Chair Paul Wood, London: HMSO.

Royal College of Nursing (2018) Standards for Advanced Level Nursing Practice. London: RCN.

Royal College of Nursing (RCN) (2019) Wake up slackers! The great nursing registration controversy https://www.rcn.org.uk accessed 6/6/2020.

Saks M (2010) Analyzing the professions: the case for the Neo-Weberian approach. Comparative Sociology 9, 887–915.

Saks M (2012) Defining a Profession: the role of knowledge and expertise. Professions and Professionalism 2 (1), 1–10.

Ten Hoeve Y, Jansen G, Roodbol P (2013) The nursing profession: public image, self-concept and professional identity. A discussion paper. Journal of Advanced Nursing 70 (2), 295–309.

Traynor M (1999) Managerialism and Nursing: Beyond Oppression and Profession. London: Routledge.

Traynor M, Buus N (2016) Professional Identity in Nursing: UK students explanations for poor standards of care. Social Science and Medicine 166, 186–194.

Tuning Educational Structures in Europe (Tuning Study) (2011) Reference Points for the Design and Delivery of Degree Programmes in Nursing. Bilbao, Spain: Deusto University Press. http://www.unideusto.org/accessed 6/6/2020.

United Kingdom Central Council for Nursing (1986) Project 2000: A New Preparation for Practice. London: UKCC.

White R (1984) Altruism is not enough: barriers in the development of nursing as a profession. Journal of Advanced Nursing 9 (6), 537–637.

Willetts G, Clarke D (2013) Constructing nurses' professional identity through social identity theory. International Journal of Nursing Practice 20 (2), 164–169.

World Health Organisation (2020) Executive Board designates 2020 as the "Year of the Nurse and Midwife" News Release Geneva Switzerland 30 January.

4 Professional identity in social work

Audrey Roulston

Introduction and chapter overview

This chapter provides a historical overview of professional identity within the context of social work. We explore what we mean by professional identity, how we measure it and the role of social work educators in terms of how it can be taught to students. In order to answer this, we need to explore various definitions of professional social work identity, to find emerging commonalities and trends. We also need to explore the findings from empirical research involving social workers and students, to establish their perceptions about how professional identity can be developed and what values or skills render the professional identity of social workers unique. We subsequently explore the challenges for educators, based on competing social work discourses, their perceived power as 'gatekeepers' to the profession and multiple identities of practitioner, researcher and educator. Empirical research conducted by the author in Northern Ireland highlights the learning activities that student social workers found most useful in terms of developing readiness for practice competence and professional social work identity (Cleak et al., 2016; Roulston et al., 2018). Undergraduate social work students who were on their first or final practice placement/practice learning opportunity (PLO) were asked the following questions: 'Overall, what did you find most helpful in assisting your learning during PLO?' and 'What would have improved your learning during PLO?' The findings offer some insights into the differing perspectives of students based on the setting and whether it was their first or final PLO as well as the perceived usefulness of specific learning activities. This chapter will conclude with some advice to curriculum developers based on the academic literature and findings from the author's empirical research.

The meaning of professional identity

According to Gibelman (1999), debates about status and identity of the social work profession have been around for over a century, since Flexner (1915) questioned if social work was a profession, and when Richmond (1917) sought to identify the skills underpinning interventions with individuals and families. A land-mark study conducted by Boehm (1957) concluded that the core activities of social work had not been authoritatively differentiated.

Since 1956 various definitions, varying in breadth and scope have emerged beginning with the Commission on Social Work Practice of the newly formed National Association of Social Workers (NASW) who proposed that the purpose of social work was to assist individuals and groups in identifying and resolving or minimising problems arising out of disequilibrium; to identify potential areas of disequilibrium… to prevent the occurrence of disequilibrium; and to seek out, identify and strengthen the maximum potential in individuals, groups and communities (National Association of Social Workers, Commission on Social Work Practice, 1956, pp. 1028–1029). Crouch (1979, p. 46) subsequently suggested that 'Social work is the attempt to assist those who do not command the means to human subsistence in acquiring them and in attaining the highest possible degree of independence'. Over the past 50 years, the NASW Task force on Labour Force have suggested several definitions, with the most recent indicating that social workers help individuals, families and groups restore or enhance their capacity for social functioning and work to create societal conditions that support communities in need (NASW, 2016). This is supported by the *Code of Ethics* (NASW, 2016, para 1), which states that the primary mission of the social work profession is to 'enhance human well-being and help meet the basic human needs of all people, with particular attention to the needs and empowerment of people who are vulnerable, oppressed and living in poverty'. This is in keeping with the global definition of social work, approved by the International Federation of Social Workers (IFSW) General Meeting and the International Association of Schools of Social Work (IASSW) General Assembly in July 2014, which states that:

> Social work is a practice-based profession and an academic discipline that promotes social change and development, social cohesion, and the empowerment and liberation of people. Principles of social justice, human rights, collective responsibility, and respect for diversities and central to social work. Underpinned by theories of social work, social sciences, humanities and indigenous knowledge, social work engages people and structures to address life challenges and enhance wellbeing.

The British Association of Social Worker's Code of Ethics for social workers in the United Kingdom was first adopted in 1975 but has been revised and updated on several occasions.

Despite fluidity within the historical overview of definitions, social work's identity and purpose is informed by a universal set of core values underpinning practice, which highlight its uniqueness from other caring professions (Risler et al., 2003). These values include social justice, human dignity and worth, respect for people, integrity and competence (Gibelman, 1999; Hawkins et al., 2001; Payne, 2005; Risler et al., 2003). These values reflect social work associations' ethical codes of conduct and enumerate social work ethics globally (Australian Association of Social Workers [AASW], 2010; British Association of Social Workers, 2002; NASW, 2008).

The broadness of the social work field is embedded within the different levels of social work: micro (i.e. individuals and families), mezzo (i.e. groups, communities and organisations) and macro (i.e. cities, policies and systemic advocacy) (Forenza and Eckert, 2018). Regardless of a social worker's practice area or level, a commitment to social justice and equitable treatment of all are common throughout the profession (Bradley et al., 2012).

The measurement of professional identity

Despite Wiles (2013) describing professional identity as an abstract construct, a number of research studies conducted with social work students or new social workers have attempted to measure professional identity. Wiles (2013) conducted qualitative research and suggested three approaches to nurturing professional identity in social work students, which included cultivating desired professional traits, facilitating collective identity and fostering an intrapersonal process towards professionalism. Levy et al. (2014) suggested that satisfaction with supervision, empathy and professional values were all related to developing a professional identity for social work students.

Forenza and Eckert (2018) conducted qualitative research with new social workers around professional identity using three qualities of healthy social identity proposed by Wenger, which were connectedness (i.e. enduring social relationships), expansiveness (i.e. the scope of social–professional identity) and effectiveness (i.e. positive or negative perceptions of identity). Findings from Forenza and Eckert (2018) indicated an inherent bond between social workers and a common language that supported social justice, empathy and strength-based practice, with participants stating that social justice was the 'hallmark of their professional identity', that it enabled them to 'address inequity, bias, oppression and other forces', and one participant believed that the 'commitment to social justice differentiated social workers from other allied health professional' (Forenza and Eckert, 2018, p. 20). Other participants found that their professional identity was easily recognisable as professional skills and values merged into everyday interpersonal relationships.

Data collected from a literature review by Ornellas et al. (2019) was analysed using qualitative content analysis to map social work across 10 countries and make cross-national comparisons of its structure, identity and development. Findings indicated that social work values were uniform across the 10 participating countries (e.g. the United Kingdom, Italy, Spain, Portugal, Brazil, Turkey, South Africa, China, India and Russia) and were based upon their respective codes of ethics, the global definition of social work (IFSW, 2014) or the IASSW. Ornellas et al. (2019) also reported that the social work value system in each country was linked to established tasks and roles of the social work profession, with some countries prioritising specific values over others. For example, in Italy interventions focused on individuals despite arguments for a more community-orientated approach (Martin et al., 2014), whereas in India, there was a shift from casework to a more macro-approach, aimed at addressing structural inequalities (Ornellas et al., 2019). It has been suggested that the implementation of neo-liberal and management principles has triggered a value crisis for the social work profession, with a stronger emphasis on management, performance and risk assessment, which is in direct conflict with government welfare policy and the values, principles or ideals of the social work profession, often leaving workers feeling powerless and ineffective (Ornellas et al., 2019).

The findings from these studies highlight the commitment of social work students and social workers to promote social justice, which some viewed as integral to their professional identity. It has been suggested that professional values are closely aligned to tasks, roles and codes of ethics, but that identity, autonomy and professional effectiveness are being compromised with the implementation of neo-liberal and management principles.

The learning and teaching of professional identity

While research has attempted to define what social work is and what social workers do, little consensus has been reached (Barnes and Hugman, 2002; Fargion, 2008; Gibelman, 1999). According to Mackay and Zufferey (2015), there are three dominant social work discourses (Dominelli, 2009; Payne, 2005; Staniforth et al., 2011): (1) the reflexive–therapeutic position or therapeutic helping approach, whereby social workers are regarded as helpers or work alongside individuals, families or groups to promote change and well-being (Dominelli, 2009; Payne, 2005; Staniforth et al., 2011); (2) the socialist–collectivist (Payne, 2005) or emancipatory approach (Dominelli, 2009), which regards social workers as agents of change, aiming to overcome oppression and foster social change (Dominelli, 2009; Payne, 2005; Staniforth et al., 2011); and (3) the individualist–reformist (Payne, 2005) or maintenance approach (Dominelli, 2009), which perceives that social workers help individuals, families or groups to navigate existing systems and access services to promote well-being (Dominelli, 2009; Payne, 2005; Staniforth et al., 2011).

The literature suggests that social work educators have the power to act as the 'gate keepers' to the profession (Moore and Urwin, 1991, p. 8; Ryan et al., 1997, p. 5) by managing entry into social work training. They are also described as 'guardians' of the profession by including or excluding students from social work training, particularly at the intersection between education and practice, when they may intervene to protect the student and the service (Agbim and Ozanne, 2007; McDonald, 2007). Qualitative research conducted by Mackay and Zufferey (2015) with 12 social work educators in two Southern Australian universities reported that the power social work educators have around who can and cannot train or qualify as social workers highlights the power of universities, and the power differentials within relationships between educators and students, which educators have to perform (McDonald, 2007). During the qualitative interviews, social work educators positioned 'social work' in contrast to and 'working alongside' less powerful people who use services. According to Mackay and Zufferey (2015), this process of identity and knowledge production indicates that institutionalised social work practices and discourses function within unequal power relations, which exist between social work practitioners and their service users, and between social work educators and students. The social work educators who participated outlined familiar knowledge, values and skills, which helped to define 'who' social workers are and 'what' social workers do and drew upon their AASW Code of Ethics. However, as Shardlow (2009, p. 37) notes, 'codes of ethics are ideals that can offer generalised and definitive answers to the dilemmas of social work, yet ethical practice is "complex, messy and imprecise" and occurs within unequal power relations'.

Furthermore, the social work educators who participated in the research described multiple identities, such as being a practitioner, researcher and educator, and their definition of the function and purpose of social work was underpinned by discourses that resonate with Dominelli's (2009) therapeutic, emancipatory and maintenance approaches. However, Mackay and Zufferey (2015, p. 656) noted that these approaches were combined rather than dichotomised. For example, to construct social work identity and practice, social work educators used the notion of 'helping' as an individualist and collectivist strategy, which did not separate therapeutic and emancipatory social work approaches (Dominelli, 2009; Payne, 2005). They described a social work practice that mediated competing, contradictory and interrelated discourses of social care, social control and social change, producing themselves as advocates for individual as well as collective social justice. The findings highlight how language and discourse constructs and informs social workers' understandings and actions, within practice and educational contexts, creating 'regimes of truth' that are socially constructed (Philp, 1979).

Findings from an empirical research conducted with social work students across Northern Ireland

This section will outline an empirical research study conducted with social work students in Northern Ireland, where the Department of Health annually commissions 260 places to study the Social Work degree at either Queen's University Belfast or Ulster University. On receipt of ethical approval from Research Ethics Committees at Queen's University (REF: EC/074) and Ulster University (REF: 16/0035), social work students who undertook a practice placement or PLO between January 2013 and May 2014 were invited to participate in a cross-sectional survey during a university recall/teaching day. The survey aimed to identify learning activities that students found 'most useful' in terms of developing readiness for practice competence and professional social work identity (Roulston et al., 2018). During the data collection period, 708 students completed their PLO, with 396 students (56%) anonymously returning a completed questionnaire.

In terms of what we meant by professional identity, the survey instrument was based on a questionnaire originally developed for the Australian context (Cleak and Smith, 2012). However, language was adapted to reflect the Northern Ireland

Framework Specification for the Degree in Social Work (Department of Health, Social Services and Public Safety and Northern Ireland Social Care Council, 2014) which highlights six key roles derived from the 'National Occupational Standards for Social Work' (Northern Ireland Social Care Council, 2011). These include maintaining professional accountability, practising professional social work, promoting engagement and participation, assessing needs, risk and circumstances, planning for person-centred outcomes and taking actions to achieve change. The National Occupational Standards outline performance criteria and core statements for skills and knowledge and are used as benchmarks for social work qualifications and ensure the provision of high-quality services.

In terms of how we measured it, a self-administered, written questionnaire collected information about the PLO (first or final); service user group (adult or children's services); setting (fieldwork, residential, hospital, day care or other) and supervision model (on-site or long-arm) as outlined in Cleak et al. (2016). Participating students were invited to rate the usefulness of 16 learning activities for developing their practice competence and professional identity using a four-point Likert scale of 'very useful', 'useful', 'not very useful' or 'not at all useful' (with an option of 'not applicable'). Learning activities were developed with reference to the key roles for social work and a review of available literature about social work placements. Two open-ended questions generated qualitative data: 'Overall, what did you find most helpful in assisting your learning during PLO?' and 'What would have improved your learning during PLO?' Information was also collected about the regularity of student engagement with the learning activities during placement, which has been reported elsewhere (Cleak et al., 2016).

Statistical analyses, which were undertaken using SPSS for Windows (Version 20), and management of missing data are outlined in Roulston et al. (2018). The learning activity rating items were coded from 1 (not useful at all) to 4 (very useful), meaning a higher score reflected a better rating. For the two open-ended questions, 311 students responded to the question: 'Overall, what did you find most helpful in assisting your learning during PLO?' and 246 students responded to 'What would have improved your learning during PLO?' Responses were analysed using thematic content analysis (Ritchie and Lewis, 2003) which involved reviewing the responses, identifying salient information and devising a framework for initial coding of emergent themes. Quotes were selected that encapsulated emerging themes or issues not already covered in the questionnaire.

Of the 396 respondents, 151 (38%) reported on their first PLO and 243 (61%) on their final PLO, with an additional two students repeating placement due to a previous fail. Fifty-four percent of students (n = 209) were in children's services, with the remaining 46% (n = 177) in adult services. Sixty-seven per cent of respondents (n = 260) were based in fieldwork settings, with the remainder in residential (n = 64; 16%); hospitals (n = 26; 7%); day care (n = 20; 5%) or 'other' settings (n = 18; 5%). Three models of supervision were recorded by respondents with 46% (n = 181) having a singleton practice teacher, 48% (n = 181) a long-arm practice teacher (with a qualified social worker as on-site facilitator) and 6% (n = 24) having a long-arm practice teacher (with an unqualified on-site facilitator).

In terms of learning and teaching professional identity, 'being given constructive feedback' was the learning activity ranked most highly (i.e. almost three-quarters of students reported that this learning activity was 'very useful' for developing practice competence and professional identity). Furthermore, 46 students referred to this learning activity in response to the open-ended question about what students found most helpful in assisting learning.

However, not all feedback was considered helpful, with some students highlighting the negative impact of receiving feedback which was not constructive. One student wanted more 'positive encouragement and constructive criticism about professional practice not personal criticism' which was echoed by another student who wanted 'more constructive feedback'.

Supervision was ranked in the top five learning activities for developing both practice competence and social work identity (Tables 4.1 and 4.2). In the qualitative comments, 140 students referred to supervision with most valuing 'regular' or 'weekly' supervision in a 'safe' or 'supportive' learning environment. 'I was well prepared for PLO and extremely well supported during my PLO by my Practice Teacher and on-site supervisor who both supervised me on a weekly basis'. Although most students found supervision helpful, 41 students recommended improved structure, consistency and objectives; avoiding frequent rescheduling; not over-emphasising

Table 4.1 Ratings of usefulness of learning activities for developing practice competence (descending order of usefulness)

Learning Activity	N	M^a	SD	% Rating As Very Useful
		Usefulness for Developing Practice Competence		
Given constructive feedback about progress	374	3.76	.48	78.3
Observe practice teacher and staff	364	3.69	.57	73.9
Discuss feelings and values about practice	376	3.68	.53	70.7
Provided with formal social work supervision	378	3.67	.56	71.7
Learn about legislation, policies and procedures	380	3.67	.55	70.0
Learn about role or function of team or organisation	378	3.67	.54	69.4
Discuss and reflect on practice skills	377	3.66	.54	69.2
Think critically and reflectively about social work's role	376	3.65	.54	67.5
Discuss and prepare for learning new tasks and skills	375	3.63	.55	65.9
Link theory and practice	373	3.57	.60	61.9
Learn about resources, systems and networks	379	3.53	.64	59.6
Have practice observed by practice teacher or staff	374	3.47	.65	54.3
Provided with reading materials and theory	368	3.44	.67	53.3
Link tasks with practice foci and key roles	370	3.40	.73	52.4
Learn about socio-demographics and service user population	371	3.36	.72	48.5
Link practice to NISCC codes of practice	364	3.36	.71	42.6

Abbreviation: NISCC = Northern Ireland Social Care Council.

[a] Higher score reflects a better rating; mean calculated to four decimal places used for ranking.

Table 4.2 Ratings of usefulness of learning activities for developing professional identity (descending order of usefulness)

Learning Activity		Usefulness for Developing Professional Identity		
	N	M[a]	SD	% Rating As Very Useful
Given constructive feedback about progress	353	3.72	.50	74.5
Think critically and reflectively about social work's role	355	3.68	.54	71.3
Discuss feelings and values about practice	355	3.67	.54	69.9
Learn about legislation, policies and procedures	353	3.66	.52	67.7
Provided with formal social work supervision	356	3.65	.59	70.5
Discuss and reflect on practice skills	353	3.65	.54	68.0
Observe practice teacher or staff	345	3.64	.58	69.0
Discuss and prepare for learning new tasks and skills	355	3.63	.55	66.2
Link theory and practice	351	3.61	.54	63.8
Learn about role or function of team to organisation	360	3.61	.58	64.6
Have practice observed by practice teacher or staff	353	3.58	.63	64.3
Provided with reading materials and theory	349	3.56	.58	60.7
Learn about resources, systems and networks	352	3.55	.63	61.6
Link practice to NISCC codes of practice	347	3.48	.71	59.7
Link tasks with practice foci and key roles	352	3.41	.74	54.0
Learn about socio-demographics and service user population	355	3.39	.71	51.6

Abbreviation: NISCC = Northern Ireland Social Care Council.

[a] Higher score reflects a better rating; mean calculated to four decimal places used for ranking.

case management and increasing opportunities to link theory to practice. Some experienced difficulties with the supervisory relationship, which was perceived as oppressive and detrimental to the learning process and highlighted a power differential between students and practice teachers. One student indicated:

> I felt that more support from my PT [Practice Teacher] would have been a big benefit. I am lucky that my on-site fulfilled some of the PT roles as I feel I would have struggled a lot more. I did not feel comfortable approaching my PT and felt significantly oppressed. I believe that if I had had a more informal, less anxious time with my PT it would have made placement easier.

As Tables 4.1 and 4.2 show, observing the practice teacher or fellow social work colleagues was highly rated. In the qualitative comments, 52 students indicated that shadowing or observing social workers exposed them to 'real world' social work. It was unfortunate that most students indicated that such beneficial shadowing opportunities were restricted to the induction. However, a minority of students reported continuous shadowing opportunities which included: 'attendance at statutory meetings to observe the role and function' or 'observing staff engaging with the young people to learn the different policies, procedures and legislation' and opportunities to hear 'how other team members deal with complex issues'. Some shared office space with hospital or fieldwork social workers, which also provided ongoing opportunities to 'listen to work conversations' and to 'listen to staff members on the phone... [or] discuss their cases' all of which shaped their professional identity.

Thinking critically and reflectively about the social work role was particularly important for developing professional identity (Table 4.2), and there were 72 students who commented on reflecting on practice, which included opportunities to discuss casework in teams or supervision. Some valued times when the team 'sat together every day and spoke about what went well and what didn't go well' and another found 'other social workers in the team were very useful for help and guidance... on how to approach cases'. Completing written tasks for the practice educator or completing academic assignments alongside the PLO caused some students stress or restricted opportunities for reflection. One student wanted: '... more time to reflect and read theory around practice issues. I believe I did not have time to do this due to the amount of written work expected in the form of both tuning-ins or evaluations and the academic assignments'. However, it is understood that written tasks demonstrate competence and promote opportunities for critical reflection on aspects of social work practice.

At the other end of the spectrum, findings highlighted learning activities which students perceived as 'least useful' for developing practice competence and social work identity (Tables 4.1 and 4.2). Less than half of students found 'linking practice to Northern Ireland Social Care Council (NISCC) (Social Care Council) standards of conduct and practice' very useful for developing practice competence (Table 4.1), with only 60% of students finding it very useful for developing social work identity (Table 4.2). In the qualitative comments, one student suggested 'more emphasis on linking practice to the Social Care Council standards', which are central to the professional registration of social workers (including students). The Standards of Conduct and Practice form the core regulatory framework for the social work profession in Northern Ireland. Standards describe the values, attitudes and behaviours expected of workers in the day-to-day role and outline relevant knowledge and skills required to demonstrate competent practice.

Just under half of the students rated 'learning about socio-demographics and the service user population' as very useful for developing practice competence (Table 4.1) and only 52% rated it as very useful for developing social work identity (Table 4.2). These findings suggest that while some students perceived links between the wider systems of their service user group and their professional identity, many did not value the usefulness of this activity.

As Tables 4.1 and 4.2 show, just over half of students reported 'linking tasks with practice foci and key roles this activity' as very useful for developing both practice competence and social work identity. According to qualitative comments, one student recommended more focus on practice and less emphasis on written tuning-in exercises or evaluations of practice, as they were deemed 'repetitive' and 'time-consuming' emphasising their perceived low level of usefulness. Despite the need to generate written evidence of competence to meet the practice foci and key roles, which are regarded as the cornerstone for assessment of competence by PLO practice educators, our results indicate that 1 in 10 students rated this learning activity as either not very useful or not useful at all. These findings suggest that some students failed to recognise the importance of generating written evidence to demonstrate readiness and competence to practice and reported it as stressful and time-consuming.

When students' mean ratings of the usefulness of each of the learning activities for developing practice competence and professional identity were compared, there was no evidence of a difference between supervision models, and no significant differences between adult and children's placements. However, differences were noted between students when rating learning activities as more useful for developing professional identity. Figure 4.1 shows that students on their final PLO, compared with students on their first PLO rated the following 10 learning activities, have practice observed by practice teacher/staff (t(349) = 2.97, p = .003); think critically and reflectively about social work role (t(349) = 2.95, p = .003); discuss feelings and values about practice (t(351) = 2.13, p = .034); learn about role/function of team/organisation (t(356) = 4.06, p < .001); learn about socio-demographic/service user (t(351) = 5.29, p < .001); learn about resources, systems and networks (t(348) = 3.82, p < .001); learn about legislation, policies and procedures (t(349) = 2.02, p = .044); link theory and practice (t(347) = 2.70, p = .007); link practice to NISCC codes of practice (t(343) = 2.93, p = .004) and link tasks with practice foci and key roles (t(348) = 2.21, p = .028).

These differences might be influenced by the different number of practice learning days completed by each cohort. For example, final PLO students would have completed 200 days of practice learning, whereas first PLO students would have

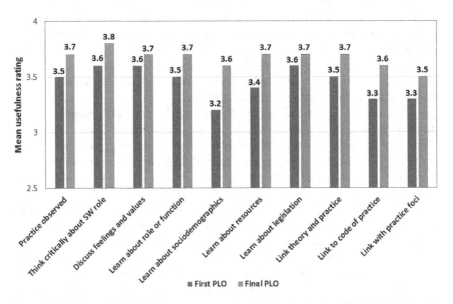

Figure 4.1 Mean usefulness of learning activities for developing professional identity by practice learning opportunity (first or final). PLO = practice learning opportunity; SW = social work.

only completed 85 days. Additionally, only final PLO students are required to have a social work practitioner based on-site, whereas first PLO students only require opportunities to periodically shadow or work with social work practitioners.

Using multivariate analysis, there was no overall difference between placement settings in the rating of the usefulness of the learning activities for developing practice competence (Wilks' Λ = .76, F(64, 1165) = 1.31, p = .057, partial η^2 = .07). However, there was a significant difference between placement settings in the rating of usefulness for developing professional identity (Wilks' Λ = .75, F(64, 1146) = 1.36, p = .036, partial η^2 = .07). As Table 3 shows, there were significant differences between placement settings for five learning activities: observing the practice teacher or other staff; being given constructive feedback about progress; discussing and reflecting on practice skills; linking theory and practice and learning about resources, systems and networks. Post hoc analyses suggest that these differences were, at least in part, due to the relatively low ratings of students in day centre settings. Students placed in day centres, compared with those in hospital settings, had lower usefulness ratings for discussing and reflecting on practice (mean difference = −.58, SE = .18, p = .018) and linking theory and practice (mean difference = −.67, SE = .18, p = .004). Students in day centres also had lower ratings for discussing and reflecting on practice than those in fieldwork placements (mean difference = −.46, SE = .15, p = .024). In addition, students in hospital settings had higher ratings for the usefulness of observing practice teacher and other staff than those in 'other' settings (mean difference = −.55, SE = .19, p = .036). There were no other statistically significant differences on post hoc analysis.

While caution needs to be exercised when interpreting these results due to the low number of students placed in day centre settings, qualitative comments suggest that some students in day care and/or supported living settings felt disadvantaged by the absence of a clearly defined social work role and the absence of a social work colleague to observe or work alongside. One student indicated that the day centre was a 'great placement for developing communication skills. However, there was no social work role as such, so I feel that my learning has been minimal'. Findings suggest that first PLO students in settings where there was no social work role model felt disadvantaged and unclear about the role of a social worker, which may have resulted in issues around readiness to practice and identity when progressing into final year.

Summary guidance to those developing a social work curriculum

This final section will draw together the key messages from empirical research findings and literature, to provide guidance to educators involved in developing the social work curriculum. As illustrated in the opening section, the meaning of professional social work identity has evolved over decades yet consistently highlights a unique set of core values to underpin practice. Namely, social justice, respect for people, integrity, competence and respecting diversity, which are embedded within the micro, mezzo and macro levels of social work. Social justice is perceived as the 'hall mark' of professional social work identity and helps one to address inequity, bias and oppression (Forenza and Eckert, 2018) through connectedness, expansiveness and effectiveness. It is important for social work educators to offer a range of learning opportunities to actively enable students not only to recognise what these core values mean from a theoretical perspective, but also how to identify and adhere to them while in practice with individuals, families, communities, groups and organisations.

As illustrated in the literature, neo-liberal and management principles have triggered a value crisis for social work by focusing on management, performance and risk assessment to the detriment of identity, autonomy and professional effectiveness. Perceived power differentials between educators and students mirror those unequal power relations that occur between social workers and service users. It is important that educators actively demonstrate ways of demonstrating core values when working with students, so that the students can replicate core values and relationship-based practice during placement.

Given the dilemmas caused by the three dominant social work discourses (Dominelli, 2009; Payne, 2005; Staniforth et al., 2011), educators (both academic and field) need to actively encourage students to navigate the different expectations in terms of the therapeutic helping approach, the emancipatory approach (Dominelli, 2009) aiming to overcome oppression and foster social change (Dominelli, 2009; Payne, 2005; Staniforth et al., 2011) and maintenance approach (Dominelli, 2009), which perceives social workers helping to navigate existing systems and accessing services to promote well-being (Dominelli, 2009; Payne, 2005; Staniforth et al., 2011).

All social work educators (academic and field) have a powerful role to act as 'gatekeepers' to the profession, by assessing the academic and professional competence of students with regards to the benchmarks highlighted in the National Occupational Standards (Northern Ireland Social Care Council, 2011) and Professional Standards of Conduct and Practice (Northern Ireland Social Care Council, 2019) or international equivalent. However, findings from the empirical research conducted by Cleak et al. (2016) and Roulston et al. (2018) highlight the importance of students developing their professional social work identity, through supervision which offers a supportive learning environment, shadowing other social workers throughout PLO and being observed, and thinking critically and reflectively through team discussions or supervision. These findings also illustrated that students reported linking their practice to social work standards or key roles least useful, despite these frameworks underpinning the core values of social work. Educators need to create a positive learning environment where students feel safe to be observed, learn from constructive feedback on their academic work and practice and think critically and reflectively about the skills, knowledge and values underpinning their practice with service users, families, groups and communities. It is acknowledged that social work agencies struggle to source sufficient PLOs to meet the high number of social work students; however, educators need to ensure that students are well supervised in teams where social workers are actively demonstrating the professional role otherwise the students will be unclear about their professional identity.

References

Agbim, K. and Ozanne, E. (2007). Social work educators in a changing higher education context: Looking back and looking forward 1982–2005. *Australian Social Work*, 60(1), 68–82.

Australian Association of Social Workers [AASW]. (2010). *Code of ethics*. Retrieved from http://www.aasw.asn.au/practitioner-resources/code-of-ethics

Barnes, D. and Hugman, R. (2002). Portrait of social work. *Journal of Interprofessional Care*, 3(2), 277–288. doi:10.1080/13561820220146702

Bradley, C., Maschi, T., O'Brien, H., Morgen, K. and Ward, K. (2012). Faithful but different: Clinical social workers speak out about career, motivation and professional values. *Journal of Social Work Education*, 48, 459–477.

British Association of Social Workers. (2002). *The code of ethics for social work*. Retrieved from http://cdn.basw.co.uk/membership/coe.pdf

Boehm, W. (1957). *Objectives of the social work curriculum of the future* (Social Work Study, volume 1). New York, NY: Council on Social Work Education.

Cleak, H. and Smith, D. (2012). Student satisfaction with current models of field placement supervision. *Australian Social Work*, 65(2), 243–258.

Cleak, H., Roulston, A. and Vreugdenhil, A. (2016). The inside story: A survey of social work students' supervision and learning opportunities on placement. *British Journal of Social Work*, 46(7), 2033–2050.

Crouch, R.C. (1979). Social work defined. *Social Work*, 24, 46–48.

Department of Health, Social Services and Public Safety and Northern Ireland Social Care Council. (2014). *Northern Ireland framework specification for the degree in social work*. Belfast: Department of Health, Social Services and Public Safety and Northern Ireland Social Care Council.

Dominelli, L. (2009). Anti-oppressive practices in context. In Adams, R., Dominelli, L. and Payne, M. (Eds), *Social work themes, issues and critical debates* (3rd edition). New York, NY: Palgrave Macmillan, pp. 49–64.

Fargion, S. (2008). Reflections on social work's identity: International themes in Italian practitioners' representations of social work. *International Social Work*, 51(2), 206–219. doi:10.1177/0020872807085859

Flexner, A. (1915). Is social work a profession? In National Conference of Charities and Corrections, Proceedings of the National Conference of Charities and Corrections at the Forty-Second Annual Session Held in Baltimore, Maryland. Chicago, IL: Hildmann. doi:10.1177/104973150101100202

Forenza, B. and Eckert, C. (2018). Social work identity: A profession in context. *Social Work*, 63(1), 17–26.

Gibelman, M. (1999). The search for identity: Defining social work – Past, present, future. *Social Work*, 44(4), 298–310. doi:10.1093/sw/44.4.298

Hawkins, L., Fook, J. and Ryan, M. (2001). Social workers' use of the language of social justice. *British Journal of Social Work*, 31(1), 1–13. doi:10.1093/bjsw/31.1.1

International Federation of Social Workers (IFSW). (2014). *Global definition of social work*. Available online at https://www.ifsw.org/what-is-social-work/global-definition-of-social-work/ (accessed 25 January 2016).

Levy, D., Shlomo, S.B. and Itzhaky, H. (2014). The building blocks of professional identity among social work graduates. *Social Work Education*, 33, 744–759.

Mackay, T. and Zufferey, C. (2015). 'A who doing what?': Identity, practice and social work education. *Journal of Social Work*, 15(6), 644–661.

Martin, L., Spolander, G., Engelbrecht, L.K. and Strydom, M. (2014). '*Social work deliverables'. Report for the implications of neoliberalism policy and management on social work and vulnerable populations*. 4 November 2014, IRSES-Marie Curie Actions, Coventry.

McDonald, C. (2007). This is who we are and this is what we do: Social work education and self-efficacy. *Australian Social Work*, 60(1), 83–93.

Moore, L. and Urwin, C. (1991). Gatekeeping: A model for screening baccalaureate students for field education. *Journal of Social Work Education*, 27(1), 8–17.doi:10.1080/10437797.1991.10672164

National Association of Social Workers. (2008). *Code of ethics*. Retrieved from http://www.socialworkers.org/pubs/code/code.asp.

National Association of Social Workers. (2016). *Social work profession*. Retrieved from https://www.socialworkers.org/pressroom/features/general/profession.asp

National Association of Social Workers, Commission on Social Work Practice. (1956). Working definition of social work practice. In Lurie, H.L. (Ed), *Encyclopedia of social work* (15th edition). New York, NY: National Association of Social Workers, pp. 1028–1033.

Northern Ireland Social Care Council. (2011). *National occupational standards for social work*. UK Commission for Education and Skills. Retrieved from https://niscc.info/storage/resources/nos_-_social_work.pdf

Northern Ireland Social Care Council. (2019). *Standards of conduct and practice for social workers*. Belfast: Northern Ireland Social Care Council. Retrieved from https://niscc.info/storage/resources/standards-of-conduct-and-practice-for-social-workers-2019.pdf

Ornellas, A., Spolander, G., Engelbrecht, L.K., Sicora, A., Pervora, I., Marinez-Roman, M-A., Law, A.K., Shajahan, P.K. and das Dores Guerreiro, M. (2019). Mapping social work across 10 countries: Structure, intervention, identity and challenges. *International Social Work*, 62(4), 1183–1197.

Payne, M. (2005). *Modern social work theory* (3rd ed). New York, NY: Palgrave Macmillan.

Philp, M. (1979). Notes on the form of knowledge in social work. *Sociological Review*, 27(1), 83–111. doi:10.1111/j.1467-954X.1979.tb00326.x

Richmond, M. (1917). *Social diagnosis*. New York, NY: Russell Sage Foundation.

Ritchie, J. and Lewis, J. (Eds). (2003). *Qualitative research practice: A guide for social science students and researchers*. London: Sage Publications.

Risler, E., Lowe, L. and Nackerud, L. (2003). Defining social work: Does the working definition work today? *Research on Social Work Practice*, 13(3), 299–309. doi:10.1177/1049731503251974

Roulston, A., Cleak, H. and Vreugdenhil, A. (2018). Promoting readiness to practice: Which learning activities promote competence and professional identity for student social workers during practice learning? *Journal of Social Work Education*, 54(2), 364–378. doi: 10.1080/10437797.2017.1336140

Ryan, M., Habibis, D. and Craft, C. (1997). Guarding the gates of the profession: Findings of a survey of gatekeeping mechanisms in Australian Bachelor of Social Work programs. *Australian Social Work*, 50(3), 5–12.

Shardlow, S. (2009). Values, ethics and social work. In Adams, R., Dominelli, L. and Payne M. (Eds), *Social work themes, issues and critical debates* (3rd ed). New York, NY: Palgrave Macmillan, pp. 37–46.

Staniforth, B., Fouché, C. and O'Brien, M. (2011). Still doing what we do: Defining social work in the 21st century. *Journal of Social Work*, 11(2), 191–208. doi:10.1177/1468017310386697

Wiles, F. (2013). 'Not easily put into a box!' Constructing professional identity. *Social Work Education*, 32, 854–866.

5 "Social workers" professional identity in its social context

A comparative analysis

Marta B. Erdos and Tomi Gomory

Introduction

Social work—underlying core values and its many different aspects

Social work as a profession has many different aspects. Those who are not social workers are often puzzled when encountering the wide variety of institutional contexts and the range of professional activities, which are considered professional social work in different countries. Social workers who do not have any international experience will often assume that whatever is identified as social work in their home country may be considered the same elsewhere. However, the practice of social work—as well as underlying theories, ideologies, and assumptions—may change according to the local history of the profession, local needs, and actual sociocultural and political contexts.

> An internationalist view proposed a unified social work as part of a professionalization project in the twentieth century to institutionalise the status and recognition of social work, but differing practices, occupational groups, contributory disciplines, social institutions incorporating social work and objectives mean that multiple potentialities exist for alternative forms of social work.

Professional identity largely depends on the sociocultural context. A professional's social network and experiences substantially shape values, attitudes, self-conceptions, and future visions on one's career. With society and social change as the focus of professional activities, sensitivity to sociocultural issues is even higher than in the case of other professions, e.g., those in engineering or medicine. The International Association of Schools of Social Work (IASSW) also emphasizes the contextual nature of social work: "*Social work's legitimacy and mandate lie in its intervention at the points where people interact with their environment*"—and this definition calls for further national and regional specifications. IASSW is a well-known resource internationally, including for Hungarian social workers (Szöllősi, 2015). Though there are striking differences among the developmental level of the profession in the different countries,

IASSW suggests some key elements that are decisive in forming social workers' professional identity:

> *Social work is a practice-based profession and an academic discipline that promotes social change and development, social cohesion, and the empowerment and liberation of people. Principles of social justice, human rights, collective responsibility and respect for diversities are central to social work. Underpinned by theories of social work, social sciences, humanities and indigenous knowledge, social work engages people and structures to address life challenges and enhance wellbeing (IASSW).*

Historical traditions and the actual social context greatly influence how social work as a profession is shaped and how a social work career and identity are formed. For quite a long time, social work was considered a semi-profession, because of its perceived diminished level of autonomy and lack of substantial research activities. Internationally, by the 1980s these two shortcomings have been amended, and semi-professional status was exchanged for a more promising label: a young and developing profession (Maschi et al., 2012; Weiss-Gal & Welbourne, 2008).

By the present comparison of practices between the United States and Hungary, we do not only want to identify the differences between the two countries—this might be self-evident—but also the strengths and limitations of each.

History of the profession in the two countries

In the United States, the profession has evolved from the early 19th century paternalistic efforts of upper class women and men in church and secular organizations to help down and out groups of the poor, the ill, and the newly landed immigrants cope with the buffeting of the severe exigencies of their lives. This "caring" began as a volunteer effort by women, known as friendly visiting (https://ssw.umich.edu/about/history/brief-history-of-social-work). Over the next 150 years or so, this helping effort of caring for individuals grew dramatically and became professionalized, growing to include men addressing all manner of problems in living, both encompassing an individual as well as a community-based perspective in a domain that has called "the Personal Problems Jurisdiction."

The very first social work training program began at Columbia University in 1898.

Blundo (2006), a representative of the broadly utilized strength-based approach, emphasized five factors in the early shift from the initial social change focus to the diagnostic approach represented by Mary Richmond. These five factors were professionalization, fear of Bolshevism after the Russian Revolution, integration of the medical model into social casework, the impact of Freudian psychoanalysis, and the contemporary faith in "reason" and "science" (linear causality) as was understood in the early and mid-20th century. This early move has its contemporary aftershocks: *"a residual tension remains among some social workers on how to integrate the objective scientific observer with the empathic counselor and passionate action-oriented reformer"* (Maschi et al., 2012:27). Olson in his important paper in 2007 points out the relationship between social justice as an original goal, and professionalization as an instrument to follow this goal, ironically now reversed. Social work's social justice project and its effort toward professionalization are currently confounded: emphasis on social justice and social rights appears to serve as a means of professionalization, rather than professionalization being the means to work for the realization of the social justice project.

In Hungary, social work as a profession followed a similar developmental path to those in the Western countries. Forms of "social care" (such as the protection of orphans and widows) appeared in Hungarian legislation as early as in the 11th century. Before modernization in the 19th century, institutionalized care was church-based. Modern, 19th century precedents were the activities of the charity organizations whose main mission was to serve the "deserving poor" and perhaps educate and control the undeserving poor in the hope that they would finally meet middle-class expectations (Pik, 1998). At the turn of the 20th century, committed Hungarian professionals introduced the settlement house model based on Jane Addams' 1889 Chicago Hull House by an early experiment in Kolozsvár in 1905 (then a Hungarian town, now part of Romania). The first successful implementation—the University Social Settlement in Budapest—took place in 1912, to be followed by a number of other settlements in the 1930s. Though educating working class people was one of their missions, they also significantly contributed to the birth of present-day community work in Hungary (Giczey, 2015).

Parallel to this development, contemporary institutionalized care was exchanged for "open care" provided in poor persons' or families' own homes. In the 1930s, however, fascist ideology gained strength and quickly spread in a milieu of deep societal despair over the significant geopolitical losses brought about by the Trianon Treaty. Unlike in Germany, where the Nazi dictatorship terminated social work practice, Hungary has continued to develop new models for assisting vulnerable families, though their activities had to be justified as serving national interests, and representing Christian values. As a satellite state of the Soviet Union after World War 2, Hungarian bona fide educational practices in the social sciences and humanities were replaced by mandating strict ideologically controlled dogmatic approaches. Ironically, Marxist theory, which is essentially a critical, economically driven problem-solving theory, was frozen into a set of dogmas, imposed by Stalinist directives. Social theorists, activists, writers, and academics who deviated from this protocol were prosecuted, imprisoned, or killed, often through the dramatic use of show trials. Hungarian poverty was severe and universal; except among some local "communist" party leaders who, as the ruling regime, very soon identified themselves fully with their previous "bourgeois" exploiters.

This dictatorship did not tolerate the existence of social work or any similar helping discipline. According to one central dogma of the era, countries following communist ideologies are inherently free of exploitation. Every single political act by the communists was asserted to serve people's equality, social welfare, and well-being. Exploitation of the working classes (by definition impossible inside the communist block thus was possible only by capitalist countries outside of it) was considered a universal explanatory principle for all types of social and mental ills. Consequently, anyone claiming that there was a high incidence of overall poverty, an unusually high rate of alcoholism, exceptionally high suicide rate, or a high incidence of other mental problems inside the communist block was considered to be a "traitor." A subsequent "soft" regime of communist dictatorship (Kádár's government) began soon after the terrors that followed the 1956 Hungarian revolution for freedom. State socialist ideologies of the era combined elements of early consumer society values with the previous communist ideologies. The system was not based on the use of open coercion but on indirect, yet powerful techniques of manipulation and social control (Lakoff, 2004; Erdős & Kelemen, 2011; Erdős, 2011).

However, the pragmatism of the Kádár regime did introduce and tolerate certain forms of social care to manage social problems that might have become a threat to the system, such as establishing school social work/child protection through Educational Centers in the 1960s, "rehabilitation" centers for alcoholics, and suicide prevention hotlines in the 1970s. Social work was done by "social caregiver" who did not necessarily have a university degree, or had teaching degrees. The first formal university-level training along social work lines was organized by an institution of higher education responsible for the training of special pedagogues. These professionals were named social organizers (Pik, 1998). A particular form of community work was included with the aim of improving adult education and promoting socialist ideology (mirror translation: people cultivators, népművelők). Both these professional titles suggest that these workers' expected readiness to control and direct people's lives, though quite a number of the professionals were actually the forerunners of today's community workers and social pedagogues.

The rebirth of social work as a profession took place during the years of the system change, shortly before 1989, preceded by the reintroduction of sociology into the system of higher education. Adapting and developing psychotherapeutic approaches in the 1980s constituted a further valuable resource (Kelemen, 2011; Buda et al., 1986). Hungarian psychotherapists had a deep interest in the personal and family consequences of lasting anomie in the Hungarian society. Social psychiatry, crisis theory, and the narrative turn were among therapists' valuable theoretical tools and helped to build a bridge toward social work. However, the shift from communication-based psychotherapy for helping the troubled of the society to the medicalized use of psychotropic drugs for controlling the "mentally ill" happened very soon, in the late 1990s (Szendi, 2005), strongly influenced by the rapid growth of the powerful pharmaceutical industry, what also impacted the nature of social workers' roles in health settings.

The first social workers were recruited from three very different groups in the late 1980s and early 1990s with different motivations and varied ideas on what social work is and should be:

- A number of "social workers" (as well as social politicians and sociologists) were former members of the ruling regime, who were motivated by a strong wish to preserve their power and status that they had consolidated in the communist era. Former party secretaries and their assistants belonged to these influential groups with a strong sense of mission to continue socialist "developments" by obtaining leading positions in social service institutions. In this respect, public perception was correct when mistaking professional social workers for "socialist" workers, socialist party members, which, as a label, has different connotations in Hungary from those in the Western societies.
- The critical intelligentsia, consisting of professional practitioners and academics in the chaos of rapid societal transformation, showed solidarity with the quickly emerging vulnerable groups: the homeless, the poor, the unemployed, and the Roma. Social workers' adherence to their core value, social justice, and their unfortunate lack of training in, or experiences of applying critical thinking principles made them susceptible to ideologies that were contrary to existing ones. However, being contrary does not necessarily mean it is actively critical, as being contrary does not mean that this substitution is a thought thru, balanced, rational, and effective reasoning.
- Other helping professionals, mainly sociologists, psychologists, and psychotherapists, quickly discovered this new area, which offered new opportunities for collaboration—or conquest (Németh, 2014).

Hungarian social workers in the 1990s mainly relied—and still rely—on European traditions involving a strong emphasis on welfare state ideologies and the related practices, such as the concept of social citizenship, social workers' mediating role between the citizen and the state, adherence to social safety, and the accompanying social services and institutions. These traditions developed in Europe after World War 2 when European citizens could experience the positive impact of strong state interventions into the self-centered and—in social terms—irresponsible sphere of economic life. Welfare state ideas and practices, flourishing up to the 1970s, demanded the presence of a strong middle class within the society, whose interests temporarily coincided with those of the less privileged. Further, welfare state ideas and developments were in sharp contrast with the previous devastations of the Nazi and communist regimes, and this protective feature made them very attractive (Kozma, 2007).

In the years of the social transition, the Hungarians hoped for a Western-type welfare system, including a system of social safety and solidarity. Welfare ideologies—a strong state that would provide for all the people—fit very well into the mental schemas of the people. However, the external and internal preconditions to establish a genuine and workable welfare system were missing. Due to economic globalization and a series of economic crises from the 1970s on, the number of the "working poor" increased. Quite recently, the highest increase was recorded in Hungary, from 5.3% in 2010 to 9.6% in 2016 in the EU member-states (https://ec.europa.eu/eurostat/web/products-eurostat-news/-/DDN-20180316-1). This trend began several decades ago, but—with moderate improvements— has continued up to now: currently, in Hungary the subsistence level is still somewhat higher than the net minimum wages (https://www.vg.hu/gazdasag/ egyutt-minimalber-es-letminimum-2-701081/). In this volatile and restrictive environment, common ground for the cooperation of middle class and vulnerable groups ceased to exist. What is more, those who might have been eligible candidates as middle-class members in Hungary—the ones with some savings—were soon impoverished in the subsequent financial crises brought about by the change of the social and political system and by global factors. Inequalities among individuals are now significant (https://www.oecd.org/statistics/Better-Life-Initiative-country-note-Hungary.pdf). The policies of the welfare state could no longer be successfully put into practice.

The idea that the introduction of social work would successfully manage the social problems that would inevitably arise in this transition period proved a mission impossible for this newly reborn profession. Social work in Hungary was not based on organically developing social solidarity of certain groups, as care and responsibility had long been perceived as a communist "state" responsibility. As a result of previous habituated state socialist discursive patterns, people (not considered citizens yet!) distanced or felt themselves alienated from state-level operations, unable, and also unwilling to make some apparently obvious cognitive connections between paying taxes and redistribution strategies, or voting and subsequently being represented by their chosen and accountable few. All these issues resulted in rapidly confounding and worsening social problems without any promising solutions. Emerging social problems that had not been previously present or acknowledged (including unemployment, extreme poverty, homelessness, substance use, the emotional and physical abuse of children, violation of human rights of many social groups [such as "politically unreliable" individuals, LGBTQ people, and persons diagnosed with mental disorders]) before the system change severely challenged the first social workers. Their enthusiasm and commitment to help often made up for the lack of effective methods and treatments. Similar to early development of social work in the United States, they borrowed ideas, methods, and techniques from the fellow helping professions.

In certain cities in Hungary—even in their city centers—one can currently encounter quite a number of potential clients of social work: homeless persons, persons with psychiatric/substance use problems, beggars (sometimes in organized beggar "mafias"), persons with physical disabilities, etc. Most of the passersby would not realize that many of these individuals are primarily the symptomatic results of untreated or mistreated social problems, for which sometimes the police may be contacted; but most often no professional response is forthcoming. Homelessness is a salient problem and is intertwined with substance use or disturbing emotional and physical behavior. Those few lay persons who have some idea of what social work might be often identify social work as a profession that could provide care for homeless persons; but they would not normally know all the other areas that are under social work's purview (Szoboszlai, 2014).

Statistical data suggest that poverty (with a high rate of material deprivation in Hungary of around 33%, Gábos et al., 2016; Eurostat https://ec.europa.eu/eurostat/web/products-eurostat-news/-/DDN-20171212-1), the challenges of an ageing society, and substance misuse (first and foremost alcoholism) are among the most urgent issues. Regional inequalities have also grown and neither employment nor a well-established system of human services is available in more remote areas (mostly rural areas where access to public and social services is poor). Most of these areas came into existence when large agricultural cooperatives as main employers in the Hungarian villages ceased to exist, and land was purchased by the lucky few (mostly, leading members of the previous socialist regime). Some of these areas can also be found in the outskirts of towns and cities where industry has ceased to exist after the transition. The Roma are definitely one of the social groups that is considered a loser in the process of social and political transition. This is due to the loss of their traditional employment areas and employment options; segregation in education accompanied by slowly changing cultural traditions (very early marriage and childbirth are perceived as a means to gain high social status, while education is sometimes seen as a form of separation from one's own culture) and discrimination in the labor market (Boros, 2017). Increasing discrimination is also associated with the social transition: the previous policy of full employment ceased to exist and acute competition for resources, including capital and employment, has begun. Prejudices served as rationalizations for ever growing inequalities.

State socialist attitudes and ideas are retained in the cultural and communicative memories of individuals. This may result in an increased susceptibility to manipulation, lack of autonomous thinking, and the dominance of rule following ideologies over balanced individual reasoning. Unlike many other communist states, Hungary has not always been a collectivistic society; rather, atomization had been a means of exercising political control (Hankiss, 1983) and has had a lasting impact on social cohesion. The idea that the state should and does provide is rather widespread; consequently, anyone suffering from some social ills must be by definition be a social outlier and an undeserving person. Fiscal issues prevail over welfare and well-being. This is supported by the well-known and often oversimplified Marxist idea of determining base (production) and superstructure of social and cultural relations (Williams, 1973). A "materialist" approach suggests that relational, social, and cultural issues are just the "surface" (the Hungarian connotations for superstructure, while base translates as "basis," "deep"), and as such, are not really important. Public perceptions that easily translate into votes during repeated elections do neither accurately reflect the reality of social problems nor of social work as a profession. The term "social" has a number of different translations in the Hungarian language. On the one hand, it not only translates as "társas," referring to human relations/communities in general, but also translates as "szociális," related to all types of human miseries. In another sense, it directly refers to communist ideologies. These latter have strong negative connotations. Social workers are szociális munkások, and not társas munkások. For quite a while, social workers were mistaken for "socialist workers," i.e., low prestige blue-collar workers in state-owned factories or socialist party members (Szoboszlai, 2014). Worker translates as munkás, which, as a term, never refers to professionals. The word munkás, as a member of the working class, was the most important or at least the most idealized class during the communist era and has subsequently lost all its positive connotations. There were a number of commentaries concerning the name choice for the profession (Darvas & Hegyesi, 2003) that have continued up to now. Today, many in Hungary would confuse a social worker for a person employed for the sake of public utility, a low-paid unskilled labor force in recent government employment programs.

Professionalization

The provocative question of whether social work is a profession at all was first raised by Abraham Flexner in 1915 in the United States by labeling it a "semi-profession," and almost the same issue was asked by József Pálinkás, President of the Hungarian Academy of Sciences in 2009. In both cases, the question resulted in joint efforts on part of the profession to become more "professional." Table 5.1 compares the levels of professionalization in the two countries.

Professionalization may refer to a set of characteristics that determine professional competencies and professional identity. It may also refer to the power, influence, and control of the given domain. When considering the process of professionalization, we seek answers to the following questions and consider the answers as particular indicators of a profession's development:

- How does the given area contribute to the functioning of the society? What is the significance of its activities in the life of the society?
- Is the area legally and publicly recognized and acknowledged as a profession?
- Have professional monopolies been formed; e.g., who is entitled to perform these activities? (Licensure and legal background)
- What are the power relations with fellow professions like? To what extent is the profession vulnerable to transient government interest?
- What are the specific professional concepts and skills; and how are these built and distributed? (system of education, research projects, and own professional terminology)
- What level of autonomy does the professional have?
- Is there a viable code of ethics? Are there any standardized procedures?
- What about levels of prestige, career planning, and salaries?
- Are there any specific institutions, services, clientele, and a specific organizational culture of the area? Are professional associations influential and able to protect the interests of the profession, those of the clients, and professionals?
- Do the representatives of the profession have their sense of own identity? (Weiss-Gal & Welbourne, 2008; Jones & Joss, 1995)

Table 5.1 Summary: Comparing levels of professionalization in the two countries

Dimension	United States	Hungary
Legal acknowledgment	Licensure and a stable legal background for professional activities.	Poor, partly due to the lack of qualified workforce. No licensure.
Public recognition, prestige	A well-known and recognizable professional area in the eyes of the public.	Very basic misunderstandings on part of the public; mistaking the professionals for simply caregiver—or for the clients themselves.
Professional monopolies	Employment with the job title "social worker" is not possible without a degree in social work but is possible with titles such as "case aide" or "social services assistant."	"Social practitioners" without a degree in social work; the area itself is divided into a number of other areas under varied labels (e.g., "community coordination," "mental health counseling," or "social pedagogy")
Fellow professions	Many associated helping professions, such as human service workers, counselors, case managers, and clinical psychologists.	Context-dependent, but an overall low recognition of social worker expertise with some promising exceptions (mainly on part of psychologists, psychiatrists, and lawyers working in the field of child protection).
Government influence	The National Association of Social Workers (NASW) serves as social work's major lobbying organization at all levels of government but the NASW's policy impact is minor, while the profession itself is highly government regulated.	High, with strong centralization tendencies.
Level of autonomy	In private practice high; in public practice low.	Low, with rapidly changing regulations and strengthening professional protocols.
Education	Around 1900: First academic-level training programs Expansion of doctoral programs in the 1960s and 1970s (Maschi et al., 2012) Council on Social Work Education (CSWE) regulates social work education's certification and curricula nationally.	Bachelor and Masters levels; a national body, the Hungarian Accreditation Committee is responsible for program accreditation. As Hungary is part of the European Higher Education Area, study programs are in accordance with European norms. Ph.D. programs are missing. A marked decline in admissions to Higher Education Institutionss (HEIs) Access to continuing professional education is poor.

(Continued)

Table 5.1 Summary: Comparing levels of professionalization in the two countries (*Continued*)

Dimension	United States	Hungary
Professional organizations	NASW regulates professional practice and social work's policy agenda.	Umbrella organizations: Hungarian Association of Social Workers, member of International Federation of Social Workers, the International Council on Social Welfare (ICSW), and the European Social Network. One of its members is the Association for the Education of Hungarian Social Workers. Both bodies have very little influence on policy decisions and on the representation of interests.
Estimated number of the professionals	Over 707,000 social workers, 0.0022 of the entire population.	No exact data are available, as social caregiver and social workers are not differentiated in the national statistics. Estimates of trained social workers vary between 12 and 20,000. Many leave for more rewarding forms of employment and very probably no more than 5000 fully qualified practitioners are present in the mainstream social sector (around 0.0005 of Hungary's population) (Szoboszlai, 2014; Farkas, 2005).
Salaries	Median income: $ 49,470=€ 44,490 per year. Obtaining an MA/DSW/Ph.D. degree increase salary levels.	Low as is usual in the state sector. Average gross salary is € 8544 per year (https://www.fizetesek.hu/fizetesek/egeszsegugy-es-szocialis-ellatas/szocialis-munkas), very near to minimum wages; differences in levels of professional education are not recognized. Project-based employment ensures higher salaries but results in the instability of one's career.
Career planning	Nothing formal.	Informal; often involves a substantial change in career (leaving the professional area); lack of Continuing Professional Development (CPD) as underpaid professionals cannot pay for the programs.
Research projects	Various state and NGO-funded research projects are ongoing in practically all areas of social work, including mental health.	Dominated by the fellow professions, mainly sociology. The Social Work Subcommittee of the Hungarian Academy of Sciences was established in 2017.

(*Continued*)

Table 5.1 Summary: Comparing levels of professionalization in the two countries (*Continued*)

Dimension	United States	Hungary
Journals, databases, etc.	Many journals.	6 journals (4 of which are also related to other fields as societal policy or social pedagogy, etc.). Not any journal containing the term "social work" in the title. Quite a number of online official information sources are available, e.g., szocialisportal.hu, tamogatoweb.hu, and szgyf.hu.
Professional terminology	Elaborate, corresponds to the many different areas of social work and has a major role in the renewal of professional concepts globally.	Distinct, well defined.
Code of Ethics	NASW Code of Ethics since 1960.	Elaborate; and in full accordance with international guidelines (first version in 1995 with regular updates: http://3sz.hu/sites/default/files/Etikai.pdf).

Jones & Joss (1995) in their seminal paper chose a different approach, and instead of concentrating on specific indicators, they focus on models of professionalism and outline a comprehensive framework of professional competencies. Their main idea is that a professional should be able to use their competencies in an ever-changing environment, and manage novel, unique, and unexpectable situations. They differentiate between four types of professionalism:

- Practical or "craft" professionalism, which denies the relevance of theories and emphasizes "common sense" knowledge. The "learning by doing" approach and refusal of theoretical knowledge results in inflexibility in novel situations: we can expect trial and error strategies as a maximum of solutions. Consequently, these "professionals" dread change: they want control and be controlled.
- There are technical experts, who do rely on systemic inquiries and consider themselves as exclusive sources of wisdom in their relationships with the clients. Their knowledge base is fragmented and there is a strong emphasis on technical rationality. Expert knowledge makes these professionals more authorities than helpers.
- Managerial experts, in addition to the earlier, emphasize efficiency, cost-effectiveness, and management issues; along with an "operative" self-image, regulations, guidelines, customer satisfaction, and organizational hierarchies.
- Reflective practitioners are characterized by a systemic–holistic approach. Their constructivist or constructionist views facilitate unique and innovative, client-centered responses that they work out in close collaboration

with their clients. Dialogue and facilitation are central to their activities. Reflective practitioners integrate their professional experiences with relevant theories and contribute to building the profession's knowledge base (Jones & Joss, 1995).

When dealing with the complexities of human life "at the points where people interact with their environments" (IASSW), only a reflective practitioner is able to help efficiently by empowering the clients and creatively resolve intervention and ethical dilemmas. A reflective practitioner is not a worker interested in controlling the client and, therefore, is possibly a persona non grata in highly paternalistic, authority-based systems. For those who want to use social problems and the underclass to manipulate citizens (Gans, 1992), the reflective practitioner is a threat. The acquisition of counseling skills, which should involve reflection by definition, might contribute to one's becoming a reflective practitioner.

Hungary situation

In the 1990s, Hungarian social workers' main professional role was perceived as the provision of subsidies for their clients. Contemporary research projects on poverty as well as some lingering state socialist ideologies suggested that providing for people is the core activity of the new professionals. Further, early social workers were aware of the traps of diagnostic approaches (e.g., blaming the victim and attributing social problems to "personality disorders") but were not at all aware of the critical and constructive messages of postmodern therapies and strength-based approaches (Blundo, 2006). Unfortunately, this was an era still dominated by psychodynamic views. On the other hand, psychologists argued that the introduction of subsidies in the frameworks of the helping process would paralyze a therapeutic process and called for the introduction of mental health counseling as a new profession (Bagdy, 1996). This is how social work lost an important area: clinical work, as well as key praxis and research methods and approaches applicable in a number of other contexts (Erdős, 2017). As an example, Darvas & Hegyesi (2003) highlighted the contradictory finding of an empirical investigation. Social work students readily attribute clients' problems to societal ills, such as exclusion and inequality, but would intervene by using psychosocial methods. No wonder: the majority of social workers are involved in direct client–helper professional relationships. It is not the social problem that contacts the helper, but the client. Clients would define their problems as deeply personal, and they would have emotions concerning these problems. First they want to be heard, then they want to be listened to, and finally they want to be understood. The lack of counseling skills in such situations is disempowering for the professional and the client, and the result is a controlling, "craftsman," or "managerial" approach in which the case is reduced to a series of actions and reactions. Where is the person in the process? What are their motivations, desires, life history? The craftsman approach readily copies the media representations that stereotype the poor as nonpersons, people without an own life story or personality (Hammer, 2004).

A reflective practitioner in social work, also trained in counseling methods, would know the limitations of social control work. Its impact is temporary and is usually sustained only up to the moment social control is sustained. It does not promote personal, interpersonal, not to mention societal changes, rather, the client is motivated to flee from the new sources of stress and end the relationship with the "helper" as soon as possible—a Dickensian out-of-door relief. Change is perhaps not always possible and there might be cases in which social control is inevitable (e.g., with certain forms of criminal behavior) but this would not justify a system where (often inconsequentially applied) control is a central issue instead of psychosocial interventions.

Control issues are related to:

- the recent introduction of a central registration system of social services to avoid parallelisms and make public spending transparent. One basic problem with the system is that the same person may need services provided by different institutions the same day, e.g., a homeless person may also have substance use problems and should utilize services at the homeless shelter and, parallel, in community care provided by a treatment center for persons with substance use disorder. This is not possible under the new system;
- standardization of social diagnosis in the system of family and child care as a precondition for services. Based on the diagnosis made by a case manager, social service institutions are obliged to introduce the proposed measures (1.01.2019. Amendments on Act 1993. III.);
- and, parallel, to the introduction of a new system of case management in family and child welfare centers, where the case manager should decide on and ensure adequate services for the client. The professional's autonomy who is directly responsible for the case is more limited in this system. Considering the available resources and the number of trained professionals, management might be reduced to a series of administrative measures (Szabó, 2017).

Currently, the professional career of a social worker is not very attractive in Hungary. Professional career models are missing; both the prestige of the profession and the salaries are very low. Therapeutic work/counseling, which are considered the most appealing segments of work, currently are not among the Hungarian social workers core activities.

Admissions to social work BA training programs have decreased to one-fifth of the original number between 2006 and 2014 (Balogh et al., 2015). As there is a shortage of a competent workforce, workload is very large, and efficient and effective forms of care are almost impossible to provide. This in turn results in further burnout and dropout. Women dominate the profession as is the case with any low pay/prestige area (Nagy, 2009). Under these circumstances, the usefulness of social work can easily be questioned; but the scarcity of resources is usually not part of the conversation.

Professional monopolies of social work are also weak: social work appears under a variety of names and in different training programs that are not considered part of social work, such as "social pedagogy," "community coordination," "mental health counseling" (with family and community specializations), and "pastoral counseling and organizational development"—just to name a few. In some of the social services, a simple postgraduate specialization (practically with any prior bachelor's degree) as a fast-track training ensures employability in a social institution (Szoboszlai, 2014). In 2018, a new and fully centralized training was introduced for the leaders of social institutions (http://emk.semmelweis.hu/szocialis_vezetokepzes/). Lifelong learning resources, such as specializations, a variety of trainings, and supervision, do exist but most of these are very costly, and as such, are rarely realistically accessible.

Currently, social institutions may be state-, church-, or NGO-based. Church-based institutions, mostly with charity-focused and social care activities, have been strengthened. Social problems that cannot be solved by benevolent individual actions—such as child poverty or homelessness—are still perceived as possible objects of charity work.

Domestic debates discuss the individual skills of the practitioner in providing direct services to individual clients or the more theoretical, abstract, and more prestigious technical expertise of policy development and implementation for the greater good. The first group often follows prescribed (and not necessarily evidence-based) procedures. This approach leads to the loss of client and practitioner autonomy and increased bureaucracy and equals to what is termed "social control work." Professionals in the second group are governed by ideas regarding social justice. These practitioners often emphasize their commitment to social work values and perceive the fight against social problems as a categorical imperative; but they may lack the necessary skills to build a resourceful social context to effectively facilitate the solutions for individuals, groups, or communities. Furthermore, there are some "social workers" who are rather remote from direct interactions with clients as well as from the idea of social justice. Practically, they are project managers, competent members of the managerial class and are principally interested in high-prestige and high pay.

Social work research as a distinct professional term is practically unknown in Hungary. Sociologists who focus on survey methods and big data analysis dominate social research. Applied research and the related qualitative research methodologies—most suitable for social work research—are largely missing. Traditions of program evaluation are very poor, and evaluation is often misunderstood as monitoring (Erdős, 2016). The idea that social work research should be an integral part of the profession and the use of adequate frameworks and methods would contribute to the skill development of the profession has recently been raised in Hungarian journals of social work (Sik & Szécsi, 2015; Szoboszlai & Patyán, 2016). Most practitioners, however, do not want to be involved in social research projects: it may be because they assume that it is not "practical" enough, e.g., it is an activity that threatens their practical "helper" identities and may interfere with administrative role-taking. Second, they might be too burdened with their professional day-to-day activities to in addition engage in time-consuming and unrewarding social work research; third, they do not see the benefits of using mainstream sociological methods in social work areas (Sik & Szécsi, 2015).

Further, and very importantly, there are no Ph.D. programs for social workers in Hungary. The social workers who want a Ph.D. degree enroll other programs such as Cultural Anthropology, Sociology, Psychology, Communication, etc., what means (at least) a double workload during their studies. This is might be due to Hungarian academic traditions that still prefer rigid disciplinary boundaries and basic research instead of transdisciplinary approaches or applied research projects. In 2017, there was somewhat of a breakthrough: the Subcommittee of Social Work within the Committee of Sociology belonging to the Section of Economics and Law of the Hungarian Academy of Sciences was formed as a new platform for future research activities.

USA Situation

More than 707,000 social workers employed in the United States. Clinical social workers are the largest professional group (over 200,000) providing mental health services exceeding all the other professions providing such services combined (https://www.socialworkers.org/news/facts/social-workers). It is also one of the fastest growing professional fields expecting an annual growth of 11%, and the median income of social workers in 2018 was $ 49, 470/year (https://www.bls.gov/ooh/community-and-social-service/print/social-workers.html). By 2019, this first effort of formalizing the act of helping into a profession has exploded with a total of 528 accredited baccalaureate, 271 master's, and 89 doctoral programs (12 DSW and 77 Ph.D.), with a total of 127,079 students in the United States (https://www.cswe.org/Research-Statistics/Research-Briefs-and-Publications/CSWE_2017_annual_survey_report-FINAL.aspx).

Social work, as can be seen from these statistics, is by now a well-established mainstream profession with excellent prospects for dramatic income, and professional growth having a very powerful political lobbying organization to aid and abet the profession's authority. That organization is the National Association of Social Workers (NASW), the largest organization of professional social workers in the world with more than 120,000 members committed to enhancing the growth and political influence of the profession on national, state, and local levels with its mission being:

> [T]o enhance the professional growth and development of our members, to create and maintain professional standards for social workers, and to advance sound social policies [and] that advocates for all social workers, nationally and locally, and works to shape public policy and advance the role of social work in effecting social change.
> (https://www.socialworkers.org/About/NASWs-Mission)

What we do not have much information about is social work's effectiveness in terms of its actual impact on the various social problems it claims to have expertise in impacting in the United States or in fact any other country. That is, is there any evidence of its professional ability in reducing the number of sufferers in the population? We appear to have no such direct data regarding the major social work fields such as poverty, mental health, child welfare, or addictions.

We know that the US poverty rate has seesawed over the 52 years between 1965 when the first serious efforts were made by implementing President Lyndon Baines Johnson's War on Poverty and 2017 to reduce the poverty rate. Regardless of the various programs that were tried over that span of time, the poverty rate has fluctuated between 15 and 12% without any correlation to programmatic efforts (see page 3 https://fas.org/sgp/crs/misc/R45397.pdf).

The field of mental health, in which social workers are the largest group of professionals providing care exceeding all other mental health workers combined, about one in five American adults are considered to be mentally ill, an epidemiological finding that has been consistent for many years, possibly suggesting that the field has not been very successful in providing effective interventions (Kirk et al., 2015).

In child welfare, the number of children in the foster care system has continued to increase, for example, in 2013, there were approximately 400,000 children in care; by 2017, this number has grown to 443,000 children (https://www.nacac.org/2019/01/18/foster-care-numbers-up-for-fifth-straight-year/).

In the field of addictions in the United States, the only national data available are from 2015 to 2018 which shows illicit lifetime drug use increased from 130,610,000 in 2015 to 134,791 in 2018 (https://www.samhsa.gov/data/report/2018-nsduh-detailed-tables). This data might suggest that these areas have not had successful programs to redress them.

Each of these social problems has increased not decreased over time despite the increased funding and programs targeting them. Possibly the interventions are not effective enough; or the preconditions to qualify a case problematic or not have been changed; or perhaps other global or national-level societal problems presented themselves.

Regarding the protocols in place for developing and assessing the level of professional education in American social work, there are two important ones. The Council on Social Work Education (CSWE) is responsible for accreditation processes, when accrediting and reaccrediting (every 7 years) schools of social work. As CSWE states:

> The Commission on Accreditation confers accreditation status on schools of social work and baccalaureate social work programs. Additionally, the commission is responsible for both formulating accreditation standards and policies, and determining the criteria and process for evaluating these standards. All of the commission's accreditation decisions are accompanied by a reasoned opinion, and the accreditation process is conducted in a manner that insures the continuation of the Council's role as the accrediting body for social work education. (https://www.cswe.org/About-CSWE/Governance/Commissions-and-Councils/Commission-on-Accreditation.aspx)

This effort to standardize the training for social work at professional programs and schools is principally done through giving formal (in writing) and informal (site visit conversation) feedback during a scheduled site visit by a CSWE team of social work academics to the evaluated social work program. The program is expected to appropriately respond to the site visit team's formal feedback by providing written explanations to the team's questions, and implement changes in their programs where appropriate. Then the instituted changes are reviewed by CSWE, and if deemed appropriate CSWE then accredits/reaccredits the program. There appears to be no research done on how well the mandated CSWE standards and competencies are taught at these professional programs or how they are translated into professional practice after graduation.

Implementing and evaluating one's professional competencies is by meeting the standards for becoming a licensed clinical social worker (LCSW). First, one is required to complete a CSWE-accredited social work program, next LCSW licensing and examination requirements, and finally to apply and gain approval for LCSW state licensure in the state one intends to practice.

As perhaps may be obvious, neither procedure assures that one will be fully skilled in practice. These approaches provide ways of acquiring the minimum skills and knowledge needed to be accepted into practice. No longitudinal studies exist as to how well such certifying procedures for social work training enhance one's skills or to what extent.

Conclusion

Social work as a profession is very sensitive to contextual factors, and especially vulnerable to political ideologies. Consequently, social workers' professional identities are determined by varied historical, cultural, and political factors, though they do share some distinct values, a common knowledge base and practical skills that guide them during their work. The area has common groundings and typical present-day conflicted areas, such as the debates over professionalization processes and the triple mandate problem, that is, tensions between client expectations, agency/government/requirements, and priorities of the profession. Dilemmas, such as help or control, or *help as control*, are global concerns (Staub-Bernasconi, 2016). Control work contradicts many central values and ideas and practices of social work, first and foremost, empowerment and client participation.

The rebirth of the profession in Hungary inevitably raised some issues that have already been solved elsewhere; and some others that are contemporary global challenges that social workers should respond to. The rhetoric of a soft dictatorship—that the state would provide and that the citizens (the people) have no particular obligations and responsibilities toward each other—severely undermined social work's possible foundations. The profession lacks public support as the notion of shared responsibility, and citizenship is largely missing from the domestic culture. Hungary had useful models to follow (those of the US and Western European countries), as well as own initiations, but these models were not always carefully adapted, evaluated, and fine-tuned—rather, they were too often changed to meet transient political and ideological preferences. In an effort to learn from international experiences, and focus more on the social justice project than the project of professionalization (Olson, 2007), most Hungarian social workers would initially emphasize the role of societal factors over psychosocial issues. This, however, impaired the efficiency of the interventions, as social workers lacked some important counseling skills; resulted in losses in professional monopolies; and in an increased vulnerability to party political orientations. There is a marked gap in certain areas in professionalization, i.e., professionals' enthusiasm and commitment are perhaps enough to build a well-established and up-to-date knowledge base for social work, but inadequate representation of interests and lack of dialogue between the professionals and the decision makers have led to low prestige, deficient working conditions, and poor recognition. Currently, the agencies focus on administration and standardized procedures, the practitioners highlight methods and skills, and the academics mostly pay attention to theoretical knowledge and international models. A feasible bridge between these currently separate areas could be built by systematic program evaluation, which could promote synergies between theory, practice, and government expectations and ensure proper feedback into professional education. In sum, social work in Hungary has been more susceptible to political machinations of the left and the right. Sometimes these political changes enhanced social work, often undermined it, but the overall picture shows that political malleability is still a danger to the profession's stability and development in the long run.

In the United States, the birth and development of social work was a more organic process, resulting from seeing some social needs that required a collective response, and the realization that private charity cannot alone ameliorate complex social societal difficulties. Though the profession's early history was challenged by some, then potentially profession destroying threats, such as the fear of Communism infiltrating its membership, and in parallel, doubts concerning the profession's status, rapid moves toward validating its professional standing soon overcame these potential barriers. Though these efforts at professionalization seemed to risk the social justice project, they instead turned social work into a strong and viable discipline while managing at the same time to keep social justice as a main focus. Currently in the United States, social work is an established and vigorous profession, with a very powerful lobby, the NASW to represent its interests. It is one of the most rapidly growing professions with hundreds of schools providing professional degrees to thousands of individuals resulting in often excellent career trajectories and salaries. The future of the profession appears bright, with more and more individuals turning to careers in social work.

Although there were some remarkable similarities in the early histories and dilemmas, such as the ones regarding professional status and worries over the use of social control and coercive methods, the political developments in each country have led to striking differences in what the profession has come to look like in each. Considering substantial differences in historical experiences and the timeframes available to establish and consolidate the profession, with 50 years less time in Hungary than in the United States, this perhaps was inevitable.

Social work thrives best in those political environments that support the freedom, autonomy, and equal rights of each member of the society, that is, democracy writ large—values that are alien to dictatorships as well as to those of today's globalized economy (Szakolczai, 2015). Freedom, autonomy, and equal rights do not only depend on legislation, traditions, and values. Freedom, autonomy, and equal rights—understood as the capacity for informed choice between viable alternatives in life, taking responsibility for oneself, for one's concern for others, and for the development of one's community—largely depend on everyone having real-time equal access to the full panoply of a society's social and environmental resources, together with the willingness of each member of the society to participate.

Social work is one of the few professions that when functioning well maintains and enhances democracy, individual and societal welfare, well-being, human empowerment, social justice, social cohesion, and solidarity.

References

Bagdy, E. (1996). A Klinikai Pszichológiai Szakkollégium állásfoglalása a mentálhigiéné, a segítő szakmák és a klinikai pszichológiai és viszonyának kérdésében. *Család, Gyermek, Ifjúság 4*, 3–7.

Balogh, E., Budai, I., Goldmann, R., Puli, E. & Szöllősi, G. (2015). *Felsőfokú szociális képzések Magyarországon. Párbeszéd.* http://parbeszed.lib.unideb.hu/file/2/5628d4c086821/szerkeszto/(1)2015_kulonszam_korrekturazott.pdf. Last accessed: 05.01.2017.

Blundo, R. (2006). Shifting our habits of mind: learning to practice from a strength perspective. In: Saleebey, D. (ed.) *The Strength Perspective in Social Work Practice*. Boston: Pearson. 25–60.

Boros, J. (2017). *Egyéni utak, társadalmi helyzetek*. Pécs: Pécsi Tudományegyetem.

Buda, B., Andorka, R., György, I. & Donga, K. (1986). *Társadalmi beilleszkedési zavarok Magyarországon*. Budapest: Kossuth Könyvkiadó.

Darvas, Á. & Hegyesi, G. (2003). Hungary. In: Weiss, I., Gal, J., Dixon, J. (eds.) *Professional Ideologies and Preferences in Social Work: A Global Study*. Westport: Praeger Publishers, 125–141.

Erdős, M.B. (2011). From ideology to eidos: recovering from state socialism in Hungary. *AUDEM: The International Journal of Higher Education and Democracy 2* (1), 5–22.

Erdős, M.B. & Kelemen, G. (2011). The finite universe: discursive double bind and parrhesia in state socialism. *History of Communism in Europe 2*, 281–309.

Erdős, M.B. (2016). *The Role of Evaluation Research in a Country in Transition*. High Wycombe: Buckinghamshire New University, 40. (Occasional Papers; 14.)

Erdős, M.B. (2017). Az erősségekre építő megközelítésben rejlő lehetőségek a klinikai szociális munka területén In: (s.n.) *Človek s duševnou poruchou ako klient sociálnej práce: Zborník z medzinárodnej vedeckej konferencie* . Ruzomberok, Kosice: Katolicka Univerzita v Ruzomberku, Teologicka Fakulta, 275–294.

Eurostat. Material and Social deprivation. https://ec.europa.eu/eurostat/web/products-eurostat-news/-/DDN-20171212-1. Last accessed: 21.03.2019.

Farkas, A. (2005). *A szociális szakma szerepe ma Magyarországon.Szociális Szakmai Szövetség* http://www.3sz.hu/tartalom/szocialis-munka. Last accessed: 01.06.2017.

Gábos, A., Tátai, A., B. Kiss, A., Szívós, P. (2016). *Anyagi depriváció Magyarországon, 2009–2015*. http://old.tarki.hu/hu/publications/SR/2016/07gabos.pdf. Last accessed: 18.10.2017.

Gans, H.J. (1992). Mire szolgálnak az érdemtelen szegények? *Esély 3*, 3–17.

Giczey, P. (2015). A settlementek esélyei Magyarországon. *Parola*. http://www.kka.hu/_Kozossegi_Adattar/parolaar.nsf/nyomtat/20323E5ED16D8656C1257F13005AC5DB? OpenDocument. Last accessed: 10.11. 2018.

Global Definition of Social Work (2014). *IASSW*. https://www.iassw-aiets.org/global-definition-of-social-work-review-of-the-global-definition/. Last accessed: 20.01.2019.

Hammer, F. (2004). Közbeszéd és társadalmi igazságosság. *Médiakutató: Médiaelméleti Folyóirat 1*, 7–24. https://mediakutato.hu/cikk/2004_01_tavasz/01_kozbeszed. Last accessed: 20.01.2019.

Hankiss, E (1983). *Társadalmi csapdák. Diagnózisok*. Budapest: Magvető.

Jones, S. & Joss, R. (1995). Models of professionalism. In: Yelloly, M. & Henkel, M. (eds.) *Learning and Teaching in Social Work. Towards Reflective Practice*. London and Bristol, Pennsylvania: Jessica Kingsley Publishers, 15–33.

Kelemen, G. (2011). *Átlendülés. Vázlatok a reflektív klinikai szociális munkához*. Budapest: Animula.

Kirk, S.A., Gomory, T. & Cohen, D. (2015). *Mad Science: Psychiatric Coercion, Diagnosis and Drugs*. London: Routledge.

Kozma, J. (2007). *A szociális munka professzionalizációja a jóléti államokban*. http://www.ncsszi.hu/files/1147.file. Last accessed: 23.01.2019.

Lakoff, G. (2004). *Don't Think of an Elephant! Know Your Values and Frame The Debate. The Essential Guide for Progressives*. Vermont: White River Junction, Chelsea Green Publishing.

Maschi, T., Youdin, R., Sutfin, S. & Simpson, C. (2012). Social work research and evaluation: foundations in human rights and social justice. In: *Social Worker as Researcher Integrating Research with Advocacy* (Chapter 1.). Boston: Pearson.

Nagy, K. (2009). Professzionalizáció- és professzióelméletek a segítő hivatások tükrében. *Esély 2*, 85–105.

Németh, L. (2014). Hová jutott a szociális szakma a rendszerváltástól napjainkig? *Esély 3*, 95–99.

Olson, JJ. (2007). Social work's professional and social justice projects: discourses in conflict. *Journal of Progressive Human Services 1*, 45–69.

Pik, K. (1998). A szociális munka története Magyarországon. A pesti és budai Jóltévő Asszonyi Egyesület. *Esély 2*, 80–90.

Sik, D. & Szécsi, J. (2015). A fókuszcsoport mint módszer szerepe a szociális munkában. *Kapocs 64*, 80–89. http://tudastar.menedek.hu/sites/default/files/sik-dorka-szecsi-judit_a-fokuszcsoport-mint-modszer-szerepe-a-szocialis-munkaban.pdf. Last accessed: 10.05. 2019.

Staub-Bernasconi, S. (2016). Social work and human rights—linking two traditions of human rights in social work. *Journal of Human Rights and Social Work 1*, 40. https://doi.org/10.1007/s41134-016-0005-0. Last accessed: 04.06.2020.

Szabó, L. (2017). Szociális munkások a terápiák világában. *Párbeszéd 2* http://parbeszed.lib.unideb.hu/file/2/596367dc68d4d/szerzo/Szabo_Lajos_Szocialis_munkasok.pdf. Last accessed: 05.04.2018.

Szakolczai, Á. (2015). Marginalitás és liminalitás. Státuszon kívüli helyzetek és átértékelésük. *Régió 23* (2), 6–29.

Szendi, G. (2005) *Depresszióipar*. Budapest: Sík.

Szoboszlai, K. (2014). A szociális munka a változások tükrében: kik vagyunk, hol tartunk és mit kellene tennünk? *Esély* 3, 87–94. http://www.esely.org/kiadvanyok/ 2014_3/2014-3_3-4_Szoboszlai_szocialis_munka.pdf. Last accessed: 30.10.2018.

Szoboszlai, K & Patyán, L. (2016). Esettanulmány a szociális munkában. *Párbeszéd 2,* 15–28.

Weiss-Gal, I. & Welbourne, P. (2008). The professionalisation of social work: a cross-national exploration. *International Journal of Social Welfare 17,* 281–290.

Williams, R. (November–December 1973). Base and superstructure in Marxist cultural theory. *New Left Review I* (82), 3–16.

6 Professional identity in teaching

Christopher Wilkins

Conceptualising teacher professional identity

Researchers' interest in the concept of professional identity is not new and has largely grown out of mid–20th century sociological and psychological interests in the relationship between notions of self and of the influence of social context on these. Mead's theory of symbolic interactionism (1934) was an influential driver of early studies of teacher professional identity in particular (but more generally in the field of professional identity). For symbolic interactionists, identity is constructed out of a sense of self, which in turn develops in response to environment, through social interactions and communications. Studies of teacher identity, therefore, have attempted to engage with the complex dynamic between 'self and context'; between internal factors such as motivation, emotion, reflection and individual agency and external ones such institutional ethos and practices, styles of leadership and pedagogical norms and expectations.

The notion that teacher identity is highly contingent on context is significant, since it has contributed to researchers' focus on the ways in which the conditions of teachers' work (system-level policy and school/classroom-level practice) shape professional identities (Nias, 1989; Flores and Day, 2006; Beauchamp and Thomas, 2009). This emphasis on context has meant studies of teachers' lives have long been prominent in the field of teacher identity, from Dan Lortie's classic *Schoolteacher: A Sociological Study* (Lortie, 1975), to more recent studies focusing on the impact of major education system reforms on teachers' working lives (e.g. Day *et al.*, 2007; Galton and MacBeath, 2008).

Teacher identity as expression of self in a professional context

Inspired by Mead's interactionism, many researchers have sought to conceptualise teacher identity as being an aspect of self-concept, the coming together of the purely personal with notions of what constitutes professional knowledge (subject, pedagogical and didactical) (Beijaard *et al.*, 2000). Rodgers and Scott (2008) saw 'self' as the vehicle by which teachers construct identity as a result of dynamic interactions with the culture of the school in which they work and with fellow teachers.

This dynamic interaction between the internal and external leads to a fusion of personal and professional identities (Day *et al.*, 2007), and in recent decades, studies of teachers' lives and identities have focused to a large extent on the tensions created by teachers attempting to reconcile the personal and professional (Wilkins and Comber, 2015). These tensions occur when the values of the individual self are at odds with schools' institutional priorities – these in turn shaped by system-level policy drivers (Pillen *et al.*, 2013). This tension between the idealistic motivation to *become* a teacher to 'make a difference' in a socially rewarding job, the more pragmatic realities of *being* a teacher lies at the heart of the process of teacher identity construction (Flores and Day, 2006), acted out through a 'negotiation of power' between individual, institutional and system interests (Wilkins *et al.*, 2012; Gu and Day, 2013).

This 'idealism–reality' dynamic in the formation of teachers' identities reflects the tension between contrasting modes of teacher professionalism, between an *authentic professionalism* resulting from a teacher's 'relationship of commitment… located within communal and internal dialogues' (Ball, 2009) and a *demanded professionalism* constructed through specific professional service-level expectations (Evans, 2008, p 36). A central theme of studies of this tension between individual teachers' professional identity and that which is demanded of them by leaders (at school and at system level) is the growth of a new mode of state regulation of education and other public services that is characterised by an increasingly intensive 'audit culture'. Ball (2003, p 216) has argued that this 'performative' mode of governance requires teachers to respond to externally imposed quantitative targets rather than their own personal beliefs and commitments, leading to judgements about the 'quality' of their work being made on the basis of supposedly hyper-rational criteria of effectiveness.

Ball (2003, p 217) also argues that the 'rational technologies' of performative systems not only reshape schools along managerialist lines but also reshape the nature of teacher identity to such an extent that life in the performative school becomes a 'struggle over the teacher's soul'. In the school where commitment to normative individual professional values (typically dominated by relational motivation, the desire to have a positive, enriching and *holistic* impact on students' personal development) comes into conflict with institutional demands to privilege the narrower goals of increased academic outcomes, professional identity in the performative school is frequently characterised in the literature as being inherently compromised (Burnard and White, 2008).

The prominence of explicit, intrusive accountability mechanisms in the school system (Cherubini, 2009; Wilkins *et al.*, 2012) can be seen as evidence of a dilution of 'traditional' professional values. Some writers argue that teaching has become a *post-professional* occupation (Hargreaves, 2000), with no space for an autonomous or collective ethical self (Ball, 2003); others have gone even further and argued that teaching has been fully de-professionalised (Ozga, 1995), with teachers reduced to mere 'classroom technician' status through the diminution of any creative, interpretive dimension to their work (Galton and MacBeath, 2008).

This pessimistic view of impoverished professional identity is not universal. Sachs (2003) argues that the 'traditional' collegial values of the profession, where teachers maintain a strong sense of self-efficacy, agency and moral purpose. A recurring theme in more optimistic accounts of teacher identity and professional values is that of the significance of teacher collaboration, focusing on the greater incidence of stability in teacher identity, and a sense of 'authenticity', in situations where a culture of *collaborative* professionalism is fostered (Hord, 1997; Katzenmeyer and Moller, 2009). Leadership commitment is seen as crucial in promoting collaboration, where school leaders are proactive in establishing the collegial ethos necessary for developing a sustainable professional learning culture (Gu and Day, 2013).

While numerous studies have addressed the part played by school leaders in nurturing collegial professionalism (Andrews and Crowther, 2006; Deal and Peterson, 2016; Hargreaves, 2019), and others have focused on the role of different approaches to school organisation and governance, as neoliberal education reforms have led to the global growth of 'quasi-autonomous public schools', such as charter schools in the United States, academies in England, independent public schools in Australia and Swedish free schools (*Friskolar*). These schools share a number of common features; they are partially liberated from the control of local/regional institutions often have greater flexibility in curriculum matters than other state schools – and in many instances are able to deviate from norms in respect of teacher pay and conditions of working. These schools can be characterised as existing in a 'third space' between the public and private; publically funded and subjected to state oversight, and although 'not for profit' organisations reflecting a neoliberal market ethos of competition, choice and entrepreneurialism (Woods *et al.*, 2007; Torres and Weiner, 2018).

This promotion of an entrepreneurial ethos into schools (a trend mirrored in other public services such as health and social care) reveals the ideological rationale for the quasi-autonomous public school model and has profound implications for teachers' professional sense of self. Although freed to some extent from direct political control, their performance is monitored as part of a punishing data-driven audit culture; the autonomy of teachers and leaders is contingent on meeting and exceeding ever more demanding targets. This in turn has led to a self-surveillance culture, with school priorities determined through a 'coercive instrumentalism' (Wilkins, 2015). In a school where a data-driven, high-stakes-accountability model dominates, the 'traditional' notion of teacher professionalism where situated learning and reflective practice shape decision-making is liable to be threatened. In the performative school, performative targets, often externally determined, replace situated learning. Instead of professional judgement creating a rationale for action, with targets determined by the rationale, the target *is* the rationale. Ball (2003, p 87) argues that this leads normative thinking founded on a critical assumption about what is effective – and ultimately to 'inauthentic practice and relationships'.

For teachers (and leaders) in such schools, a number of studies have found that the competitive, market-oriented ethos emphasises 'performance and product'

(Moore and Clarke, 2016), privileging of cohort-level outcomes data over the less tangible holistic development of students, and creates a normative consensus on what constitutes effective/efficient practice – the uncritical acceptance of pedagogic strategies and techniques as being 'what works' (Rizvi and Lingard, 2010).

Working in the entrepreneurial school has a significant impact on teachers' professional identity, as the commitment to abstract notions of public service and being a transformative influence on students is largely subsumed by a commitment to the institution and its goals. It is common to hear principals of academies in England (or the CEOs of multi-academy trusts) talk of doing things '…the xxxxx Way'; embracing every aspect of teachers' work, from specific language used to start/end lessons and prescribed ways of giving feedback to students, to dress codes – typically for academies, this will be described as 'professional' or 'business' dress.

Teacher identity and the assessment of professional competence

In the decades between 1980 and 2000, both researchers and policymakers interested in teacher professionalism were preoccupied by debates about the nature of teachers' work and what constitutes professional knowledge. As a consequence, similar attention has been given to how teachers' competence can best be nurtured, sustained and measured. In doing so, a distinction is often been drawn between *demanded* or *prescribed* professionalism (defined by service-level expectations framed as skills, knowledge, competencies) and *enacted* professionalism (defined by how teachers act – how they think about their professional actions) (Evans, 2008).

This distinction lies at the heart of the tensions outlined in the previous section, as the service-level expectations have increasingly dominated the terrain. For some, the growing dominance of 'demanded' professionalism in the increasingly managerialist culture of school systems has had a positive impact; Coles and Southworth (2005) interpret this as a *collegial* professionalism with the power to have a transformative impact on schools. This collegial professionalism is characteristic of the distributive leadership model (Gronn, 2000) in which responsibility for setting – and working towards – institutional priorities is dispersed throughout the school, through an expanded tier of 'middle leaders'. However, the prevailing view of educational researchers in the 1990s and 2000s was a less positive one, warning of an inexorable drift towards de-professionalisation of teachers, in which a 'new professionalism' emerged as a form of occupational control (Ozga, 1995; Whitty, 2001). The concept of new professionalism is one which is highly fluid, being contingent on specific demands being made by system leaders (either leaders within schools or at local/national governmental level) (Helsby, 1995).

Prior to the era of 'new professionalism', teachers' work was largely judged by their 'enactment' of professionalism, with a general acceptance that their professional growth came through the development of a collective understanding of what it actually means to be a teacher, through the development of shared values and a shared commitment to ways of working and to what constitutes effective practice.

With the arrival of the concept of the new professionalism, from the late 1980s onwards, these largely internally generated values and purposes began to be displaced by external forces. In this new era, accountability began to displace autonomy, performance management largely replaced peer evaluation – and a discourse of 'teacher competency' started to undermine the primacy of teacher self-efficacy.

Above all, teacher competency has become perhaps the single most significant aspect of teachers' work. To take England as an example, performance management was only made statutory in 2007 (Evans, 2011), but the shift towards a competency model long before this, led by reforms of initial teacher education (ITE) in the 1980s to prescribe the 'competencies' expected to be evidenced for beginning teachers to be awarded Qualified Teacher Status. These competences were further codified as 'standards'; first in 1998, with the most recent iteration being the Teachers' Standards published in 2011 (DofE, 2011). The discourse of competency and standards is a highly performative one, reshaping assumptions about teacher professionalism and so with significant implications for notions of teacher identity. Beck (2009) viewed this discourse as a form of 'pedagogic reformation' (after Bernstein), in which prescribed standards revealed the determining principles of the government's pedagogic orientation (p 7). Beck's (2009, p 8) analysis of teacher standards highlights their performative nature, manifest not only in their content but also in the reductive discourse of the rubrics that accompany them, suggesting becoming an effective, or 'competent', teacher is simply a matter of acquiring a corpus of (state prescribed) knowledge alongside technicist skills.

This focus on performative professionalism has had significant consequences for both pre-service teacher education, with the emergence of quantitative models of assessment of practical teaching competence, and for the assessment of serving teachers' competence, with developmental appraisal largely supplanted by performance management (Evans, 2011). The effect of this shift from a formative, developmental framing of teachers' work to a performative discourse has, for both Beck and Evans, led to a significant 'reshaping' of teacher professionalism. Beck (2009, p 8) notes that this discourse is 'profoundly reductive' and has led to a technicist model of professionalism limited to '…the acquiring of trainable expertise', and Evans, when describing the tensions created by the mismatch between the 'demanded professionalism' of teaching standards and the 'enacted professionalism' generated by teachers' own interpretation of what it means to be a teacher, quotes Cribb's (2009) notion of 'ironic role distancing' to describe the ways in which teachers respond to the ethical dilemmas created when institutional priorities demand they act in ways which run counter to the values central to their teacher identity (Evans, 2011, p 863).

This 'role distancing' resonates with Ball's notion of 'inauthenticity' of practice as a result of the struggle of the teachers' soul in the performative system (Ball, 2003). Numerous writers have examined the adverse impact on teachers' self-efficacy – and therefore the stability of their professional identity – of the intrusive performance management and high-stakes-accountability present in performative schools (Day *et al.*, 2005; Galton and MacBeath, 2008; Cherubini, 2009; Moore and Clarke, 2016).

This negative portrayal of teacher professionalism in decline is not a universal one, however. Michael Barber's work on school effectiveness has been highly influential with policymakers, arguing that the shift towards competency-based models of teacher professionalism, what he terms *informed* professionalism, is prerequisite of 'world-class' education systems. Barber suggests that the teaching profession is inherently resistant to change (Barber and Sebba, 1999), and that school leader autonomy, frameworks for teacher training curriculum and rigorous performance management systems to govern the quality of teachers' work are essential elements of driving improvement through change (*ibid.* p 185). Tellingly, perhaps, Barber and Sella argue that this approach reflects developments in other sectors, including business, and speak approvingly of governmental efforts to 'modernise' the teaching profession, including improving rewards for successful teachers and an 'intolerance of incompetence' (*ibid.* p 187).

Barber's notion of informed professionalism is essentially argued for a fundamental cultural shift in teacher professionalism. This shift was from a professionalism of 'values/principles' to one of 'evidence', from input to outcomes, from received wisdom to best practice informed by evidence from data and from a focus on teachers as producers to students as 'customers/citizens' (Barber, 2004, p 32). Again it is easy to detect in Barber's work the conscious coupling of teacher professionalism with entrepreneurial, private sector norms (see, for instance, his foregrounding of the need for 'a committed, high quality, flexible workforce'; Barber and Sebba, 1999, p 187).

Teacher identity and teacher development: the process of identity construction

The changing nature of teacher professionalism and teacher identity over the past 30 years has inevitably had significant implications for the ways teacher identity develops from the beginning (in the pre-service preparation phase – often referred to as ITE). The chapter has outlined the key trends in conceptualising teacher professionalism and teacher identity, particularly focusing on the impact of the global spread of neoliberal policies and practices in education (as well as other public services). Neoliberalism in the public sector is typically characterised by the deployment of 'high-stakes'-accountability frameworks, intensive inspection mechanisms and the creation of a marketised environment where market levers (parental choice, diversified service provision etc.) are deployed to incentivise success and sanction underperformance (Wilkins, 2011, p 392).

Studies of beginning teachers in this environment have highlighted the tensions inherent in becoming a performative teacher, negotiating the tensions between personal values/motivations and school cultures and institutional priorities (Cherubini, 2009; Wilkins, 2011; Lloyd and Davis, 2018). Given the importance of teacher motivation in teachers' development of strong, stable professional identities, there is evidence of these tensions leading to destabilisation of identity, and raised levels of teachers leaving the workforce (OECD, 2005; Galton and Macbeath, 2008; Ryan, *et al.*, 2017), and higher levels of 'drop-out' in ITE programmes (Hobson *et al.*, 2009; Foster, 2018).

The characterisation of the learning to become a teacher in neoliberal performative systems is often a conflictual one (Burnard and White, 2008), in which the development of professional values of criticality, reflexivity and situated learning is incompatible with the realities of practice being driven by externally imposed, data-driven institutional priorities, and as a consequence, creativity and interpretative aspects of the teachers' role being squeezed out – or at best pushed to the margins (Galton and MacBeath, 2008) by 'inauthentic' practice driven by the 'terrors of performativity' (Ball, 2003).

As noted earlier, however, that more traditional, inquiry-oriented professionalism can be maintained, particularly where teachers are empowered to keep a focus on the 'moral purpose' of teaching (Sachs, 2003). Others have noted the importance of the strong, stable professional identity, pointing out that this can be nurtured more effectively when a collaborative culture is promoted by school leaders (Hord, 1997; Katzenmeyer and Moller, 2009). This focus on collaboration underpins the extensive body of research examining the potential for professional growth offered where school leaders support a whole-school 'professional learning culture' (Stoll and Louis, 2007; Gu and Day, 2013).

Within the professional learning community ethos, proponents argue there is more opportunity for sustained, holistic early career support, so minimising the risk of the conflict between 'ideals/values' and 'real world priorities' leading to a destabilisation of professional identity.

Teacher identity and teacher preparation: the reshaping of professionalism in 'school-led' teacher education systems

The relationship between teachers' professional identity and the situated culture of individual schools is a significant one. 'Becoming a teacher' (as opposed to merely 'learning to teach') is as much as anything a process of socialisation, with new teachers finding ways of reconciling their preconceived ideas about what being a teacher would be like with the lived reality (Kyriacou *et al.*, 2003; Cherubini, 2009). In order for this to be a process *supportive* of identity development rather than one of simply negotiating (and reducing) tensions, both the new teacher *and* those who are responsible for their training and development need to both recognise and adapt to specific micropolitical contexts (Ketchermans and Ballet, 2002; Wilkins *et al.*, 2012).

In recent decades, the growth of competency- and standard-led approaches to teacher professionalism has been accompanied by a turn away from a theoretically based university-led teacher education towards a more practically focused 'training' model. This reorientation of teacher preparation, often disparagingly dismissed as an 'apprenticeship' model, has been perhaps most apparent in the ongoing reforms of the English teacher education system (Furlong, 2005, 2013). However, it is a trend by no means restricted to England; the phenomenon is widespread throughout Europe and beyond (Fitzgerald *et al.*, 2010; Beach and Bagley, 2013; Helgevold and Wilkins, 2019).

The debate around the comparative merits of 'traditional' university-led models of ITE and newer school-led models largely echo the arguments that have persisted about traditional and post-performative constructions of teacher professionalism (Wilkins, 2011). Critics of school-led approaches argue that these adopt a misleadingly simplistic notion of what constitutes effective teacher preparation; that it requires little more than an apprenticeship in which novices learn from 'experienced and skilled masters' (Mutton *et al.*, 2017, p 16). While proponents of school-led approach argue that the 'close to practice' nature of school-led programmes brings some benefits (Carter, 2015), there is no significant empirical evidence as yet (given the relatively recent emergence of these models) of the effectiveness of school-led ITE.

Alongside the rising profile of school-led approaches to teacher education, many education systems across the globe have also increased attention paid to the curriculum *content* for teacher education. This, of course, is directly aligned with the trend for more instrumental, competency-based models of performance management; once the skills and knowledge deemed necessary to be a competent teacher have been articulated, developing a curriculum with the express purpose of ensuring new recruits to the profession are focused on acquiring these is the inevitable next step.

So, while the school-led system is perhaps not established enough to be able to confidently detect the ways in which it is shaping teacher professional identity, there is sufficient evidence from research into the influence of wider aspects of education reforms to suggest that the tensions between 'traditional' models of values-driven *enacted* professionalism and 'modern' *demanded* professionalism will continue to be a significant issue of concern. For school leaders and teacher educators alike, there is a clear need to create the conditions in which teachers (new and experienced) are able to reconcile these tensions and develop the stable sense of self that will allow them not only to stay in the teaching profession but also to continue to grow professionally.

References

Andrews, D., and Crowther, F. (2006) Teachers as leaders in a knowledge society: encouraging signs of a new professionalism, *Journal of School Leadership*, 16(5), 534–549.

Ball, S. (2009). Education reform, teacher professionalism and the end of authenticity. In Simons, M., Olssen, M. and Peters, M. (Eds) *Re-reading Education Policies: Studying the Policy Agenda of the 21th Century* (Rotterdam, Sense, 667–682).

Ball, S.J. (2003) The teacher's soul and the terrors of performativity, *Journal of Education Policy*, 18(2), 215–228.

Barber, M., and Sebba, J. (1999) Reflections on progress towards a world class education system, *Cambridge Journal of Education*, 29(2), 183–193.

Barber, M. (2004) The virtue of accountability: system redesign, inspection, and incentives in the era of informed professionalism. *Journal of Education*, 185. 7–38.

Beach, D., and Bagley, C. (2013) Changing professional discourses in teacher education policy back towards a training paradigm: a comparative study, *European Journal of Teacher Education*, 36(4), 379–392.

Beauchamp, C., and Thomas, L. (2009) Understanding teacher identity: an overview of issues in the literature and implications for teacher education, *Cambridge Journal of Education*, 39(2), 175–189.

Beck, J. (2009) Appropriating professionalism: restructuring the official knowledge base of England's 'modernised' teaching profession, *British Journal of Sociology of Education*, 30(1), 3–14.

Beijaard, D., Verloop, N., and Vermunt, J. (2000) Teachers' perceptions of professional identity: an exploratory study from a personal knowledge perspective, *Teaching and Teacher Education*, 16, 749–764.

Burnard, P., and White, J. (2008) Creativity and performativity: counterpoints in British and Australian education, *British Educational Research Journal*, 34(5), 667–682.

Carter, A. (2015) *Carter Review of Initial Teacher Training (ITT)* (London, Department for Education).

Cherubini, L. (2009) Reconciling the tensions of new teachers' socialisation into school culture: a review of the research, *Issues in Educational Research*, 19(2), 83–99.

Coles, M.J., and Southworth, G. (2005) *Developing Leadership: Creating the Schools of Tomorrow* (Buckingham, Open University Press).

Cribb, A. (2009) Professional Ethics: whose responsibility? In Gewirtz, S., Mahony, P., Hextall, I. and Cribb, A. (Eds) *Changing Teacher Professionalism* (London, Routledge, 31–42).

Day, C., Eliott, B., and Kington, A. (2005) Reforms, standards and teacher identity: challenges of sustaining commitment, *Teachers and Teacher Education*, 21(5), 563–577.

Day, C., Sammons, P., Stobart, G., Kington, A., and Gu, Q. (2007) *Teachers Matter: Connecting Lives, Work and Effectiveness* (Maidenhead, OUP).

Deal, T.E., and Peterson, K.D. (2016) *Shaping School Culture* (San Franscisco, John Wiley & Sons).

DofE. (2011) *Teachers' Standards* DFE-00066-2011, *accessed online 10/12/19 at* https://assets.publishing.service.gov.uk/government/uploads/system/uploads/attachment_data/file/665520/Teachers__Standards.pdf.

Evans, L. (2008) Professionalism, professionality and the development of education professionals, *British Journal of Educational Studies*, 56(1), 20–38.

Evans, L. (2011) The 'shape; of teacher professionalism in England: professional standards, performance management, professional development and the changes proposed in the 2010 White Paper, *British Educational Research Journal*, 37(5), 851–870.

Flores, M., and Day, C. (2006) Contexts which shape and reshape new teachers' identities: a multi-perspective study, *Teachers and Teacher Education*, 22(2), 219–232.

Foster, D. (2018) *Teacher Recruitment and Retention in England*, Briefing Paper 7222 (London, House of Commons Library) Accessed 12/12/19 at researchbriefings.files.parliament.uk/documents/CBP-7222/CBP-7222.pdf.

Furlong, J. (2005) New Labour and teacher education: the end of an era, *Oxford Review of Education*, 31(1), 119–134.

Furlong, J. (2013) Globalisation, neo-liberalism and the reform of teacher education in England. *The Educational Forum* 77, 1, 28–50.

Galton, M., and MacBeath, J. (2008) *Teachers under Pressure* (London, Sage).

Gronn, P. (2000) Distributed properties: a new architecture for leadership. *Educational Management Administration and Leadership*, 28(3), 317–338.

Gu, Q., and Day, C. (2013) Challenges to teacher resilience: conditions count, *British Educational Research Journal*, 39(1), 22–44.

Hargreaves, A. (2000) Four ages of professionalism and professional learning, *Teachers and Teaching: History and Practice*, 6(2), 151–182.

Hargreaves, A. (2019) Teacher collaboration: 30 years of research on its nature, forms, limitations, and effects, *Teachers and Teaching*, 25, 603–621.

Helgevold, N., and Wilkins, C. (2019) International changes and approaches in initial teacher education. In Wood, P., Larssen, D., Helgevold, N. and Cajkler, W. (Eds) *Lesson Study in Initial Teacher Education: Principles and Practices* (London, Emerald Publishing Limited, 1–15).

Helsby, G. (1995) Multiple truths and contested realities: the changing faces of teacher professionalism in England. In Day, C., Fernandez, A., Hague, T. and Moller, J (Eds) *The Life and Work of Teachers* (London, Falmer).

Hobson, A., Giannakaki, M., and Chambers G. (2009) Who withdraws from initial teacher preparation programmes and why? *Educational Research*, 51(3), 321–340.

Hord, SM. (1997) *Professional Learning Communities: Communities of Continuous Inquiry and Improvement* (Austin, SEDL).

Fitzgerald, T. et al. (2010) Bureaucratic control or professional autonomy? Performance management in New Zealand schools, *School Leadership and Management*, 23, 91.

Katzenmeyer, M., and Moller, G. (2009) *Awakening the Sleeping giant: Helping Teachers Develop as Leaders* (Thousand Oaks, CA, Corwin Press).

Ketchermans, G., and Ballet, K. (2002) The micro-politics of teacher education: a narrative biographical study on teacher socialisation, *Teaching and Teacher Education*, 18, 105–120.

Kyriacou, C, Kunc, R., Stephens, P., and Hultgren A. (2003) Student teachers' expectations of teaching as a career, *Educational Review*, 55(3), 255–263.

Lloyd, M., and Davis, J.P. (2018) Beyond performativity: a pragmatic model of teacher professional learning. *Professional Development in Education*, 44(1), 92–106.

Lortie, D.C. (1975) *Schoolteacher* (Chicago, IL University of Chicago Press).

Moore, A., and Clarke, M. (2016) 'Cruel Optimism': teacher attachment to professionalism in an era of performativity. *Journal of Education Policy*, 31(5), 666–677.

Mutton, T., Burn, K., and Menter, I. (2017) Deconstructing the carter review: competing conceptions of quality in England's 'school-led' system of initial teacher education, *Journal of Education Policy*, 32, 1, 14–33.

Nias, J. (1989) *Primary Teachers Talking: A Study of Teaching as Work* (London, Routledge).

OECD. (2005) *Teachers Matter: Attracting, Developing and Retaining Effective Teachers* (Paris, OECD).

Ozga, J. (1995) Deskilling a profession: professionalism, de-professionalisation and the new managerialism. In Busher, H. and Saran, R. (Eds) *Managing Teachers as Professionals in Schools* (London, Kogan Page).

Pillen, M., Beijaard, D., and Brok, P. (2013) Professional identity tensions of beginning teachers, *Teachers and Teaching: Theory and Practice*, 19(6), 660–678.

Rizvi, F., and Lingard, B. (2010) *Globalizing Education Policy* (London, Routledge).

Rodgers, C., and Scott, K. (2008) The development of the personal self and professional identity in learning to teach. In Cochran-Smith, M., Feiman-Nemser, S., McIntyre, D. and Demers, K. (Eds) *Handbook of Research on Teacher Education: Enduring Questions and Changing Contexts* (New York, Routledge, 732–755).

Ryan, S.V., Nathaniel, P., Pendergast, L.L., Saeki, E., Segool, N., and Schwing, S. (2017) Leaving the teaching profession: the role of teacher stress and educational accountability policies on turnover intent, *Teaching and Teacher Education*, 66, 1–11.

Sachs, J. (2003) *The Activist Professional* (Buckingham, OUP).

Stoll, L, and Louis, K. (2007) *Professional Learning Communities: Divergence, Depth and Dilemmas* (Maidenhead, OUP).

Torres, C., and Weiner, J. (2018) The new professionalism? Charter teachers' experiences and qualities of the teaching profession, *Education Policy Analysis Archives*, 26(19), 1–28

Whitty, G. (2001) Teacher professionalism in new times. In Gleeson, D. and Husbands, C. (Eds) *The Performing School* (London: Routledge).

Wilkins, C. (2011) Professionalism and the post-performative teacher: new teachers reflect on autonomy and accountability in the English school system, *Professional Development in Education*, 37(3), 1–21.

Wilkins, C., Busher, H., Kakos, M., Mohamed, C., and Smith, J. (2012) Crossing borders: new teachers co-constructing professional identity in performative times, *Professional Development in Education*, 38(1), 65–78.

Wilkins, C. (2015) Education reform in England: quality and equity in the performative school, *International Journal of Inclusive Education*, 19(11), 1143–1160.

Wilkins, C., and Comber, C. (2015) 'Elite' career-changers in the teaching profession, *British Educational Research Journal*, 41(6), 1010–1030.

Woods, P., Woods, G.J., and Gunter, H.M. (2007) Academy schools and entrepreneurialism in education, *Journal of Education Policy*, 22 (2), 237–259.

7   Changes of academic identities in UK universities

George Brown and Sarah Edmunds

Introduction

Academics are significant members of the professions for they provide broad education and initial training for many other professions. This chapter provides a brief,
accessible introduction to the identities of academics whether they are vice chancellors (VCs), senior staff or lecturers. However, identity is a slippery concept so at
the outset it might be helpful to readers if we provide our conceptions of academic
identity and organisational identity of universities. Later in the chapter, we return
to the theme of the relationship between professional and academic identities.

Put simply, academic identity is concerned by how academics see themselves
and how others see them. They grow out of earlier personal identities. They are
not fixed entities (see Figure 7.1). Changes in academic identity are described,
wherever possible in terms of demographics, perceptions by others and self-
perceptions. All of these change as the identity and functions of universities and
the university system change.

Capturing the organisational identity of universities is a little trickier. For the
purposes of this chapter, we use a continuum with traditional collegiality at one
end and at the other extreme, the full force of neoliberalism. Collegiality is primarily concerned with collaboration between staff and students and joint decision-
making. Its focus is on learning for all aspects of life not merely employment.

---

*Identities are inextricably linked with roles and task of universities and its con-
stituents. Their identities are shaped by their histories. A useful analogy for the
changes in personal identity are layers as in Matrioska (Russian) dolls. For individuals, the most inner layer is genetic and neurological characteristics which, to
some extent, we share with lower primates. The next layers are our childhood and
schooling, then the experiences of studying and life at university. For staff, there is
an added layer shaped by their jobs, which may have changed, or they may have
changed jobs. All of these are influenced by the gradual introduction of neoliberalism in the identities of universities by government policies in the past 100 years.*

Figure 7.1 A useful analogy of identity.

It may be characterised as broad knowledge seeking and exploration. At the core of neoliberalism is private ownership to pursue profits for its stakeholders. In universities, it focuses on marketisation and its concomitant, consumerism. Learning is to be paid for by individuals, not through taxes, and it is primarily for preparation for employment. The middle ground is occupied by universities which contain elements of neoliberalism and the legacy of collegiality. These elements have very powerful effects on the university system, the universities and their staff. Figure 7.2 provides a summary of the main characteristics of neoliberalism

---

Strong neoliberalism in universities

- Emphasis on selling degree courses to students as customers.
- Increasing private provision in universities and the number of private universities.
- Minimal governmental control of private-funded universities.
- Tight control via government of public-funded universities.
- Measurement of outputs used to control funding e.g. graduates entering employment.
- Efficiency gains through redundancy and increasing working loads of staff.
- High salaries for VCs often designated as CEOs.
- Senior academic staff such as Heads of Departments (HoDs) and pro-vice-chancellors (PVCs) are relatively permanent posts.
- Increasing control of staff (e.g. weakening employee security of tenure).
- Reducing staff rights (e.g. limiting trade union activity and security of pensions).
- Competition with other universities (e.g. League tables).

Strong collegiality in universities

- Emphasis on collaboration between staff and students.
- Knowledge seeking, exploration and sharing, including exploration of evidence and values.
- Decision-making and control is primarily an internal responsibility.
- Emphasis on education rather than training.
- Organisational change based on experiences and reflections of staff and students.
- Marginally higher salaries for VCs and senior staff.
- Senior positions such as HoDs and PVCs rotate.
- VC is *primus inter pares* rather than the chief executive.
- Cooperation between universities (e.g. joint teaching and research activities).

Figure 7.2 Comparison of neoliberalism and collegiality.

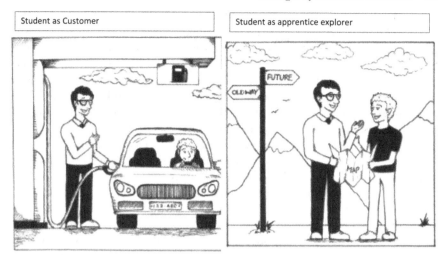

Figure 7.3 Two different perspectives.

and collegiality in universities. Figure 7.3 illustrates, in a light-hearted way, a key difference of the two approaches to working with students.

Changes in identity of universities in the UK

Until the Further and Higher Education Act of 1992, universities were defined as institutions that had a royal charter which granted the power of awarding degrees. In the 19th century, there were only seven such universities in Britain and Ireland. By the onset of World War 1 (WW1), there were 21 universities. By 1970, there were 39 universities and in 1992, polytechnics, colleges of advanced technology and central institutions swelled the numbers to approximately 83. By 2018, there were 162 universities or colleges. Of these, 136 were members of Universities UK (Universities UK, 2018a,b). These changes *per se* inevitably brought about changes in the roles, demands and identities of universities and their staff.

A short history of the changes

In the 19th and early 20th centuries, many of the newer universities and university colleges grew out of mechanics institutes. All the universities were small. For example, the entire University of London had only 2000 students. The universities received funding from philanthropists and local education authorities but very little funding from government. The government did not want to be involved and the universities did not want government's involvement. These universities saw their main function as teaching part-time and full-time students through the mode of lectures and, in the sciences demonstrations rather than practicals. Doing research was a personal predilection prior to WW1. But by 1916, the loss of staff and students because of the traumas of WW1 and the recognition that Britain was lagging behind its main competitors, Germany and the United States, awoke the government from its slumbers. It began to recognise the contribution that universities could make to research and training in war machines such as munitions, tanks and aircraft, in disease control and social work. The government began to look ahead to the contributions that universities could make to industry, business and communities after WW1 (Taylor, 2018).

Twelve days after WW1 ended (23 November 1918) a meeting between government ministers and leading academics formulated a plan which led to the post-war development of the expansion of universities. Research, including the establishment of PhDs (Simpson, 1983) and new subjects such as Russian, Spanish, Aeronautical, Electrical and Automotive Engineering, emerged. More women were allowed to enter the professions except veterinary medicine and theology. Courses in dentistry, social work, medicine, veterinary medicine and teaching were modernised. New teaching methods such as seminars, laboratory practicals and projects were introduced (Taylor, 2018 cit. op. Wilkinson). The government provided more funding. But there was a price. In return for funding, the government demanded more control: the university system was established.

The University Grants Committee and the Committee of VCs and Principals were founded to oversee the quality and finances of universities, the negotiating body and the forum for discussions of policy in the new Higher Education (HE) system. The seeds of tight governmental control were sown. But they did not begin to germinate until over 70 years later and did not come to fruition until a further 30 years.

There was little change in the identity of universities in the interwar years. In post-World War 2, there was initially more generous funding to universities. The Anderson Committee (1960) introduced mandatory grants and travel allowances for students which continued in the 1960s and 1970s. Many more students had access to HE and consequently the assessment procedures changed but lecturing remained part of the core identity of lecturers. On the eve of the Robbins Report (1963), universities were still small, relatively elitist and predominantly male. Post-Robbins, more new universities were established, and student numbers increased. In the 1980s and 1990s, there was a profound change in identity of the HE system begun by Baroness Thatcher's *kulturkampf* of universities in 1981 and continued by the recommendations of the Dearing Report (1997). Further details are provided by Collini (2012) and in the section on changes in student identity.

The year 1989 witnessed the end of the UGC. It was replaced by the Higher Education Funding Councils in 1992. These were buffers against excessive governmental control but they only survived for 26 years (Scott, 2015). In England, HEFCE was abolished. Its regulatory functions were taken over by the Office for Students (see OfS, 2019). It is claimed that it is not a government body but one which advises the government through the Department for Education. Nonetheless, it is in close propinquity of ministerial offices. A similar fate befell the Research Councils which were established in the 1960s and in 2018 replaced by UK Research and Innovation (UKRI, 2019).

New regulatory frameworks were introduced by the government in the late 20th and early 21st century: Research Excellence Framework (REF), the Teacher Excellence Framework and Student Outcomes (TEF) and the Knowledge Exchange Framework (KEF) (see Wonkhe, 2017).

REF replaced the Research Assessment Exercise in 2014. It now purports to be concerned with economy, society, public policy, culture and the quality of life. Measuring impact in some of these areas may prove troublesome (Watermeyer, 2016; Wilkinson, 2017). A consultation exercise on a new REF scheduled to begin in 2021 has already begun (REF, 2021). This may stimulate further guidelines on measuring the impacts of research. In 2014, TEF replaced some of the functions of the Quality Assurance Agency. It is now primarily concerned with outcomes that lead to graduate employment or entry to postgraduate courses. Institutions that perform well on these criteria may charge marginally higher fees. The latter are being used to determine funding and tuition fees through the use of the categories 'gold', 'silver' and 'bronze'. The Higher Education Policy Institute has produced a favourable report on TEF (Beech, 2017). It reports some collaboration between staff and students, joint research and between universities. But its statistical procedures have been criticised by the Royal Society of Statistics (RSS, 2018). There are also some concerns that measures based on student satisfaction may not be taking into account biases towards males and BME lecturers. KEF England was established in 2017. Its primary concern is improving industrial strategies which will benefit the economy. At the time of writing (early 2019), it has not published any briefings or papers. Its work will overlap and, perhaps, conflict with the work of REF. These new frameworks have consequences on funding for research and teaching and therefore the roles and identities of academics.

An additional change to HE is advocated by the well-grounded Auger Report (2019). It recommends changes in funding, the reorganisation of higher and further education under the umbrella of 'tertiary education'; more emphasis on technical education rather than academic education, and on generic skills for improving the future economy. If the recommendations are accepted by government, then one can expect further change in the identities of universities and academic staff.

Underneath these frameworks, one can discern the influence of market forces described earlier. But it could be argued that the future is relatively unknown so rather than preparing students for immediate employment, we should be preparing them for an unknown future as some large employers and advocates of collegiality suggest (Bowden & Marton, 1998). The discussion by Brown et al. (2003) is also relevant to this theme.

In summary, there have been seismic changes in the identity of the HE system in the UK in the past 100 or more years. The degree of control the government has over universities has increased considerably. This control is based largely on a neoliberal ideology (Mahony & Weiner, 2017 cit op), sometimes labelled 'academic capitalism' (Jessop, 2017). Put more simply, it is based on the notion that education is a commodity to be bought by individuals and sold by universities.

The government's main function in HE is currently to control public universities tightly but apparently at a distance. As the university system changed, the identity of the universities themselves changed and therefore the identities of those who work or study in universities changed (Williams, 2013). Willetts (2017) in a comprehensive and well-written book provides an insider's view of government policies and a broad historical sweep of changes in British Society, the HE system and universities. He argues cogently for changes in UK universities and their funding.

Figure 7.4 provides a heuristic model of these changes. There are some interactions across boundaries of identities. It is not an atomic model in which the nucleus has the strongest force. It also provides an indication of the sections of this chapter.

Identities of academic staff

Vice chancellors

Overall, there are 35 Heads of Universities who are women and 127 men (Universities UK, 2018a, b). These include one black woman, Dame Valerie Amos, who was appointed Head of School of Oriental and African Studies in 2015 (Oshu, 2018). There are now three VCs of the top 50 universities who are BME (see https://www.diversitylink.co.uk/resources.php: http://www.thecolourofpower.com/colour-of-power).

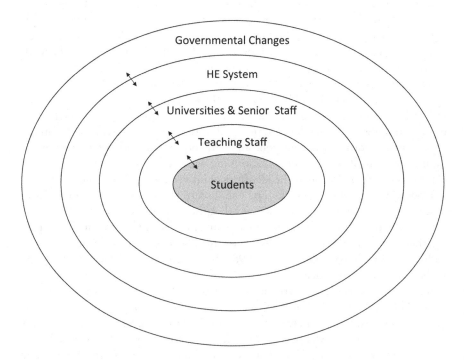

Figure 7.4 Changes in organisational and personal identities.

Fifty-five percent of VCs come from backgrounds in the sciences, social science, engineering and medicine and its allied subjects (HESA, 2019), perhaps because of their experience in managing large research projects or occupying posts as senior staff.

In 2017–2018, 54 VCs received more than £300,000 p.a. The report from the Office for Students (OfS, 2019) suggests that calls for pay restraint have had little effect. The Head of OfS, Nicola Dandridge, defended their approach.. '*It is not for the Office for Students to set a vice-chancellor's pay. We understand that running a university is a significant and complex task, and it is right that those who excel in their roles should be well rewarded,*' she said.

These salaries are comparable with many CEOs in business and industry. Nonetheless, the gap between their salaries and those of lecturers has caused disquiet which is reflected in views of the perceived identities of VCs by their academic staff (Hall, 2017). That shift in the perceived identities of VCs from Academic Leader to Chief Executive was, in part, due to the Jarratt Report (1985) based supposedly on case studies. It was aided by the introduction of league tables of universities in the UK imported from the United States in 1993. Collini (2012) in a trenchant critique of developments in universities suggested that VCs, as CEOs, keep a nervous eye on their league tables as much as football managers do.

We did not find any research on how VCs see themselves but the reflections of Professor *David Burgess* (Burgess, 2008) and Professor *Shearer West* (West, 2018), the VC of Nottingham, on her first year in office provide some interesting insights of the complex identity and roles of a VC.

Senior staff in universities

There are approximately 500 senior staff in universities. They usually have the titles of Deputy VC (DVC) and PVC. Like the Heads of UK universities, their salaries are well above those of lecturers and most HoDs. Only 45% earn less than £345,000 (Glassdoor, 2018).

PVCs and DVCs are, and always have been, almost exclusively drawn from the ranks of established academics. Most are professors and typically have an Oxbridge, London or Civic University pedigree. Only a small minority of academics become PVCs much before their 50th birthday. Most were, and still are, men.

In a nutshell, their identities are based on their roles and tasks of strategic and operational management (Shepherd, 2014). From the research report by Smith et al. (2007), it can be inferred that PVCs present a more collegiate identity to less senior staff at formal meetings and with individual colleagues and try to avoid presenting a management identity. With external agencies, they tend to present a management identity. However, as they are perceived is influenced by how VCs see them, whether as a close colleague with whom to discuss policy and strategies, or merely as a facilitator of their VC's vision and an initiator of action to achieve that vision. Whatever their perceived identity by VCs they share with them a cross-institutional perspective which influences their self-identity.

Heads of departments

We have been unable to trace detailed demographics of HoDs *per se* in universities but Alexander & Arday (2015) provide a wide perspective. There is also an earlier insightful article by Deem (2003). She reports the views of a sample of HoDs and other senior staff on gender identities and how their self-portrayals of being consultative and people-focussed differ from those of their managed staff (including lecturers, secretaries, technicians and porters) who saw them as increasingly managerial and showed little concern for stress levels of employees. Some used aggressive management. She also reports on how males saw females as managers and vice versa. There were mixed views.

'Lecturing' staff

By 2017, the number of all academic staff (including senior staff) involved directly in teaching, and research had increased to 206,870 compared with 212, 835 non-academic staff (HESA, 2018). Of these approximately 45% were female (Oshu, 2018). Women were less likely to have higher academic ranks even when age, qualifications, number of publications, number of children, time to devote to teaching and research are taken into account (Santos & Dang Van Phu, 2019). As the authors of this study state: '*Put simply, two people who have similar, or even identical credentials and personal circumstances except for one being a man and the other being a woman, are likely to have different academic ranks, with the man having a higher rank than the woman.*'

The vast majority of lecturing staff are white followed by Chinese and other Asians. We found no reports of how their ethnic identity influenced the perceptions of others. But minority ethnic groups did have reservations about the university system in the UK (ecu.ac.uk, 2011; Bhopal, 2014, 2015, 2016). We found no statistical data on social class identity of lecturing staff but one can safely assume that the majority of academic staff, as reported in the section on VCs, are from middle-class backgrounds and occasionally from upper class or upward social mobility backgrounds. The student–staff ratio in universities ranges from approximately 11:1 to 21.5:1 (Complete University Guide, 2019). These differences are likely to have affected differentially the workloads and identities of academic staff.

Clegg (2008) discussed these changes in self-identity of academics from a postmodernist perspective. Her study provided a review and a qualitative study of changes in lecturers' perspectives. More recently Mahony & Weiner (2017) provide a useful review of the effects of neoliberalism upon identities of academics. They argue that the emphasis by the UK government on 'students as customers' has shaped the identity of academic staff through its effects on both their senior staff and their students. Their qualitative study indicates that heavier loads on academic staff are the result of greater demands by students for 'value for money', course and teaching satisfaction, stronger guidance and support in writing assignment and for university education to be primarily a gateway to better jobs. The list is formidable. Similar findings from their review and qualitative research are provided by Wong & Chiu (2017). They point out that changes in governmental policy, institutional and student demands have reshaped the identities of academic staff. Their qualitative study was based on the remembered self-identities as lecturers, before and after the implementation of higher fees, in two London-based post 1992 universities. They concluded that changes in governmental policies had changed radically the identities of lecturers through its effects on senior staff and students. It is not surprising that job satisfaction among academic staff was low in the UK (Coates & Goedegeburre, 2012) and the mental health of some staff is deteriorating (Morrish, 2019). One can surmise with confidence that the identity of lecturing staff has changed.

The shift is characterised as a change from academic managers to managed academics by Winter (2009) due to tensions in academic and commercial identity (Winter & O'Donohue, 2012). These changes may be summarised in the simple equation:

Teacher + Researcher + Junior Manager Identity = Academic Identity.

'Teacher' includes providing student support such as workshops and tutorials on how to get good grades as well as teaching a subject and providing prompt feedback. 'Researcher' includes doing and monitoring research, 'Junior Manager Identity' includes course design, data entries and student evaluations and recruitment activities such as visits to schools and open days. Research, because it generates income as well as a measurable outcome in the form of the number and location of articles, is usually seen as the higher priority.

In summary, Wood & Feng (2017) suggest that lecturers are often regarded as accountable service providers by students, academic staff themselves and senior staff. As one of our older colleagues observed mournfully *'We used to be a vocation then we became a profession. Now we are service providers.'*

There is plenty of research on students' views of lecturers, but little on how lectures see themselves (but see Figures 7.3 and 7.5). In one study of expectations of South Asian students and academic staff of each other, it was argued that the discrepancy may be traced to differences between Confucian and Socratic cultures (Kingston & Forland, 2008) (see also Hofstede, 1980). Their account implies that universities and staff need to change their perceived identity of these students so that the perceived identities of academic staff by students change.

On a wider front, it has consistently been shown that students perceive effective lecturers as systematic, stimulating and friendly (Ryans, 1960; Marsh, 1987). More recently the study by Wood & Feng (2017) showed that from students' perspective, the characteristics of good lecturers were those who had good subject knowledge, used inspirational teaching methods, were willing to help students, had a touch of humour and provided speedy feedback. Similar findings were found in a study of Chinese students (Bailey, undated) as one student said:

Nice and kind, always ready to help students to solve their problems. Also must be good at teaching.

In the 1970s, one of the authors gave seminars[i] on counselling personal tutorial students. One of the tasks he used was

Write down whatever comes into your head immediately when I ask this question. The question was 'What are you?' Some of the answers were:-

I'm a Yorkshireman. I'm a historian. I'm a Catholic and an English Teacher. I'm a senior lecturer in physics. I'm an engineer. I'm a Jewish academic from Germany now a little Anglicised. I am a lecturer in Adult Education and working class. A female lecturer in engineering wrote 'I am a woman in a man's world.' One newly appointed lecturer wrote 'I am a microbiologist and a knowledge-seeker!' The responses give some indication of variations in self-identity of lecturers.

i 'Seminars' have connotations of sowing seeds of knowledge – part of collegiality. Later in the 1980s, it was more fashionable to use the term 'workshops' which has connotations of industry and employment.

Figure 7.5 Some self-identities of lecturers.

Views of academics and employers

There is little research on how employers see academics or vice versa. Large employers prefer graduate from Oxbridge or Russell Group Universities (THES, 2015). UCAS (undated) claim that *'a significant number of employers consider UK graduates lack basic skills in numeracy and literacy, problem solving, communication, teamwork, analytical thinking, self-management, and resilience (able to cope with change and pressure in the workplace)'*. This is not the view taken by Clarke (2018) who argues that students develop a graduate identity from the courses they take. These courses are usually based on learning outcomes relevant to employability. But this graduate identity does not itself guarantee graduate employment. Other aspects of identity such as social class, gender, ethnicity, social networks and university status maybe more influential. Furthermore, an earlier report indicated only 13% of UK employers reported that they participated with universities in the development of these skills (Flash Eurobarometer, 2010). It seems that they considered these skills primarily, if not wholly, the initial responsibility of universities.

Subject identity

This section is rather different from previous sections that were predominantly concerned with the identities of academic staff. Subjects also change their identities and, like staff identities, subjects have these features:

- All subjects in universities have some things in common.
- Some subjects have more in common.
- All subjects have unique characteristics.

The corollary of this principle is the broader the generalisation, the more probable are exceptions.

For example, history in the Arts and histology in the Sciences are both studied, taught and researched in universities but they have different conceptions of valid research methods and very different approaches to research and publications. Within these subjects, there are also differences in approaches and methodologies.

The most frequently cited discussion of subject differences in the 20th century was Snow's views of the two cultures of Arts and Sciences (e.g. Snow, 1959). However, his views seem to be more redolent of his reservations of the lack of understanding of Science by Arts-educated senior civil servants than the differences between Arts and Sciences (Jardine, 2010). A better distinction is provided by Ricoeur (1981) who was interested in the differences between scientific and personal understanding (see Figure 7.4). It serves as a useful distinction between Sciences and Arts and some approaches in field biology, psychology and the social sciences.

Soon after Ricoeur's publication, Becher (1989) wrote 'Academic Tribes and Territories' based on a comprehensive review and his own empirical research of semi-structured interviews with 221 academics from 12 disciplines.

On the basis of his research, he developed four dimensions: *Hard v Soft, Pure v Applied, Convergent v Divergent and Urban v Rural.* These dimensions embrace both the 'territory' (subject area and epistemology) and the 'tribes' (personnel and social organisation) who inhabit the territory. It is difficult to map these four dimensions on a two-dimensional page but some of his findings are given in Table 7.1. It should be noted that these dimensions are continua not rigid categories. There are variations within subjects as well as between subjects.

Table 7.1 Examples of dimensions of subject identities

Hard (clear, determinate answers can be found)	Mixture	Soft[a] (no clear determinable answers: subject to belief systems and opinions)
Chemistry, Mathematics, Pharmacy, Physics	Biology, Mechanical Engineering, Economics, Geography	History, Law, Modern Languages, Sociology
Applied (leads to immediate practical outcomes)	*Mixture*	*Pure (does not lead to immediate practical outcomes)*
Mechanical Engineering, Law, Pharmacy	Synthetic Organic Chemistry, Economics	Biology, Physical Chemistry, Physics
Convergent (tightly knit)	*Mixture*	*Divergent (loosely knit)*
Economics, History, Physics, Mathematics	Biology, Chemistry, Law	Geography, Mechanical Engineering, Modern Languages, Pharmacy, Sociology
Urban (capital intensive)	*Mixture*	*Rural (labour intensive)*
Biomedical Sciences, Control Engineering, Physics	Mathematics, including Statistics and Applied Mathematics	Chemistry, History, Economics, Modern Languages, Sociology

Source: Based on *Becher (1989)*.

Becher also examined the cultures of disciplines and how they are influenced by national cultures and the social organisation within university departments. His study also revealed the differences in perception of academics of their own and other subjects. Even within their own specialities, they reported that there were national differences in research identities. More details of this work may be found in Becher & Trowler (2002), Trowler et al. (2012) and Trowler (2014).

A recent study (Rosewell & Ashwin, 2018) considered the self-perceptions of their subject identities by 35 academics in one UK university. Their use of IPA (interactive phenomenological analysis) revealed multilayer identity within the broad framework of teacher, researcher and academic. Those who viewed their predominant identity as a teacher were concerned with helping their students to understand and passing on their interest and love of their subject.

Being a researcher included knowledge creation and transmission. The creative process was a voyage of discovery. Its transmission was for official recognition. The identity of being an 'academic' went beyond the identity of researcher or teacher to being self-focussed, a contributor to knowledge and perhaps more than just a job. However, there were gender differences. The majority of males regarded being an academic as just a job, whereas females regarded being an academic as the core of their self-identity. A similar view was common among early career academics (Churchman & King, 2009).

It is interesting to speculate why subject identity rather than teaching identity is strong. A possible first-order explanation worth pursuing is early socialisation in a subject – because most academics study their subject in postgraduate studies. There certainly does seem to be differences in attitudes among lectures in Arts and Sciences (Brown & Daines, 1981) which probably still persist.

Finally, although the identities of academics in other countries are outside the brief of this chapter, the text edited by Barnett & Di Napoli (2008) considers, *inter alia*, identity changes in universities in other countries; Evans & Nixon (2015) provide a European perspective, and Dugas et al. (2018) provides a cautionary note on the effects of neoliberalism on academic identities.

Academic staff training and development

Soon after WW1, academic staff training and development was a recurrent theme in official reports and conferences. Their recommendations were ignored by most universities and their academics (Matheson, 1981; Nisbett & McAleese, 1979; Partington, 1965). The Hale Report (1964), a major precursor of staff development, led to various recommendations and exhortations by the AUT, CVCP and the NUS. These continued to be ignored by universities and their academics. A common myth was that university staff need not be trained: their subject knowledge was sufficient (Brown, 1977). This myth persisted until the 1980s and it may still be found, in various guises today.

Polytechnics (post 1991 universities) and their staff were more receptive of the need for training in teaching. The recommendations by the CNAA (Council for National Academic Awards) led to the establishment of educational development units in the late 1970s, whereas in universities staff development remained peripheral even though the Robbins Report (1963) had recommended training.

In 1985, Brown and Atkins (Brown & Atkins, 1985) published the results of a survey of academic staff training and development in universities. Their recommendations contributed to the development of Staff Development Units and subsequently to policies in most universities (Brown, 1994). These provided voluntary short courses on teaching and allied activities for all staff but were strongly recommended for new staff. Eventually they led to professional qualifications, often called Postgraduate Certificates in Higher Education (PGCHEs) in teaching and a requirement in most universities for probationers. The courses grew out of the recommendations of UCOSDA (Universities and Colleges Staff Development Association), now defunct, and the ILT (Institute of Learning and Teaching, 2000–2004). The ILT became the Higher Education Authority (HEA), a statutory body, for the formal approval of PGCHEs. HEA went on to develop more advanced qualifications in teaching and management and to become a provider of short courses and publications on aspects of the work of academics. For more advanced qualifications, they required the submission of reflective portfolios. HEA was incorporated into Advance HE in 2018. SEDA (Staff Educational Development Association) which grew out of SCEDSIP (Standing Conference on Educational Development Services) followed similar procedures of accreditation so it is not uncommon for senior academics and staff developers to become fellows of both these organisations (FHEA, FSEDA). These courses and organisations have stimulated a plethora of texts and articles on teaching, learning, assessment, leadership and academic management. SEDA also has an active online community of practice.

Two areas which might enhance staff development are teaching and research in different subjects. For example, seminars and tutorials in Arts require a different approach to those in the physical sciences. Pedagogical research on methods of teaching subjects (known as 'Didactics' on the European continent) would inform and enhance teaching development.

Senior academics are also now expected to attend courses in management training. Some of these are provided under the auspices of Universities UK, by individual universities or the SRHE (Society for Research in Higher Education). The latter since its foundation in 1965 has been a major influence on the training and development of all academics through its journals, reports, publications of texts and short courses.

All of these developments have contributed to changes in the identity of academic staff.

Academic and professional identity

We now return briefly how comfortably academic identity fits the concept of professional identity. The answer depends on what is considered as professional and academic identity. Originally the professions were only Law, Medicine and the Church. Currently, the term has been extended to any group that has received training, a formal qualification, has approved membership of an official organisation and abides by its light regulatory framework. The framework provides a guide to professional competence which may be regarded as the ability to perform to an acceptable standard in a given context. This new definition extends the notion of professional identity. It can be applied to many others, including funeral directors and stage designers. But it cannot yet be applied to academic identity for only academics in their early careers who are required to have a licence to practice in academe and the tight regulatory frameworks surrounding academics (and the health professions) could be regarded as de-professionalisation.

End notes

Our endnotes provide a summary of the chapter, some suggestions for future research and our concluding remarks.

Summary of chapter

In this chapter, we have provided *our* overview of the changing identities of the university system, universities and its constituents: students and academic staff, including VCs and senior staff. It has not considered changes in identities of Computing Services, Finance Department, Libraries, Registrars, Human Resource Managers, Staff Development Units or their staff, although their identities will almost certainly have changed with the advent of neoliberal policies, nor have we considered the complex relationships between self and identity or language and identity.

In reviewing the literature, we have drawn on three overlapping sources of evidence, historical perspectives, conceptual analyses, often postmodernist-based, and empirical research. The historical evidence have enabled us to map the changes in organisational and personal identity changes. The conceptual approaches have revealed different perspectives and the empirical reports contain both qualitative and quantitative data of reported changes in organisational and personal identities. All of these are important when considering changes in identity. But one should bear in mind that in a brief chapter, one has to be selective and not everyone will agree with our selection. We stress these in our views. Other writers and readers will have different views shaped by their values and belief systems. It is also worth noting that the current rapid changes in governances in the UK in 2019 are likely to change the identities of staff and students yet again.

Suggestions for future research

Values influence the collection and interpretation of evidence, so future researchers may wish to explore how values shape the forms of measurement and methods selected (Greenbank, 2003). For example, REF values citation indices as measures of impact. But an article might be cited frequently not because of its likely impact but because it is weak in methodology or conclusions. Nor does REF take into account replication of studies even though some may change the knowledge landscape. More fundamentally, it could be argued that impact is about changes in institutions or individuals so citations are, at best, proximal variables that might lead to impact – but not necessarily in the near future. Informal observations suggest that social media and the ubiquity of computers and smart phones almost certainly brought about changes in perceived and self-identities of students and staff. It can be argued that they have extended the notion of marketing identities, with presenting oneself favourably for different audiences. But informal observations need to be turned into qualitative and quantitative research.

The increasing power and connectivity of computers has also led to an increase in the use of analytics (the fashionable term for computated statistical analysis). They do have their uses in both neoliberalism and collegiality for support for executive decisions. They are also useful tools for governments, their agencies and universities. But they can result in remote decisions which may not tally with the realities of the work of staff or students and the decisions may render changes in academic identities that do not necessarily benefit universities. So more attention to qualitative studies, within universities and by non-governmental organisations, is desirable. They would leaven findings in analytics.

Beneath the reported changes in identity, one can detect the conflicts and benefits of the traditional identity of universities as transmitters, preservers and creators of knowledge and the neoliberalism identity of privatisation and commodification (Robertson, 2007). Within universities, a neoliberal approach has alerted universities to efficiency measured in terms of financial benefits but it can be myopic. Collegiality has been shown to increase morale and develop long-term academic values (Bolden et al., 2012). But hierarchical forms of consultation can retard innovation and are cumbersome. For example, in a predominantly collegiate-oriented university, it may take 3 years or more from the initial proposal for a curriculum reform or research project to be approved by the final decision-making committee. By which time the proposal may have been overtaken by other events. Case studies of the balance of the benefits of collegiality and neoliberalism in universities could be beneficial to the whole HE sector. Our conjecture is that universities which have strong characteristics of both are most likely to be more productive and have higher group morale.

The concept of collegiality itself needs expanding. Currently, it is confined to developments *within* universities. But there are likely to be both neoliberal and collegiate benefits to more cooperation *between* universities and in particular, if universities share national or international centres of research. These might be more efficient and productive. Such an enterprise would benefit staff and research students and, ultimately others, but their development and value to the HE sector and communities need to be explored.

Neoliberal policies have not only affected universities directly but also indirectly through their effects on economic and social structures. Schools are increasingly subject to neoliberal policies (Mishuria, 2014). As the gap between rich and poor widens, there are reported increases in social and health problems in the UK (and other countries) which affect the poorer populations and individuals (Wilkinson & Pickett, 2009, 2018; Bayliss & Mattioli, 2018). These together with their limited access to health, community facilities such as libraries, family support and adequate schooling are likely to influence recruitment, attitudes, values and identities of both students and staff in universities. Research on these issues will be complex and challenging but sorely needed.

Concluding remarks

At the heart of the problem of identities of universities, their constituents and their contexts is the issue of individual freedom versus control. Allowing people to do as they choose with little responsibility or concern for the university in which they work or the communities and the society in which they live is likely to lead to anarchy, dubious ideologies, such as Social Darwinism or the immorality of taxes, and consequently the neglect of many citizens. If profits benefit only a small minority in a country the situation is likely to be exacerbated. The question 'Cui bono?' is apposite. On the other hand, if collegiality slips into rigid control in a community or society then it is likely to lead to passive obedience, lack of initiative and, like extreme neoliberalism, to corruption. The message is clear: *in via media* is the better option. But where that middle path is depends on one's initial viewpoint. For us, a softer neoliberalism combined with collegiality within universities and care of communities is the preferred option. It remains to be seen whether our preference will become the route taken by universities, or neoliberalists will continue to shift the roles and identities of universities, their staff, other organisations and the wider communities. We are not entirely optimistic.

Acknowledgements

We wish to thank Jacob Kempton and Kathleen Lagan for their assistance with the figures; Elizabeth Brown and Gary Dench for their patience and Roger Ellis for keeping us on the right pathway towards publication.

References

Alexander, C. & Arday, J. (2015) (eds) *Aiming Higher: Race, Inequality and Diversity in the Academy* London: Runnymede.
Anderson Committee (1960) *Awards to Students at Universities and Comparable Institutions: Consideration of Recommendations* Not digitised. REF T227/1466 Available at Kew: The National Archives.
Auger Report (2019) *Review of Post-18 Education and Funding* London: HMSO.
Bailey, C. (undated) *"The UK Lecturers Don't Teach Me Anything": Chinese Students' Expectations of Their Teachers and Implications for UK HE Providers.* University of Wolverhampton Available at https://pdfs.semanticscholar.org/39d1/32b3dcccd933e551b5c2900bc334e5d09911.pdf Accessed 6 February 2019.
Barnett, R. & Di Napoli, R. (2008) (eds) *Changing Identities in Higher Education: Voicing Perspectives* Abingdon: Routledge.

Bayliss, K. & Mattioli, G. (2018) *Privatisation, Inequality and Poverty in the UK: Briefing Prepared for UN Rapporteur on Extreme Poverty and Human Rights Sustainability Research Institute*, University of Leeds Accessed 12 June 2019.

Becher, T. (1989) *Academic Tribes and Territories: Intellectual Enquiry and the Cultures of Disciplines* Milton Keynes: Open University Press and SRHE.

Becher, T. & Trowler, P. (2nd ed) (2002) *Academic Tribes and Territories*Milton Keynes: Open University Press and SRHE

Beech, D. (2017) *Going for Gold: Lessons from the TEF Providers HEPI Report* Available at https://www.hepi.ac.uk/wp-content/uploads/2017/10/FINAL-HEPI-Going-for-Gold-Report-99-04_10_17-Screen.pdf Accessed 13 May 2019.

Bhopal, K. (2014) *The Experience of BME Academics in Higher Education* Leadership Foundation Available at https://eprints.soton.ac.uk/364309/1/__soton.ac.uk_ude_personalfiles_users_kb4_mydocuments_Leadership foundation paper_Bhopal stimuls paper final.pdf Accessed 16 April 2019.

Bhopal, K. (2015) *Race, Inequality and Diversity in the Academy* London: Runnymede Trust, Soton Press Available at https://eprints.soton.ac.uk/374244/1/__userfiles.soton.ac.uk_Users_slb1_mydesktop_Aiming Higher.pdf Accessed 16 April 2019.

Bhopal, K. (2016) *The Experience of Black and Minority Ethnic Identities* London: Routledge.

Bowden, J. & Marton, F. (1998) *The University of Learning: Beyond Quality and Competence in Higher Education* London: Kogan Page.

Bolden, R., Gosling, J. & O'Brien, A. et al (2012) *Academic Leadership: Changing Conceptions, Identities and Experiences in UK Higher Education* London: Leadership Foundation.

Brown, G. (1977) Myths of staff training and development. *Impetus*, 6:2–8.

Brown, G. (Chmn) (1994) *Staff Development for Teaching: Towards a Comprehensive and Coherent Policy* Sheffield: UCoSDA.

Brown, G. & Daines, J. M. (1981) Can explaining be learnt? Some lecturers' views. *Higher Education*, 10(5):573–580.

Brown, G. & Atkins, M. (1985) Academic staff training in British universities: results of a national survey. *Studies in Higher Education*, 11(1):29–42.

Brown G., Rohlin, M. & Manogue, M. (2003) Collaborative learning, collegiality and critical thinking in Sweet, J., Huttly, S. & Taylor, I. (eds) *Effective Teaching and Learning in Medical, Dental and Veterinary Education* London: Kogan Page.

Burgess, R.D. (2008) The myth of a golden age? Reflections of a vice-chancellor in Barnett, R. & Di Napoli, R. (eds) *Changing Identities in Higher Education: Voicing Perspectives* Abingdon: Routledge.

Clarke, M. (2018) Rethinking graduate employability: the role of capital, individual attributes and context. *Studies in Higher Education*, 43(11):1923–1937, Accessed 24 June 2019.

Clegg, S. (2008) Academic identities under threat? *British Educational Research Journal*, 34:329–345.

Collini, S. (2012) *What are Universities for?* Harmondsworth: Penguin Books.

Churchman, D. & King, S. (2009) Academic practice in transition: hidden stories of academic identities. *Teaching in Higher Education*, 14:507–516.

Coates, H. & Goedegeburre, L. (2012) Recasting the academic workforce: why the attractiveness of the academic profession needs to be increased and eight possible strategies for how to go about this from an Australian perspective. *Higher Education*, 64(6):875–889.

Complete University Guide (2019) Available at https://www.thecompleteuniversityguide.co.uk/league-tables/rankings?o=Student-Staff+Ratio&v=wide Accessed 6 March 2019.

Dearing Report (1997) *Higher Education in the Learning Society Main Report* London: Her Majesty's Stationery Office.

Deem, R. (2003) Gender, organizational cultures and the practices of manager-academics in UK universities. *Gender, Work and Organization*, 10(2):133–136.

Dugas, D., Stich, A.E., Lindsay, N., Harris. L.N. *et al.* (2018) 'I'm being pulled in too many different directions': academic identity tensions at regional public universities in challenging economic times. *Studies in Higher Education*:239–259 Accessed 19 April 2019.

ecu.ac.uk (2011) https://www.ecu.ac.uk/wp-content/uploads/external/annual-review-2011 Accessed 16 April 2019.

Evans, L. & Nixon, J. (eds) (2015) *Academic Identities in Higher Education: The Changing European Landscape* London: Bloomsbury.

Flash Eurobarometer (2010) *Employers Perception of Graduate Employability* Accessed 10 June 2019.

Glassdoor (2018) Glassdoor.ac.ukhttps://www.glassdoor.co.uk/Salaries/uk-pro-vice-chancellor-salary-SRCH_IL.0,2_IN2_KO3,22.htm Accessed 17 April 2019.

Greenbank, P. (2003) The role of values in educational research: the case for reflexivity. *British Educational Research Journal*, 29(6):791–801, Published online 2010.

Hale Report (1964) *Report of the Committee on University Teaching Methods* London: HMSO.

Hall, R. (2017) *University Staff: VCs are too 'far away from the day to day reality'* Report of a Guardian Survey 10th May 2017 Accessed 18 March 2019.

HESA (2018) *Higher Education Statistics: UK 2016/7* Accessed 26 February 2019.

HESA (2019) *Higher Education Statistics: UK 2017/8* Accessed 26 February 2019.

Hofstede, G. (1980). *Culture's Consequences: International Differences in Work-Related Values* Beverly Hills, CA: Sage.

Jardine, L. (2010) *C.P. Snow's Two Cultures Revisited* The 2009 C.P. Snow Lecture, given in Christ's College by Professor Lisa Jardine. 14 October 2009 http://www.christs.cam.ac.uk/cms_misc/media/Publications_Christs_Magazine_2010_web.pdf Accessed 18 April 2019.

Jarratt Report (Chmn) (1985) *Report of the Steering Committee for Efficiency Studies in Universities* London: Committee of Vice-Chancellors and Principals.

Jessop, B. (2017) On academic capitalism. *Critical Policy Studies*, 12(1):104–109.

Kingston, E. & Forland, H. (2008) Bridging the gap in expectations between international students and academic staff. *Journal of Studies in International Education*, 12(2):204–221 Accessed 12 June 2019.

Mahony, P. & Weiner, G. (2017) Neo-liberalism and the state of higher education in the UK. *Journal of Further and Higher Education*, 43(4):560–572 Accessed 23 February 2019.

Marsh, H.W. (1987) Students' evaluations of university teaching: research findings, methodological issues, and directions for future research. *International Journal of Educational Research*, 11(3):253–388.

Matheson, C.C. (1981) *Staff Development Matters: A review 1961–81* Coordinating Committee for the Training of University Teachers, CVCP.

Mishuria, A. (2014) *The Neo-liberalisation Policy Agenda and Its Consequences for Education in England: A Focus on Resistance Now and Possibilities for the Future* Policy Futures in Education Volume www.wwwords.co.uk/PFIE Accessed 1 June 2019.

Morrish, L. (2019) *Pressure Vessels: The Epidemic of Poor Metal Health Amongst Higher Education Staff* Occasional Paper 20, London: Higher Education Policy Institute.

Nisbett, J. & McAleese, R. (1979) Staff development in universities in Teather, D. (ed) *Staff Development in Higher Education* London: Kogan Page.

OfS (2019) Office for Students Available https://www.officeforstudents.org.uk Accessed 11 May 2019.

Oshu, S. (2018) *How far Have Women Come in Higher Education Advance HE* Available at https://www.ecu.ac.uk/blogs/far-women-come-higher-education/ Accessed 6 March 2019.

Partington, P. (1965) Staff Development and EHE in Gray, H. (ed) *Changing Higher Education* London: SED Salford and UCosDA.

REF (2021) Available at (https://www.ref.ac.uk/publications/draft-guidance-on-codes-of-practice-201803/) Accessed 13 May 2019.

Ricoeur, P. (1981) *Hermeneutics & the Human Sciences* Cambridge: Cambridge University Press.

Robbins Report (1963) *Higher Education Report of the Committee Appointed by the Prime Minister under the Chairmanship of Lord Robbins* London: Her Majesty's Stationery Office.

Robertson, S.L. (2007) 'Remaking the World': neo-liberalism and the transformation of education and teachers' labour in Weis, L. & Compton M. (eds) *The Global Assault on Teachers, Teaching and their Unions* New York: Palgrave.

Rosewell, K. & Ashwin, P. (2018) Academics' perceptions of what it means to be an academic. *Studies in Higher Education* Published online 2018 Available at https://www.tandfonline.com/doi/abs/10.1080/03075079.2018.1499717 Accessed 8 April 2019.

RSS (2018) *Teaching Excellence Framework* Available file://localhost/at https/::www.rss.org.uk:Images:PDF:influencing-change:2018:RSS-Evidence-Dept-Education-Teaching-Excellence-Framework_final-21May-2018.pdf Accessed 8 March 2019.

Ryans, D.G. (1960) *Characteristics of Teachers* Washington, DC: American Council of Education.

Santos, G. & Dang Van Phu, S. (2019) Gender and academic rank in the UK. *Sustainability*, 11:31–76 Accessed 6 June 2019.

Scott, P (2015) Abolishing the Higher Education Funding Council for England would remove valuable 'arm's length' regulation of the sector. *The Guardian* 29 November 2015 Accessed 24 February 2019.

Shepherd, S. (2014) The rise of the career PVC. *Leadership Foundation Magazine Autumn*, 36:10–13.

Simpson, R. (1983) *How the PhD Came to Britain* Milton Keynes: Open University Press.

Smith, D., Adams, J. & Mount, D. (2007) *UK Universities and Executive Officers: The Changing Role of Pro-Vice-Chancellors Final Report* Higher Education Policy Unit University of Leeds.

Snow, C.P. (1959) *The Two Cultures and the Scientific Revolution* Cambridge: Cambridge University Press.

Taylor, J. R. (2018) *The Impact of the First World War on British Universities: Emerging from the Shadows* Basingstoke: Palgrave Macmillan.

THES (2015) *Graduate Employability: Top Universities in the UK Ranked by Employers 2018* https://www.timeshighereducation.com/student/best-universities/graduate-employability-top-universities-uk-ranked-employers-2018.

Trowler, P. (2014) Depicting and Researching Disciplines: strong and moderate essentialist approaches. *Studies in Higher Education*, 39(10):1720–1731. DOI: 10.1080/03075079.2013.801431 Available at https://www.tandfonline.com/doi/abs/10.1080/03075079.2013.801431?journalCode=cshe20 Accessed 29 April 2019.

Trowler, P. Saunders, M. & Bamber, V. (2012) (eds.) *Tribes and Territories in the 21st Century: Rethinking the Significance of Disciplines in Higher Education* Abingdon: Routledge.

UCAS (undated) *What are Employers Looking for?* https://www.ucas.com/careers/getting-job/what-are-employers-looking Accessed 23 June 2019.

UKRI (2019) *United Kingdom Research and Innovation* Available at https://www.ukri.org Accessed 11 May 2019.

Universities UK (2018a) *Higher Education in Numbers* https://www.universitiesuk.ac.uk/facts-and-stats/Pages/higher-education-data.aspx Accessed 21 March 2019.

Universities UK (2018b) *Pattern and Trends in UK Higher Education 2018* https://www.universitiesuk.ac.uk/facts-and-stats/data-and-analysis/Pages/Patterns-and-trends-in-UK-higher-education-2018.aspx Accessed 10 May 2019.

Watermeyer, R. (2016) Impact in the REF: issues and obstacles. *Studies in Higher Education*, 41(2):199–214.

West, S. (2018) *Vice Chancellors Blog* Available atfile://localhost/ https/::www.nottingham.ac.uk:about:vice-chancellor:blog:blog-014.aspx Accessed 4 April 2019.

Wilkinson, C. (2017) Evidencing impact: a case study of UK academic perspectives on evidencing research impact. *Studies in Higher Education*, 44(1):72–85.

Wilkinson, R. G. & Pickett, K. (2009) The spirit level. *Why More Equal Societies Almost Always Do Better* London: Allen Lane.

Wilkinson, R.G. & Pickett, K. (2018) *The Inner Level: How More Equal Societies Reduce Stress, Restore Sanity and Improve Everyone's Well-being* London: Allen Lane.

Willetts, D. (2017) A *University Education* Oxford: Oxford University Press.

Williams, J. (2013) *Consuming Higher Education: Why Learning Can't be Bought* London: Bloomsbury Press.

Winter, R. (2009) Academic manager or managed academic? Academic identity schisms in higher education. *Journal of Higher Education Policy and Management*, 3(2):121–131.

Winter, R. & O'Donohue, W. (2012) Academic identity tensions in the public university: which values really matter? *Journal of Higher Education Policy and Management*, 34(6):565–573.

Wong, B. & Chiu, Y.T. (2017) Let me entertain you: the ambivalent: role of university lecturers as educators and performers. *Educational Review*, 71(2):218–233.

Wonkhe (2017) *A New Framework is Born: Meet KEF* Available at https://wonkhe.com/blogs/a-new-framework-is-born-meet-kef/ Accessed 16 April 2019.

Wood, M. & Feng Su (2017) What makes an excellent lecturer? Academics' perspectives on the discourse of 'teaching excellence' in higher education. *Teaching in Higher Education*, 22(4):451–466 Accessed 18 April 2019.

8 Evolving professional identities in healthcare

The case of associate professions

Damian Day

Introduction

At the time of writing in later 2019, the United Kingdom (UK) was in the midst of a snap general election. The issue that prompted the election was Brexit, the UK's decision to leave the European Union. That decision had been taken, in the form of a referendum, in 2016. Healthcare, specifically the National Health Service (NHS), was one of the key campaigning issues: various parties were promising more nurses, more doctors and more hospitals, at a time when the NHS was struggling to fill some posts and maintain services. The National Health Service (NHS)'s (2019) *Interim People Plan* makes it clear that some healthcare professionals are increasing prioritizing lifestyle over work, resulting in part-time working and early retirement in many cases. Added to that is the reshaping some roles and making others less relevant. Taking the supply of medicines as an example, the traditional face-to-face transactional model between a community (high street) pharmacist and a patient is still a reality for many people, but other options are now available and are gaining market share. Some medicines supply companies act as intermediaries between a prescriber (probably a doctor) and a patient: they take receipt of a prescription, dispense it and bring it to your door. Others act as prescribing services themselves: after collecting some health data, a remote pharmacist will prescribe a medicine which will then be delivered to you.

Technology is reshaping service delivery as well, assisting healthcare professionals in many cases but threatening to make other roles redundant in the not too distant future. Finally, it is generally accepted that the Brexit decision itself caused significant number of European-trained healthcare professionals to leave the NHS and, in many cases, the UK. This is most acute in nursing, where the Interim People Plan acknowledges there will be a significant shortfall in the supply of nurses unless steps are taken to reverse the current decline.

Reshaping the healthcare workforce

What does the current situation mean for the way in which healthcare professions are being reshaped? One clear theme is the recognition that traditional disciplinary boundaries will not hold fast in the future. To use medicine supply and use as an example again, the historic – and slightly crude – demarcation between roles was that doctors prescribed medicine, pharmacists supplied medicine and offered some advice to patients about the medicine and nurses counselled patients on the medicine's use. Since 2006, after some additional training both nurses and pharmacists have been able to prescribe medicines independently (without reference to another prescriber, usually a doctor), counsel a patient on the use of the medicine and also monitor their long-term health. Depending on your perspective, this either allows highly trained healthcare professionals to operate to the fullest extent of their licence or it breaks the indispensable bond between a patient and their doctor.

The reshaping of traditional disciplinary boundaries has had another important effect: the widespread introduction of multi-professional clinical teams and the recognition within the NHS that there will 'undoubtedly need to be growth in all the established professions – and in some new professions – to meet future demand' [National Health Service (NHS), 2019, p 3]. Consequently:

> This transformation of our workforce is already underway in some parts of the NHS. But we must now accelerate our efforts to create a more flexible and adaptive workforce, further developing our people to make the best use of their talents, as well as getting the most value from critical new roles such as physician and nursing associates and our wider workforce of volunteers, carers and partners. This will mean supporting and enabling health professionals to work in new ways that make better use of the full range of their skills.
>
> [National Health Service (NHS), 2019, p 32]

In primary care, networks of healthcare are coalescing around general practitioner (GP) practices, where doctors are supported by practice nurses, and practice pharmacists, and then linking to other health and social care providers in the same geographical area. On the one hand, the networks are a vehicle for allowing healthcare professionals to be used as affectively as possible, on the other they are bringing a wider range of services closer to people and away from pressurized secondary care centres, particularly hospitals. The underpinning principle identified in the Interim People Plan is subsidiarity, both in respect of delegating activity from the centre to the local area and also in delegating activity from one professional, where it has resided historically, to others. In some case, the professions are well established ones which are being repurposed – pharmacists working in GP practices, for example – but in other cases the professions are new (or at least new to the NHS in their current form). Two emphasized in the Interim People Plan are Nursing Associates and Physician Associates:

> We will continue to develop the new nursing associate role, as part of our expansion of the nursing workforce. This role acts as a bridge between the unregulated healthcare assistant and the registered nurse. Our new nursing associates will be a vital part of the wider health and care team, providing

valuable support to registered nurses and enabling them to focus on more complex clinical duties. They are educated to work with people of all ages and in a variety of settings across health and social care, including in hospices, in community nursing teams and nursing homes, and in acute inpatient, mental health, learning disability and offender health services.

[National Health Service (NHS), 2019, p 40]

and

Physician associates, as generalist healthcare professionals trained to a medical model, will increasingly become an indispensable part of our primary and acute care teams. We estimate there will be over 2,800 physician associate graduates by the end of 2020, rising to over 5,900 by the end of 2023. The government's commitment to regulate physician associates is a significant step towards maximising their capability and embedding this critical role in our workforce.

[National Health Service (NHS), 2019, p 43]

Associate professions and professionals

Nursing associates, physician associates and pharmacy technicians are examples of professions that have arisen in part to allow more established professions to work in as efficient a way as possible and using their experience, knowledge and skills to the fullest extent. As has been mentioned, the roles are comparatively new to the NHS in their current configuration but do have longer histories. In some respects, nursing associates are similar to the historic 'enrolled nurses', who worked in healthcare teams under the supervision of registered nurses (nurses); and physician associates performed and do perform similar roles to the new one in the US military and remote/rural areas, where access to a doctor can be difficult. Finally, technical roles have existed in pharmacy for some time and predate the current registered[1] pharmacy technician role.

Rather than viewing these roles as subsets of and subsidiary to other professions, this chapter suggests they should be considered as a layer of professions in their own right with a shared set of characteristics. A helpful place to start is the UK's Office for National Statistics' (ONS) Standard Occupational Classification hierarchy. It classifies doctors, dentists, pharmacists, nurses and midwives as 'professional occupations' and paramedics, dispensing opticians, pharmaceutical (pharmacy) technicians, medical and dental technicians and health associate professionals as 'associate professional and technical occupations'. A key difference between the two groups being the 'practical application of an extensive body of theoretical knowledge...' vs 'experience and knowledge of principles and practices necessary to assume operational responsibility and to give technical support to Professionals and to Managers, Directors and Senior Officials' (see Table 8.1).

Table 8.1 Office for National Statistics' Standard Occupational Classification Occupation Definitions

Office for National Statistics' Standard Occupational Classification	
Occupation Definitions	
Professional Occupations	*Associate Professional and Technical Occupations*
Job description:	Job description:
This major group covers occupations whose main tasks require a high level of knowledge and experience in the natural sciences, engineering, life sciences, social sciences, humanities and related fields. The main tasks consist of the practical application of an extensive body of theoretical knowledge, increasing the stock of knowledge by means of research and communicating such knowledge by teaching methods and other means.	This major group covers occupations whose main tasks require experience and knowledge of principles and practices necessary to assume operational responsibility and to give technical support to professionals and to managers, directors and senior officials.
Most occupations in this major group will require a degree or equivalent qualification, with some occupations requiring postgraduate qualifications and/or a formal period of experience-related training.	The main tasks involve the operation and maintenance of complex equipment; legal, business, financial and design services; the provision of information technology services; providing skilled support to health and social care professionals; serving in protective service occupations and managing areas of the natural environment. Culture, media and sports occupations are also included in this major group. Most occupations in this major group will have an associated high-level vocational qualification, often involving a substantial period of full-time training or further study. Some additional task-related training is usually provided through a formal period of induction.
22 Health professionals	32 Health and social care associate professionals
2211 Medical practitioners	3213 Paramedics
2213 Pharmacists	3216 Dispensing opticians
2215 Dental practitioners	3217 Pharmaceutical technicians
2231 Nurses	3218 Medical and dental technicians
2232 Midwives	3219 Health associate professionals

Perspectives on associate professional roles[2]

One of the more intriguing aspects of these new roles is that in some respects – on paper, perhaps – they seem to be quite similar to their linked 'professional occupation'. Discussing them with education and training leads the differences emerged in discussion through examples rather than by a close reading of text (which we will do in the following section). To build on the ONS definition in the previous section, some common themes did emerge:

1   *Filling natural gaps as established professional roles are upskilling*: Education and training leads view associate professional roles as the consequence of a shift in emphasis in traditional professional roles: for example, doctors should be

able to focus more on complex patients with co-morbidities, allowing pharmacists to manage patients with less complex needs and also managing the medicines dispensing process. As pharmacists develop their skills as clinicians managing less complex patients, while they might be managing the medicines prescription service, its technical and operational aspects can be managed and undertaken by pharmacy technicians. A clear illustration of the subsidiarity principle at work.

2 *Very little difference in the core skills of professionals and associate professionals*: When pressed, education and training leads found it difficult to identify major areas in which the core skills of associate professionals differed significantly from that of their closest professional counterparts. The difference they felt was the degree of autonomy enjoyed by the different groups and differing scopes of practice, to which we will return.

3 *Associate professional roles and assistants*: We should not forget that relationships are not only between associate professionals and professionals but also between associate professionals and support staff. Community pharmacy illustrates the point well, in that the more established relationship would be between a pharmacist and an assistant in the dispensary or a counter assistant. With the introduction of the pharmacy technician, assistants are finding it difficult to understand the role because while pharmacists are legally responsible for dispensing medicines, most other functions can be undertaken by pharmacy technicians. This includes triaging patients, taking medical histories, running some clinics and managing the pharmacy in the pharmacist's absence. Rebalancing roles across the pharmacy team has been embraced by some but others find it confusing.

4 *Emphasis on tasks*: In general, the view of education and training leads was that associate professional roles were slightly more task-based and less holistic than professional roles but, accepting that, they felt that in time there would be scope to introduced advanced roles at the associate professional level as well.

5 *Generic vs specialist*: Finally, there was a view that the skills of associate professionals were more generic, on the whole, than those of professionals.

Taken together it could be argued that associate professionals are part of a general move to a more nuanced and progressive hierarchy of roles, along the lines of Figure 8.1.

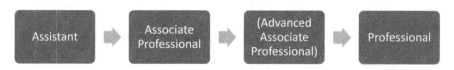

Figure 8.1 A move to a more nuanced and progressive hierarchy of roles.

Examining an associate professional role in greater depth

One of the problems in comparing roles of any complexity is their variety: as professionals develop, they grow into roles, become more or less specialist and/or decide on any number or routes from being a day 1 novice to advanced specialist or generalist. For this reason, the most reliable point of comparison between professions is the point of initial registration and the education and training leading up to it.

For pharmacists and pharmacy technicians, the domains for initial education and training are the same:

Domain 1: Person-centred care
Domain 2: Professionalism
Domain 3: Professional knowledge and skills
Domain 4: Collaboration

If we take the first domain, person-centred care, the coverage is remarkably similar, but that could be because what is being described is mainly generic and could apply to most healthcare professions (although that is an important point in itself).

Domain 1: Person-centred care

Note:
Student pharmacist learning outcomes are not italicised
Pharmacy technician trainee learning outcomes are italicised

- Work in partnership with patients, carers and the public to support and empower them when making decisions about their health and well-being – DOES[3]
- Take into consideration factors that affect people's behaviours in relation to health and well-being – SHOWS HOW
- *Involve, support and enable every person when making decisions about their health, care and well-being – DOES*
- *Listen to the person and understand their needs and what matters to them – DOES*
- *Give the person all relevant information in a way they can understand, so they can make informed decisions and choices – DOES*
- *Obtain relevant information from people – including patients, carers and other healthcare professionals – and use it appropriately – DOES*
- Proactively support people with the safe and effective use of their medicines and devices – DOES
- *Optimise a person's medicines to achieve the best possible outcomes – DOES*
- *Recognise adverse drug reactions and interactions and respond appropriately – DOES*
- *Advise people on the safe and effective use of their medicines and devices – DOES*
- Understand and meet their legal responsibilities under equality and human rights legislation and respect diversity and cultural differences

- Take responsibility for ensuring that person-centred care is not compromised because of personal values and beliefs – DOES
- *Recognise and value diversity and respect cultural differences – making sure that every person is treated fairly whatever their values and beliefs – DOES*
- Adapt their approach and communication style to meet the needs of each person – DOES
- *Adapt information and communication to meet the needs of particular audiences – DOES*
- Effectively promote healthy lifestyles using evidence-based techniques and take appropriate actions – DOES
- *Effectively promote healthy lifestyles using available resources and evidence-based techniques – KNOWS HOW*
- Take action to safeguard people, particularly children and vulnerable adults – DOES
- *Understand how to safeguard people, particularly children and vulnerable adults – KNOWS HOW*

Pharmacy technician trainees only

- *Apply the principles of information governance and ensure patient confidentiality – DOES*

In the second domain, we see a similar degree of convergence with just four learning outcomes unique to pharmacists:

Pharmacist students only

- Demonstrate the values, attitudes and behaviours expected from a pharmacist – DOES
- Recognise their own future role as a responsible and accountable pharmacist who understands the legal and ethical implications in the environments in which they work – DOES
- Critically evaluate and use national guidance and clinical evidence to support safe, rational and cost-effective procurement and use of medicines, devices and services – DOES
- Understand and address the importance of infection control and management in populations, environments and individuals – SHOWS HOW

In that group, the first learning outcome could apply equally to pharmacy technicians and there is no reason the third and fourth could not apply as well. It is only the second that can apply solely to pharmacists because what supports it is the legally binding 'responsible pharmacist' – the person who is responsible for the safe and effective running of a pharmacy. Whatever the day-to-day reality is, that role is reserved to the pharmacist.

It is really only in the third domain, professional knowledge and skills, where there is any significant divergence:

Pharmacist students only

- Understand and apply the science of pharmacy – DOES
- Understand and apply the principles of clinical therapeutics and make effective use of medicines – DOES
- Recognise and apply the principles of pharmacovigilance – DOES
- Critically evaluate the evidence base to improve practice and systems and the quality of care – DOES
- Engage in research activities and understand how research is applied to practice – DOES
- Identify and use appropriate diagnostic or physiological testing techniques to apply to clinical decision-making – DOES
- Demonstrate effective consultation skills – DOES
- Demonstrate effective diagnostic skills to decide the most appropriate course of action – DOES
- Undertake safe and appropriate physical examination and use clinical skills to apply to clinical decision-making – DOES
- Apply the legal and professional requirements around the management of information and to ensure patient confidentiality – DOES
- Use current and developing technologies and data to support the health of people by the safe and effective delivery of pharmaceutical services – DOES
- Use technology to improve the understanding of health problems, health and care services and interventions – DOES
- Implement appropriate strategies in relation to the misuse of drugs – DOES

This set of learning outcomes is where the significant scientific basis of pharmacist initial education and training is described and also it highlights the importance of research. It includes consultation skills, diagnostic skills and clinical examination but in doing so creates a dilemma. A pharmacy technician (and a counter assistant, for that matter) could demonstrate consultation and diagnostic skills sufficient to sell Anadin rather than Paracetamol to someone who is hypertensive but would not be able to make more complex decisions about patient care. The same is true of pharmacists, whose consultation and diagnostic skills would be unlikely to cover the full range of paediatric, adult, psychiatric and geriatric conditions dealt with by a doctor. The dilemma is how to deal with the nuances between the roles – this is discussed in the next section.

Scope of practice

In the previous section, we have seen the closeness of the curriculum for professionals and their cognate associate professions, which does prompt one to consider the differences in the roles. Part of the answer may be that the initial education and training of some associate professions is at a lower academic level than their cognate professional groups. For example, while pharmacists are educated to master's level (level 7 in the English and Welsh qualifications hierarchy), pharmacy technicians are educated to level 3, the vocational equivalent of the school-leaving qualification for an 18-year-old. Added to that professionals and associate professionals are discussed in the same context but without a clear understanding of the distinction between them. Taking physician associates as an example, the Faculty of Physician Associates states 'Physician associates (PAs) are a relatively new member of the clinical team, seen as complementary to GPs rather than a substitute… By employing a PA, it does not mitigate the need to address the shortage of GPs or reduce the need for other practice staff. They can help to broaden the capacity of the GP role and skill mix within the practice team to help address the needs of patients in response to the growing and ageing population.' [Royal College of Physicians, Faculty of Physician Associates (FPA), 2012]. Therefore, they add to the skills mix with some but not all of the skills of a doctor. There are a few differences which are common to associate professional groups compared to professional groups but not a great many. An example would be the ability to prescribe medicines, which doctors, pharmacists and nurses can do[4] but pharmacy technicians, nursing associates and physician associates cannot[5]. In some jurisdictions, the boundaries of a profession seem to be quite clearly and tightly defined: a pharmacist example would be the core curriculum in Japan which lists 1070 'small behavioural objects' [Pharmaceutical Society of Japan (PSJ), 2018]. In the UK, however, the difference between professional roles is dealt with by requiring adherence to a common code of professional conduct but then distinguishing between roles by referring to 'limits of competence' or 'scope of practice' as being the distinction between roles: 'Nurses, midwives and nursing associates uphold the Code within the limits of their competence. This means, for example, that while a nurse and nursing associate will play different roles in an aspect of care, they will both uphold the standards in the Code within the contribution they make to overall care.' [Nursing and Midwifery Council (NMC), 2018, p 4]. Returning to pharmacy and the education and training of pharmacy technicians, this is dealt with in learning outcomes thus:

- Recognise and work within the limits of their knowledge and skills and seek support and refer to others when needed – DOES (pharmacist student)
- *Recognise and work within the limits of their knowledge and skills and refer to others when needed* – DOES (pharmacy technician trainee) [General Pharmaceutical Council (GPhC), 2017]

There are similar statements in equivalent standards for other professional and associate professional roles.

In the final section, we consider the implications of this approach for job roles and the skill mix within healthcare.

Conclusion: the changing skills mix

Some healthcare associate professionals are well established and have recognized, bounded roles. While acknowledging that, all roles are being challenged and boundaries pushed as the NHS tries to make the most of its resources. The associate professional challenge is that while many roles are similar to other, more established professional roles, the associate professionals tread a line between being an autonomous professional and one who refers to other professionals in certain circumstances. The extent to which this occurs depends on the experience of the associate professional and the context in which they are working.

It is clear from discussing the new roles with education and training leads that there is a need and a purpose for the roles but if the discussion turns to tasks, it becomes far more difficult to define the boundaries between professions and to define precisely what it is associate professionals cannot do, other than things which are reserved in law to other professionals. To ask a slightly different question, is there much difference between a highly experienced associate professional and a minimally competent professional? These kinds of issues are challenging professional groups and employers alike. The challenge is partly one of skill mix but also financial, as average salaries of associate professionals, no matter how experienced, as significantly lower than those of professionals. As an example, a GP practice dispensing service may once have been staffed by doctors writing prescriptions, many of them low risk, repeat prescriptions, but now that service may be managed by pharmacists and pharmacy technicians, saving both time and money.

An overarching issue is the extent to which roles can be stretched or created and the consequences of that for safe delivery of a service, delegation and accountability, particularly when something goes wrong. There is no firm evidence that delegation and subsidiarity are putting patients at risk, but it is legitimate to ask whether that could be the case if the expertise of professionals was stretched ever further if recruitment problems persist. For now, we should view that issue in perspective: it is still the case that medical roles are undertaken overwhelmingly by doctors (there are c.150,000 doctors in the UK and less than 10,000 physician associates) and for nursing roles the figures are c.320,000 nurses and c.1500 nursing associates. Nevertheless, as it is clearly the NHS's strategic intention to embed and expand these roles, the balance between professions will change over time.

In this chapter, we have considered an approach to discussing the emergence of new roles in relation to established ones and it is an approach not normally taken. While we have considered examples from healthcare, the same is true in most areas – accountancy and law being just two examples. The wider context has been discussed as well – including the changing needs of the public, automation and the use of technology. While the public may not notice too much of a difference in the way healthcare is provided – they may still collect their medicine from a pharmacy or visit a GP practice for healthcare advice – the way in which the service is being configured behind the scenes may change considerably.

Notes

1. At the time of writing, pharmacy technicians had been registered with the General Pharmaceutical Council for 8 years, since 2011, it had been agreed recently that nursing associates should be registered with the Nursing and Midwifery Council and legislation was being prepared to allow Physician Associates to be registered by the General Medical Council.

2. I am grateful to colleagues at the University of Central Lancashire, University of Worcester, St George's Medical School, Birmingham City University and GPhC accreditors for sharing their views with me.
3. 'Does', 'shows how' and 'knows how' refer to outcome levels in Miller's Triangle of Clinical Competence.
4. Pharmacists and nurses after additional post-registration training.
5. Although this may change for physician associates, once they are regulated by the General Medical Council.

References

General Pharmaceutical Council (GPhC) (2017) *Standards for the Initial Education and Training of Pharmacy Technicians.* Retrieved November 20 2019 from https://www.pharmacyregulation.org/standards

National Health Service (NHS) (2019) *NHS Interim People Plan.* Retrieved November 2019 from https://improvement.nhs.uk/resources/interim-nhs-people-plan/

Nursing and Midwifery Council (NMC) (2018) *The Code, Professional Standards of Practice and Behaviour for Nurses, Midwives and Nursing Associates.* Retrieved November 10 2019 from https://www.nmc.org.uk/globalassets/sitedocuments/nmc-publications/nmc-code.pdf

Pharmaceutical Society of Japan (PSJ) (2018) *Model Core Curriculum for Pharmacy Education.* Retrieved November 20 2019 from https://www.pharm.or.jp/kyoiku/pdf/corecurri_eng180426.pdf

Royal College of Physicians, Faculty of Physician Associates (FPA) (2012) *Physician Assistant Managed Voluntary Register Competence and Curriculum Framework.* Retrieved November 12 2019 from https://www.fparcp.co.uk/about-fpa

9 Professional identity and competence to practise in medicine

Adrian Furnham

Introduction

This chapter will attempt to assess the way in which the medical profession and patients define, determine, regulate and evaluate competence in doctors. The concept of competence is both multidimensional and remains ambiguous, which makes any analysis of this issue problematic. Furthermore, it has numerous synonyms such as sufficiency, capacity and adequacy, none of which quite tap the subtlety of the actual concept of competence as applied to professional quality assurance. Moreover, the concept gets expanded to cover new areas such as the current interest in cultural competence.

As a consequence, a lot has been written about a 'competency-based medical curriculum'. Indeed, Albanese et al. (2009) suggested that building a competency-based curriculum is about maintaining quality control and relinquishing control to students in the face of challenges like declining availability of teaching patients and over-burdened faculty, instituting quality control and relinquishing control will be necessary to maintain high quality.

Many professionals attempt to instil, by formal and informal socialisation and education, a certain degree or level of competence in a large number of specific, profession-related skills. These skills are usually assessed by a formal examination. The central question is which skills, how best to instil and measure them.

There are essentially three ways of teaching/training people: classroom/ward teaching using traditional teaching methods; active learning through practice and assignments; and personal coaching. We are now also seeing the emergence of e-learning and teaching. Most doctors are trained by all four methods. One question for those in medical education is how to use different methods to achieve maximum competence at minimum cost to the taxpayer. This question is at the heart of the issue for academics, politicians and members of the general public.

The concept of competence

Psychologists tend to assess people in term of ability, motives and traits. Human resource specialists on the other hand talk about individual differences in terms of capability, competency, experience, know-how, potential and proficiency. Most organisations now have *competency frameworks* that are used to make decisions about appraisal, recruitment, selection and training. These are often described in great detail, and it is unclear how the individual difference competencies originate, how trainable/malleable they are and whether they change over time.

It has been noted that the term competence, with its allusion to *mere* sufficiency and adequacy, sounds dated in a world that demands excellence and outstanding performance. Some argue that people can only infer competence from *seeing incompetence*. On the other hand, dictionary definitions do stress that competence is an ability, skill or know-how: something done in an efficient and effective or adequate way. Many organisations still use it as the way to describe salient individual differences that define salient behaviours at work. For all sorts of reasons, they seem to prefer not to talk about cognitive ability or personality traits.

Although there may be difficulties with the technical definition of competence, there are even more when it comes to incompetence. Furnham (2000a,b, 2008) considered the following half dozen alternative or opposite meanings:

Not having the competencies: This involves not having the abilities, traits or motivation to behave competently. Whether these are learned or inherited is, of course, crucially important but the salient point for the definition is that the crucial, specified (core) competencies are missing.

Not applying the competencies: The definition suggests that a person has the necessary skills, abilities and traits needed for competence but chooses not to exercise them. This may be an individual or collective act. For instance, 'work-to-rule' is a possible sign of volitional incompetence. On the other hand, it is possible, but unlikely, that people have latent competencies but do not 'apply' them through lack of awareness, but lack of self-confidence, or lack of opportunity.

Having irrelevant or redundant competencies: People may have been recruited and selected for a particular set of competencies that are now redundant. Jobs change as do the skills and attitudes required to do them. It is therefore possible that a person who was once competent becomes less so over time.

Being too competent for a job: Most people have experienced being 'overqualified' for a job. Jobs that are dull, routine, tedious or repetitive can wear down talented and skilled individuals who then perform them badly.

Being deliberately incompetent: There are reasons why individuals or groups choose to behave in ways that are less than competent. There are often feelings of anger, vengeance or inadequacy resulting from some perceived inequality at work. They may perform poorly in order to demonstrate the importance of their job (when competently executed) to customers, colleagues or superiors.

Not practising the competencies: Because competencies are related to abilities and skills, they require practice. If not exercised, they can become rusty and hence a competency becomes an incompetency.

McClelland (1973) argued that the term competency should replace the term skill, which was too narrow. Thus, one may have the skill to drive a bus but lack the competency to deal with passengers. He argued that the only comprehensive way to identify competencies is through behavioural event interviews. Further, standard job analysis methods, which focus on minimum competencies, leave things out, particularly how outstanding individuals work. Therefore, strategic planning, as a competency, needs to be backed by a competence for influencing so that plans can be 'sold' to others.

According to McClelland, the core competencies of an organisation are embedded in the organisation's systems, motives, mechanisms and processes. Core competencies may, he argued, represent unique sources of an organisation's competitive advantage.

McClelland's ideas have been criticised for various reasons. Competencies concern past, not future behaviour, and they concern success in the past, not necessarily the future, which may be quite different. Also, behavioural interview methods are often unfair to minorities or women who have not had the same developmental experiences as white males. It is also very expensive to transcribe long interviews for what may be a poor epistemic or practical yield.

There seem to be as many definitions of competency as there are people who talk about them. The British define competencies in terms of something that managers can do – a demonstrable behaviour or, an outcome. Some American writers believe a competency is a 'higher order' trait, skill, motive or disposition that distinguishes between average or superior managers. Competency has been used as an *adjective* and a *noun*. Thus, one can be a competent strategic planner or have marketing competency. Supposedly, one can also draw up a definitive list of required competencies – a discrete and definitive set of knowledge, values and skills. One may have areas of competence – that is parts of a job (or skills) – that one does well.

Mansfield (1999) defined the term as meaning 'people who are *suitable for work*, *sufficiently skilled* for the work they do, *fit* for work and *efficient* in their work!' He suggests the term implies a barely acceptable level, or threshold, of ability (suitable, sufficient) but also rather more than that (fit, efficient). In short, competent people are efficient and effective: incompetent people are not.

> To have a degree is still taken to be an important signal of general capacity. To be experienced is a valued characteristic in selection for employment. In some cultures, to be white or male — or both — is taken to be sufficient evidence of capability. The competency movement seeks to change the tradition by asking a simple question. People may have degrees, they may be experienced, they may be thought reliable – but what can they actually do? How they learned to do it, how long they have been doing it, and what kind of person they are, are seen as subordinate.
>
> (Mansfield, 1999, p. 28).

Yet, as Furnham (2008) has noted, there is confusion over the term for various reasons. Consider the following three issues:

1   *Singular or plural*: Nouns are divisible into counted nouns and uncounted nouns. The former has simple plurals: manager – managers; article – articles. Competence is an uncounted noun. Thus, we have *the* competence of managers not a competence, which confuses a task performed or any underlying trait or ability. It does not mean a set standard of behaviour. At present, competence is taken to mean what a person is like, how they do things and what they can do – all of which are conceptually distinct. Thus, some, supposedly competency-based assessments, look at the *former* two factors to decide whether people have the 'competencies' needed to do the job well, while others use the *latter* two factors to decide whether they have the ability or potential to do the job.
2   *Adequate or excellent*: There is some confusion about whether the term refers to barely capable or extremely good. One approach focuses on abilities and characteristics that may have good comparative norms; hence, it is easy to talk about levels of excellence. A second approach looks at what people should be able to do in order to execute the job competently, not what they are like. A good manager has the skills/knowledge to complete the job and characteristics of a particular team. Having particular characteristics will not ensure success nor will a job analysis say much about personal characteristics. Thus, the adequate/excellent debate needs to be dropped.
3   *Inputs and outputs*: Most competency approaches have focused on how things are done; on outcomes of activities rather than on the underlying state or disposition that determines the activity. The emphasis is on the resultant behaviour, not on traits or processes.

The three central features in assessing any sort of professional competence are essentially the following.

First, what is the range of knowledge and skills that the professional should have? This, of course, requires a demarcation of that which is, and that which is not, salient for competent practice in the job or profession. Furthermore, this may require making a list of necessary but not sufficient skills and knowledge or a list of some sort (rank-ordered) of the most important or desirable skills. This is, of course, a complex and value-laden task that often remains implicit in professional socialisation and is never, or rarely, openly discussed, partly because historical precedents have defined the issue.

Second, once the domain of requisite knowledge and skills has been specified, it is important to establish a cut-off point to separate the competent (though barely) from the incompetent. With most, but not all professions, competence is a continuous variable (like height) rather than a discrete variable (like sex). It therefore becomes important to decide what are the criteria of specifying competence, because in doing so, it is possible to know whether the person does or does not reach these criteria.

Third, it is important to develop a means to assess, evaluate or measure these criteria, both in order to confer professional status and a licence to practise and also to check the development of these skills over time so as to plot their gradual (or rapid) decline or improvement. There is, in the social sciences, a large battery of possible assessment devices available, each with its own strengths and weaknesses and it becomes important to select one or more that competently measure competence!

Despite the clear relevance and importance of professional groups to specify the aforementioned three criteria of competence, conceptual and empirical work in this field is patchy. Various reasons may account for this – the problem is difficult and complicated – but above all, it is frequently value-laden and politically sensitive, hence avoided. Second, one branch of a profession may have quite different ideas from another as to the solution to the abovementioned problems. Finally, the results of such investigations into professional competence often turn up so many problems that for many, they are best avoided by obfuscating the problems of evaluation in the first place.

Essays on professional competence are as numerous as they are diffuse. There appears to be no agreement as to the domain of skills required nor the best way of assessing them. Early studies used patient surveys, analysis of personal case record and observational techniques as well as critical incident technique. These studies suggested that competence concerned efficacy of diagnosis, provision of care and developing relationships.

Despite all this work, the term competence appears and needs to be frequently used possibly because it is too vague or an all-encompassing term, or possibly because there remains no general agreement as to its various components.

The medical profession

There is a great deal of debate as to what exactly a profession and a professional is. It is usually agreed that the professional should create, organise and transmit the knowledge, which should be difficult to acquire and even mysterious. Also, the professional should be accepted as the final arbiter in disputes over the validity of any technical solution lying within his area of expertise or competence.

Sociologists have argued that the recent history of medicine can be seen as a series of struggles among certain group alliances over the definition and treatment of illness. Historical dominance by physicians has meant that occupational groups who have more recently developed in the medical field have been forced to seek their mandate of operation, not only from their clients and the state but also from the physician organisations in every country. Groups seeking to establish a unique diagnostic role have encountered greatest opposition from those that have been prepared to purchase a limited form of autonomy by recognition of the physician's superior role. This issue may be summed up by a distinction between those professions to whom physicians have devolved jurisdiction and those who are thought of as having appropriated it. The quite different historical experiences of nurses and social workers illustrate this distinction.

The century has seen the rise of a number of largely hospital-based semi- or paraprofessions, which have all attempted to establish some control over a particular category or aspect of illness, its treatment and over a particular technological apparatus or process. Each has a history of conflict and compromise, and of co-operation with the other professional or paraprofessional groups. Each has, quite naturally, attempted to achieve the status of a profession in order to establish their autonomy and self-regulatory abilities. The degree of conflict between these groups is therefore likely to be a function of the similarity between those groups in terms of their training, their clientele and the services they offer.

Various professions have been studied within this historical framework: doctors, nurses, midwives and dentists. Similarly, other medical practitioners, variously labelled paramedical, limited practitioners, marginal practitioners and quasi-practitioners, have been studied in terms of their history, training and status. A number of theoretical studies have also attempted to compare various healthcare groups in terms of their professionalism, which has been defined in a number of ways. Thus, from the sociological perspective, there appear to be a number of reasons to expect differences in the perceptions of various medical and paramedical professions. That is, the conflict between groups is likely to be manifest in their intergroup perceptions.

In an early study, Furnham et al. (1981) set out to determine similarities and differences in the perception of different medical and allied healthcare professionals. They found, first, that the professionals evaluated and perceived each other negatively if in competition over a field of specialization, a treatment method or a particular client group. This appeared to be true particularly of GPs and social workers, as well as occupational and physiotherapists. Second, it was demonstrated that in nearly every case, the groups tended to value or perceive themselves, more positively on each dimension than any other group. Thus, there is a tendency on the part of individuals of certain groups both to perceive themselves favourably in comparison with others, and to perceive certain other groups, namely those who threaten the expansion, position or prestige of one's own group in particularly negative terms. That is, a health professional is likely to have a specific constellation of perceptions because of their particular interests.

However, there is very little doubt within the minds of laymen, or indeed, in the analyses of sociologists, that medicine is a profession. Yet there are numerous dimensions or categories in the profession of medicine that differ radically from one another. For instance, on a discriminant analysis, territory map of nine medical specialities, Furnham (1986) showed that all specialities fall into four quadrants based on two dimensions: soft–hard and general–specific. Thus, general practice is seen as soft (scientifically) and general in the sense that it deals with various aspects of the patient, while surgery is hard (scientifically) yet neither general nor specific. Similarly, general practice and psychiatry are both on the extreme of one dimension (soft) yet at almost opposite ends of the other (general).

Despite these various specialisations, all medical students have to go through the same basic training. Students are selected, taught, trained and examined in much the same way as in every other profession. However, once they decide to specialise, they are, in Great Britain, required to sit the exams of the appropriate Royal College, such as that of general practice, surgery, psychiatry or gynaecology and obstetrics. Concerning what and how the different colleges assess competence of candidates is beyond the scope of this chapter, which will concentrate on general practice.

It seems that in Great Britain, of all the various branches of medicine, general practitioners are among the most concerned with evaluating competence. There could be many reasons for this. They may be the most frequently accused of incompetence by the public and peers and hence feel it in their best interests for various 'in-house' procedures. On the other hand, being a relatively new college, they may be highly self-critical and keen to establish their academic and professional credibility by careful quality assurance. It also may be that because assessment of competence is particularly difficult in general practice, compared say, to surgery, that they have particular attention to this issue. Whatever the reason, there is a fairly long tradition of competence assessment in general practitioners.

Competent doctors

There are a number of papers where practitioners from various backgrounds list competencies in their area (Yazdani & Akbari-Framad, 2016). For instance, Beliveau et al. (2014) suggest physicians should have six basic competencies: professionalism, patient care and procedural skills, medical knowledge, practice-based learning and development, interpersonal and communication skills and a system-based practice. Earlier Epstein and Hundert (2002) defined medical professional competence as '*the habitual and judicious use of communication, knowledge, technical skills, clinical reasoning, emotions, values, and reflection in daily practice for the benefit of the individual and the community being served*' (p. 226).

Fernandez et al. (2012) in a very thorough and thoughtful paper on the many and varying conceptions of competence concluded,

> There is agreement that competence is composed of knowledge, skills and other components. Although agreement about the nature of these other components is lacking, attitudes and values are suggested to be essential ingredients of competence. Furthermore, a clear divergence in conceptions of how a competent person utilises these components is apparent. One view specifies that competence involves selecting components according to specific situations, as required. A second view places greater emphasis on the synergy that results from the use of a combination of components in a given situation (p. 357).

Saravia (2017) noted that it may be easier to define incompetence than competence. He listed various possible markers: typical scenarios where a hospital or licensing board may allege that a physician is incompetent are as follows: a lack of skills; deficiencies in knowledge; impairments due to substance abuse, psychiatric or health conditions; attaining a certain age; a long leave of absence;

being disruptive and interfering with other medical professionals' patient care; misdiagnosis of a patient's condition; overprescribing of controlled substances; inadequate medical records; practicing outside of the specialty area; and failing to meet specialised standards of practice leading to adverse outcomes.

There are also many papers which are concerned with who and what should be measured to judge a doctor competent (Santos et al., 2017) and the role of supervisors in the competence assessment process.

There is always the concern about being up-to-date and what to include in an already overstretched curriculum. For instance, Boulet and Durning (2019) suggest team-work and business knowledge may be added to increase the concept of medical education and competence. Another new 'competence' which has been suggested by a few is 'cultural competence' which is the ability to deal with diverse groups in terms of their age, ethnicity, gender, migrant and socio-economic status (Sorensen et al., 2017).

Those interested in competence assessment have been concerned with whether there is much of a difference between self-perceived and objectively measured competence. Indeed Katowa-Mukwato and Banda (2016) showed form their research 'the negative correlation between self-perceived and objectively measured competence demonstrated the inability of students to assess and rate themselves objectively due to fear that others may know their weaknesses and realize that they are not as competent as expected at a specific level of training' (p. 122).

There are various national perspectives on doctor competence. The American Board of Medical Specialities suggested six perspectives:

1 *Professionalism*: Demonstrate a commitment to carrying out professional responsibilities, adherence to ethical principles and sensitivity to diverse patient populations.
2 *Patient care and procedural skills*: Provide care that is compassionate, appropriate and effective treatment for health problems and to promote health.
3 *Medical knowledge*: Demonstrate knowledge about established and evolving biomedical, clinical and cognate sciences and their application in patient care.
4 *Practice-based learning and improvement*: Able to investigate and evaluate their patient care practices, appraise and assimilate scientific evidence, and improve their practice of medicine.
5 *Interpersonal and communication skills*: Demonstrate skills that result in effective information exchange and teaming with patients, their families and professional associates (e.g. fostering a therapeutic relationship that is ethically sound, uses effective listening skills with nonverbal and verbal communication; working as both a team member and at times as a leader).
6 *Systems-based practice*: Demonstrate awareness of and responsibility to larger context and systems of healthcare. Be able to call on system resources to provide optimal care (e.g. coordinating care across sites or serving as the primary case manager when care involves multiple specialties, professions or sites).

The British Royal College of General Practitioners has the following definitions:

The workplace-based assessment (WPBA) component of the MRCGP exam is designed to test GP trainees' competence in 13 key areas derived from the core RCGP curriculum statement 'Being a GP'.

Competence means having the abilities, knowledge and skills necessary for professional practise. Our framework for WPBA is made up of 13 competences:

1 Communication and consultation skills – communication with patients and the use of recognised consultation techniques
2 Practising holistically – operating in physical, psychological, socio-economic and cultural dimensions, taking into account feelings as well as thoughts
3 Data gathering and interpretation – for clinical judgement, choice of physical examination and investigations and their interpretation
4 Making a diagnosis and making decisions – a conscious, structured approach to decision-making
5 Clinical management – recognition and management of common medical conditions in primary care
6 Managing medical complexity and promoting health – aspects of care beyond managing straightforward problems, including management of co-morbidity, uncertainty, risk and focusing on health rather than just illness
7 Organisation, management and leadership – an understanding of the use of computer systems to augment the GP consultation and primary care at individual and systems levels, the management of change and the development of organisational and clinical leadership skills
8 Working with colleagues and in teams – working effectively with other professionals to ensure good patient care, including sharing information with colleagues
9 Community orientation – management of the health and social care of the practice population and local community
10 Maintaining performance, learning and teaching – maintaining performance and effective Continuing Professional Development (CPD) for oneself and others
11 Maintaining an ethical approach to practice – practising ethically, with integrity and a respect for diversity
12 Fitness to practise – the doctor's awareness of when his/her own performance, conduct or health, or that of others, might put patients at risk, and taking action to protect patients
13 Clinical examination and procedural skills – competent physical examination of the patient with accurate interpretation of physical signs and the safe practice of procedural skills

Each country has tried to provide a comprehensive definition of medical competency. Some are more comprehensive than others. These are always in flux, under debate and challenged but there are very clear patterns.

Medical education

As with most professions, the licence to practise, which is in a sense the profession's certificate of competence, is bestowed after the successful completion of a set of examinations at the end of a specified period. The issue of what standards are required to be reached is the core subject of medical education. Medical students are trained at medical schools for about 5 years and work in hospital for 1 year as 'preregistration housemen' under careful supervision, usually arranged as 6 months' medicine and 6 months' surgery.

Not all evaluations of medical education are damning or general. To a large extent, the plethora of articles in this area is concerned with two specific topics. First, many authors have been especially interested in the relevance of the various disciplines taught to medical students. To a large extent, this is a debate between *theoretical purists* and *applied pragmatists*. The former advocate a thorough, albeit somewhat hurried, grounding in the fundamental principles of the discipline, while the latter are concerned with teaching only those principles and skills that are necessary to, and relevant in, practice. It is frequently the argument of the purists that the 'from-first-principles' approach allows a proper understanding of the problem and that the applied approach produces only technicians unable to fully comprehend and, therefore, respond to, all the subtle changes necessary. The pragmatists, on the other hand, complain that students are bombarded by detailed facts that are completely irrelevant to the practice of everyday medicine. Thus, to both camps, incompetence may result from not following their approach.

A second, frequently debated issue is the best method of assessment. Numerous writers have considered the various advantages and disadvantages of multiple-choice questions, compared to more traditional essay-type questions and the oral examination or viva voce (McGuire, 1966). The results are somewhat equivocal, no doubt because the authors are attempting to achieve rather different objectives. Very few studies are longitudinal, attempting to assess how an examination method predicts knowledge or skills at a much later point in time.

As with nearly every avenue of human endeavour, there are recurrent themes in the discussion about medical education. Many years ago Metcalfe (1983) has listed four 'unresolved issues' in medical education. The *first* is 'education vs. training', which is concerned with the relevance of the knowledge provided. A *second* related issue is whether subjects like anatomy or even psychology should be taught 'as pure discipline' or 'as applied to medicine'. *Third*, there is an important debate on the balance of teaching between 'diagnosis vs. management', i.e. whether so much time should be dedicated to diagnoses rather than effective, efficient and patient-centred management. *Finally*, the unresolved issue of 'curing vs. caring', which relates to the issue that many major illnesses and diseases cannot be cured. He argues that there is, therefore, a large mismatch or list of discrepancies between the pattern of undergraduate learning/education and the graduate doctor's task/practice.

Metcalfe (1983) lists six 'cardinal' discrepancies'. These include the selection of 'convergent' scientific thinkers, rather than 'divergent' thinkers more suited to problem-solving in clinical medicine. Second, students are first encouraged to use inductive problem-solving and then hypothetical-deductive routines, but are not helped over this transition. Third, students are taught on inanimate learning material or 'undressed, horizontal, non-autonomous patients' but have to practise on live, autonomous patients. Fourth, learning takes place in a doctor-controlled environment, while most medical care takes place in a patient-controlled or neutral environment. Fifth, students are taught in 'high certainty areas' but are required to practise in 'low certainty areas'. Finally, much clinical practice requires calm both for decision-making and for transmission to patients.

There is no shortage of critics of medical education, all of whom lament the training that potential 'certified-competent' doctors get. Yet few have suggested why these criticisms are not taken seriously. There are a number of obstacles to change. These include the perceived threat to status and teaching time of established departments, a natural conservatism in the medical profession, the intransigence and lack of motivation for clinical teachers to change and a general hostility towards innovations, particularly that recommended by social scientists!

There has been much debate about medical education, more particularly about assessment. Govaerts et al. (2018) propose a model note, '*Assessment polarities and tensions are likely to surface with the continued rise of complexity and change in education and health care organisations. With increasing pressures of accountability in times of stretched resources, assessment tensions and dilemmas will become more pronounced.*' (p. 72).

While different countries use slightly different approaches with different emphases, all agree on the importance of multiple methods of assessment (Yielder & Moir, 2016).

Watling and Ginsburg (2019) noticed, '*four trends in education research: (i) shifting perspectives on assessment; (ii) shifting perspectives on feedback; (iii) increasing attention on learners' perceptions of assessment and feedback, and (iv) increasing attention on the influence of culture on assessment and feedback.*' (p. 76).

Overall then, although many would no doubt deny it, medical education, as traditionally conceived and executed frequently, does not produce medical professionals competent to practise. Clearly, much of their learning to be competent must be done after formal, examinable and medical education. One of the major problems for any evaluation of medical education is that definitions of competence or expectations of professional skill differ from one group to another.

Performance management

The Royal College of General Practitioners (London) has been particularly concerned with carrying out medical audits or, what they more recently term, performance review. In a sense, this can be seen as not so much a licence to practise medicine but a check-up on the quality or competence of licensed performance and practice as general practitioner, i.e. the efficacy of people qualified.

However, interesting and merit-worthy many of these suggestions are for performance review, not all were clear about precisely what to review or how. An exception is Schofield and Pendleton (1986) who specified four areas of performance to be measured-professional values, accessibility, clinical competence and ability to communicate. More importantly, they described a six-part, assessment method:

1 Study of the practice profile, which comprised a completed questionnaire circulated to the assessors in advance of the visit, which recorded the salient features of the practice.
2 Direct observation of the practice premises, its facilities and equipment and the way it functions.
3 Discussion with the ancillary staff and with other members of the practice's healthcare team.
4 Inspection of individual clinical records and any registers of indexes the practice possesses.
5 Review of the videotape of a series of the doctor's recent consultations, together with the relevant records, and with his summary.
6 An interview with the doctor to elicit his views and understanding on a variety of topics, including material derived from randomly selected records of his patients.

However, much of this work on performance review is ongoing. No agreed published set of criteria or methods are available. As Schofield and Pendleton (1986) have noted, four questions must be answered before that occurs. Are the areas of performance and criteria accepted as crucial to the provision of good quality care? Is the method of assessment valid and reliable? Are practice visits an effective method of identifying strengths and weaknesses and producing changes? Finally, how can this procedure be introduced into the existing structure of general practice?

In other words, it is recognised that a post-training evaluation of performance (medical audit) should be done. The merits of such a system are obvious: it could act as a motivator to individual doctors, it could identify areas of competence and incompetence, strength and weakness and educational need and it could determine a clear baseline standard against which any change could be measured. Clearly, it is a bold and imaginative act to even attempt to institutionalise an extensive, critical, post-examination review of medical competence in a number of areas among general practitioners.

Communicative competence

Until recently, little or no attempt was made to train doctors to communicate more effectively with their patients. It was, and for some still is, assumed that this skill or set of skills is no more than common sense, which, anyway, will be acquired or improved by practitioners 'on the job' with increasing experience. Yet it has not been denied that these skills may be directly related to such things as diagnosis and patient compliance (Furnham et al., 1980).

Over the past 20 years, there has been considerable interest in social skills training and research (Argyle, 1981; Furnham, 1985, 2008). The underlying message of this approach is that the ability to communicate efficiently and effectively is a skill that can (and must) be taught and learnt. Many individual skills make up social competence, which is thought of as the ability to produce the desired effects on other people in social situations. Much of the research in this field has concentrated on groups who, for one reason or another, do not possess these skills such as mental patients (schizophrenics and neurotics), addicts (particularly alcoholics), criminal offenders (recidivists, delinquents), disturbed adolescents and handicapped people.

McGuire (1981) has attempted to specify the range of communication or social skills that doctors need, but which they do not appear to acquire during professional training. First and foremost are history-taking skills, which are so clearly relevant in diagnosis. McGuire (1981) reviewed numerous studies on junior and experienced, hospital doctors and general practitioners and showed that there is a consistent lack of certain key, history-taking skills that are not compensated for, or acquired with, greater experience or postgraduate training. He also argues that doctors lack skills of exposition in the giving of information and advice to patients. The reasons why these crucially important skills are not acquired are manifold:

1 The time-honoured apprenticeship method is inappropriate, both because the models are not very good and also because social and psychological aspects are ignored.
2 Doctors are assumed to possess these skills despite the considerable evidence that they do not.
3 Doctors cannot acquire these skills, believing that they cannot be learnt – either one has them or not.
4 The use of these skills will only create problems in that practising them would lead to patients disclosing difficult-to-handle problems.
5 The skills are assumed to have no important effect on care despite the considerable evidence to the contrary.

McGuire (1981) believes that these five objections are misplaced and that one should develop more effective skill-training methods for doctors that would identify deficiencies, measure performance and provide feedback.

An interest in communication or interpersonal-skills courses for medical students or, indeed, qualified doctors has attracted evaluative research. Despite the importance, relevance and efficacy of communication-skills training, it appears that the profession as a whole, and general practice in particular, still has not laid down any rules for the training or assessment of communicative competence in doctors.

Patients' perspectives on clinical competence

Various organisations and individuals have attempted to help clients/patients assess the clinical competence of their doctors. In the case of individuals, they have frequently become dissatisfied with the professional advice that they have been given. In the case of organisations such as the Consumers' Association, the Health Education Council and the Patients' Association, encouraging patient assessment may be a very effective and efficient way of maintaining regular checks on clinical competence.

Various books and pamphlets are available on patients' rights. King et al. (1985) have written a useful handbook for the layman/patient subtitle 'A family guide to dealing with your GP'. In this book, there is a section on clinical competence that follows, in out a Royal College of General Practitioners booklet entitled 'What sort of doctor?' This has four sections: accessibility, clinical competence, communication skills and values, which are divided into two subdivisions, the practice and the doctor him/herself. After the relevant chapter, the authors provide a questionnaire, which is simple and straightforward, but useful for patients to use in assessment. The 19 items used to assess the GP by the patient are set out as follows:

Your doctor

a   *Accessibility.* (Can you get to see him?)

1	Does he provide enough surgeries?	Yes	No
2	Can you usually see your doctor within 2 days?	Yes	No
3	Can you get to speak to your doctor on the telephone?	Yes	No
4	Will your doctor do home visits?	Yes	No
5	Are his appointments at least 5 minutes long?	Yes	No

b   *Clinical competence.* (Does he know his stuff?)

1	Is your doctor a Member or Fellow of the Royal College of General Practitioners?	Yes	No
2	Does your doctor examine you thoroughly from time to time?	Yes	No
3	Are you always given a prescription? (You probably should not be)	Yes	No
4	Is your doctor mean with antibiotics and tranquillisers?	Yes	No

c   *Communications.* (Can you talk to him?)

1	Does your doctor listen?	Yes	No
2	Does your doctor make you feel rushed?	Yes	No
3	Is your doctor often interrupted?	Yes	No
4	Does your doctor ask what you think about your problem?	Yes	No
5	Does your doctor ask you what you are worried about?	Yes	No
6	Does your doctor give you plenty of information?	Yes	No
7	Does your doctor let you decide with him how your problem should be handled?	Yes	No

d *Professional values.* (What does he regard as important?)

1   Is your doctor interested in you as a person?   Yes   No
2   Is your doctor enthusiastic about health?   Yes   No
3   Is your doctor involved in health matters in the community? Yes   No

This questionnaire is, no doubt, not meant to be exhaustive or psychometrically sophisticated. It is simply meant to aid patients to consider four aspects of competence in their doctor. As such, it appears to be a useful exercise providing a client checklist. There are, of course, numerous dangers in using this as an assessment device. First, there are various constraints on the individual doctor and practice (i.e. size, location, demography of catchment), about which individual doctors can do little. Second, it is important to know various salient features about the clients (demographic and psychographic details as well as medical history) in order to establish which subgroups find which features of general competence more, or less, important. For instance, if there are reliable sex, age or ethnic differences in what patients expect of their doctor, the responses one may get on such questionnaires probably reflect more about the patient profile than the doctor's competence.

Patients' preferences

Given a choice of medical practitioner or specialist what would a patient choose? Presumably, patients choose who they like and trust: those they believe to be both approachable and competent. In three studies examining choice of doctor (GP and specialist), dentist and counsellor Furnham and colleagues investigated preference as a function of age, sex and country of origin/nationality (Furnham & Swami, 2008, 2009; Furnham et al., 2006). They noted that practitioner choice, as opposed to allocation is associated with greater patient satisfaction with the consultation, improved disclosure of information to the practitioner, and more positive patient–practitioner relationships.

Much of the literature on patient preferences for practitioners has focused on a few demographic factors. There is a well-established finding for same-sex practitioners of general medical care particularly when patients present with intimate health concerns. Female practitioners appear to be judged to have better personal and emotional skills than male practitioners and patients also report more participatory consultations with female practitioners.

Patients also show a preference for practitioners from their own ethnicity. This may influence patient–practitioner communication and promotes patient feelings of participation in the consultation. Patients, however, seem more accepting of practitioners from ethnic groups other than their own, especially if the practitioner displays a positive personal manner.

Professionals' amount of experience is obviously an important factor. This is usually expressed by considering the age of the professional but the results of studies are more equivocal. Some studies suggest that practitioner age does not influence patient preferences (e.g. Furnham et al., 2006), but other work suggests that patients prefer older practitioners because they are seen as having better interpersonal skills and are more thorough in the consultation compared with younger practitioners. Some patients perceive younger practitioners as more up-to-date and as having better technical and explanatory skills. There is clearly seen to be a trade-off between experience/knowledge and interpersonal skills.

Some studies have looked at factors like practitioner certification, training location and experience (Bornstein et al., 2000). Patients prefer practitioners with better qualifications and experience, but also that such factors may be more important than demographic factors.

Overall the Furnham studies showed a strong matching or similarity effect: people preferred practitioners like themselves: same sex, age group and nationality. The results beg the bigger question of whether client/expert similarity has an effect on therapeutic outcome. It is difficult to conduct appropriate studies looking at the efficacy of different therapeutic interventions, and most of these studies have compared various types of therapy against one another. Few have examined whether practitioner and client factors (notably demographics) have a direct or even placebo effect on outcomes.

Few professionals would wish to have their competence evaluated exclusively by their clients. Nevertheless, patients' perspectives on clinical competence can add a great deal to an objective assessment of a doctor's general competence to practise medicine.

Conclusion

This chapter has attempted to discern what approach medicine has adopted and defined the concept of competence. It appears that the profession approaches the idea of a general practitioner's unique set of skills by examining formal medical education and, to a lesser extent, in-service training. Inevitably there have been a number of changes over the years as technology has developed, as well as the rise of specific specialities. There have also been changes in medical education as well as patients' access to medical information on the web and indeed their own medical file.

There are many criticisms of traditional, formal, medical education that suggest it does not always lead to sufficient competence to practise medicine. However, there appear to be a number of attempts at medical schools throughout the world to address their syllabi, teaching and examining format to produce better practising doctors. While there are clear similarities between the medical regulatory bodies in different countries, there are clearly many similarities. All experience the same tension with regard to the delivery of exemplary education, training and assessment within a constrained and often diminishing budget. Population increases in the third world and increasing longevity in the first world, combined with universally increasing patient expectations, has put and will put a lot more pressure on universities and health regulatory bodies to deliver competent and motivated medical practitioners.

References

Albanese, M., Mejicano, G., Anderson, W., & Gruppen, L. (2009). Building a competency-based curriculum. *Advances in Health Science Education, 15*, 439–454.

Argyle, M. (ed) (1981). *Social skills and health*. London, Methuen.

Beliveau, M., Nishimura, R., & O'Gara, M. (2014). Physician competence. *Methodist Debakey Cardiovascular, 10*, 50–52.

Bornstein, B., Marcus, D., & Cassidy, W. (2000). Choosing a doctor: an exploratory study of factors influencing patients' choice of a primary care doctor. *Journal of Evaluative Clinical Practice, 6*, 255–262.

Boulet, J., & Durning, S. (2019). What we measure… and what we should measure in medical education. *Medical Education, 53*, 86–94.

Epstein, R., & Hundert, E. (2002). Defining and assessing professional competence. *JAMA, 287*, 226–235.

Fernandez, N., Dory, V., Ste-Marie, L-J., Chaput, M., Charlin, B., & Boucher, A. (2012). Varying conceptions of competence. *Medical Education, 46*, 357–365.

Furnham, A. (1985). Social skills training: a European perspective. In L. L'Abate and M. Milan (eds), *Handbook of social skills training and research*. New York, Wiley.

Furnham, A. (1986). Career attitudes of preclinical medical students to the medical specialities. *Medical Education, 20*, 286–300.

Furnham, A. (2000a). *The hopeless, hapless and helpless manager*. London, Whurr.

Furnham, A. (2000b). *Managerial competency frameworks*. London, Career Research Forum.

Furnham, A. (2008). *Personality and intelligence at work*. London, Routledge.

Furnham, A., King, J., & Pendleton, D. (1980). Establishing rapport: interaction effects and occupational therapy. *British Journal of Occupational Therapy, 43*, 322–325.

Furnham, A., Pendleton, D., & Manicom, C. (1981). The perception of different occupations within the medical profession. *Social Science and Medicine, 15*, 289–300.

Furnham, A., Petrides, K.V., & Temple, J. (2006). Patient preferences for medical doctors. *British Journal of Health Psychology, 11*, 439–449.

Furnham, A., & Swami, V. (2008). Patient preferences for psychological counsellors: evidence of a similarity effect. *Counselling Psychology Quarterly, 21*, 361–370.

Furnham, A., & Swami, V. (2009). Patient preferences for dentists. *Psychology, Health and Medicine, 14*, 143–149.

Govaerts, M., van der Vleuten, C., & Holmboe, E. (2019). Managing tensions in assessment. *Medical Education, 53*, 64–75.

Katowa-Mukwato, P., & Banda, S. (2016). Self-perceived versus objectively measured competence in performing clinical practical procedures by final year medical students. *International Journal of Medical Education, 7*, 122–129.

King, J., Pendleton, D., & Tate, P. (1985). *Making the most of your doctor: a family guide to dealing with your GP*. London, Methuen.

Mansfield, R. (1999). What is 'competence' all about?. *Competency, 6*, 12–16.

McClelland, D. (1973). Testing for competency rather than intelligence. *American Psychologist, 28*, 1–14.

McGuire, C. (1966). The oral examination as an assessment of professional competence. *Journal of Medical Education, 41*, 267–274.

McGuire, P. (1981). Doctor-patient skills. In M. Argyle (ed), *Social skills and health* (pp. 55–81). London, Methuen. 1986; 'Social skills training for health professionals'.

Metcalfe, D. (1983). The mismatch between undergraduate education and the medical task. In D. Pendleton and J. Hasler (eds), *Doctor-patient communication* (pp. 227–232). London, Academic Press.

Santos, P., Alves, L., & Simoes, J. (2017). What distinguishes a competent doctor in medical education?. *International Journal of Medical Education*, 8, 270–272.

Saravia, A. (2017). Determining whether a physician is competent to practice medicine. *MD Magazine*, September.

Schofield, & Pendleton, D. (1986). What sort of doctor?. In D. Pendleton, T. Schofield and M. Marinker (eds), *In pursuit of quality* (pp. 168–179). Exeter, Devon Press.

Sorensen, J., Norredam, M., Dogra, N., Essink-Bot, M-L., Suurmond, J., & Krasnik, A. (2017). Enhancing cultural competence in medical education. *International Journal of Medical Education*, 8, 28–30.

Watling, C., & Ginsburg, S. (2019). Assessment, feedback and the alchemy of learning. *Medical Education*, 53, 76–85.

Yazdani, S., & Akbari-Farmad, S. (2016). Proving the meta-model of development of competency the meta-ethnography approach. *Journal of Medical Education*, 15, 65–74.

Yielder, J., & Moir, F. (2016). Assessing the development of medical students' personal and professional skills by portfolio. *Journal of Medical Education and Curriculum Development*, 3, 9–15.

10 The future starts now – the identity and competence of doctors and the impact of accreditation

Julie Gustavs and Theanne Walters

Introduction

Identity and competency are central tenets of a doctor's practice and key hallmarks of the medical profession. In this chapter, we briefly define the concepts of identity and competence. We draw on the works of the French philosopher Michel Foucault to trace the impacts of knowledge/power (Foucault and Gordon 1980) on changing doctor identities and competence. Our focus is to explore how accreditation standards development and, in turn, curriculum development respond to and shape shifts in doctor identity and competence, at an individual practitioner and an institutional level. We show the multilevel impacts on professional identity formation and competence of doctors at an individual level and at the broader level of the medical and healthcare professions and service provision. We conclude by setting out future plans for accreditation review to better equip doctors to keep pace with change on the horizon.

The Australian Medical Council – our institutional context

Over the past three decades, as the standard-setting body and accreditation agency for the continuum of medical education in Australia and New Zealand, the Australian Medical Council (AMC) has played a thought leadership role within Australia and New Zealand. The AMC has worked extensively in partnership with international agencies to foster quality improvement to assist medical education providers and their members navigate change and remain current in a world where the pressures and priorities are manifold.

Current AMC accreditation standards comprise eight key domains. The standards focus on key concerns of identity and competence at an individual practitioner and institutional level: ensuring that the institution considers the context of the education program and manages stakeholders and partners to ensure that those impacted by the medical education programs are an integral part of decision-making. In addition, broadly, the AMC accreditation standards ensure that the purpose and outcomes of training are well understood, as well as, ensuring educational elements are in place in programs, including curriculum development, teaching and learning, assessment and evaluation. These elements play a key role in determining what skills, knowledge and behaviours doctors of the future should exemplify, how they should be supported to gain such skills, how judgements will be made about their competency and readiness for practice and how at an individual and organisational level continuous improvement cycles will be maintained.

To ensure these standards are met the AMC engages in accreditation processes which focus on rigorous self-examination and peer review with the aim of supporting medical education providers to improve their educational programs at an organisational level with downstream impacts on doctor identity and competence.

In this chapter, we explore how the AMC accreditation standards have changed over time, but first, we briefing define the concepts of identity and competence and look at the theoretical thinking tools of genealogy (Foucault) to make sense of how these standards can operate as technologies which impact change in doctor identity and competence formation.

Part 1: theories of identity and competence

Current theories of identity stress that concepts of identity do not remain stable over time are multifaceted, relate strongly to learning and are shaped by communities of practice (Wenger 1998). Equally, rather than being seen as a concept which operates exclusively at the individual level, identity is multilayered with individuals and the spaces in which they work: the family, the hospital, the community all impacting and shaping each other in ways which determine what comes to count as true, and how we are to prioritise future practices and activities.

Equally, contemporary theories of competence focus on the interactions between individuals and contexts. The work of Stephenson (1999) is particularly useful in explaining how professional practice evolves in stages from stable and known contexts, to being able to take on increased responsibility for problem-solving and leadership in situations where challenges are less knowable and increasingly complex. Central to competence is deliberate practice (Ericsson 2006) and the need to consider both formal and informal learning in the crafting of expertise in a particular field of practice (Eraut 2004).

Part 2: genealogy and the tracing of changes in discourse of the 'good doctor'

In this next section, we draw on the work of Foucault with his concepts of knowledge/power and genealogy in pointing to the ruptures in *episteme* (systems of thought and knowledge), which determine shifts in conceptions of who is considered to be a 'good' and competent doctor throughout time. We draw on Foucault's thinking as a means of showing how power comes into play to shift practices forward, and to change what counts as 'true' and acceptable ways of being and doing. Foucault's focus on power dimensions is a way forward in consolidating our theoretical thinking tools to inform our understanding of how shifts in identity and competence in medicine are being shaped and reshaped over time.

Knowledge/power

Foucault's concept of knowledge/power is useful in helping us to understand that what counts as 'true' and acceptable behaviour is in constant flux and negotiation. Foucault's theorising challenges the idea of power being concentrated in structures and bodies or even held by key agents, he argues that power is embodied and enacted rather than possessed and constitutes agents rather than being deployed by them. His theorising has major implications for understanding identity formation because he shows us that rather than identity being something ready-made or assured because of our role or standing, it is constituted through the choices we make in the everyday, with actions and reactions shaping outcomes. In his work, he identifies that the 'self' is defined by a continuous discourse of shifting communication of oneself to others. Others listen to our words and make sense of them in relation to their consistency and juxtaposition with our actions and reactions to everyday choices. This makes up who we are and who we are seen to be. Knowledge/power is a useful thinking tool in research on doctor identity and competence because it allows us to trace everyday behaviour of doctors to establish some key persona and archetypes of what it is to be a 'competent doctor'.

Genealogy

Foucault argues that not all is possible at any given time. The contexts and times in which we live shape us. Through his methodology of genealogy, he traces the shifts in meaning, priorities and methods within society over time. Foucault's work traverses analysis of many of our institutions – including hospitals, schools, asylums, prisons and judicial courts. He is fascinated with how these institutions have come into being and how they are organised to manage the people within them. Through challenging the notion of power being a negative force, proposing in its stead that power is pervasive – shaping and reinforcing the very institutions in which we live and work – he also makes a broader comment about how historical shifts in episteme and sense-making occur in these institutions. In his work, Foucault draws parallels between the underlying mechanisms of control – identifying three main methods of control:

- **Hierarchical observation** is the authoritative and hierarchical gaze to ensure that individuals are conforming to the norm.
- **Normalising judgement** involves establishing a standard norm that individuals must measure up to a certain level and those unable to reach the set level are deemed 'abnormal'.
- **Examination** is a modern technology of power, which enables decisions of what is good and acceptable and what does not meet the grade through cognitive measurement and review of performance (as opposed to 'old technologies' focused on punitive measures of corporal punishment.).

These control mechanisms have a clear impact on individuals and at a broader organisational level as they determine what is the norm, what is abnormal, who and what is to be rewarded and shunned – these mechanisms determine membership within organisations and sectors. They shape professional identities and social and professional norms about what it takes to be deemed competent.

Genealogy is a useful thinking tool in this chapter as it allows us to see that shifts have occurred in what it is to be a competent doctor over time shaping the accreditation standards and peer review processes which shape what counts as a 'good doctor' and professional institution. We identify key shifts in public discourse and expectations over time, which relate directly to changes in the AMC accreditation standards. We argue that further disruptions to these conceptions on the horizon.

Part 3: accreditation processes as mechanisms of control over doctor identity and competence

In this section, we explore the power of accreditation processes to prioritise and shape the behaviour of doctors and their professional institutions: medical schools, hospitals and specialist colleges.

Accreditation plays a powerful role in bringing about change within medical education and the profession, maintaining standards and seeking to plot a course to address future challenges, which require developments in and changes to professional knowledge, skills and attributes.

Drawing on Foucault's thinking, we see that accreditation works as a powerful technology of control through hierarchical observation, normalising judgement and examination. Here we stress again, control is not to be seen as a negative force but one that helps the profession to maintain its currency and relevance to community and societal needs. Accreditation achieves this purpose through peer review processes, which holds doctors accountable to their peers' judgements about what constitutes a quality medical education program and therefore what learning they need to engage in to qualify as doctors and maintain their currency and ongoing membership. In the last 20 years, who constitutes 'peers' has been widened to capture perspectives of those entering the profession, junior doctors, as well as the community and patients, and a broad base of clinicians from different fields within medicine and other health professions. Gender and cultural diversity within the panel of experts who assess programs is also considered necessary.

Central to the power of accreditation is the core quality standards against which the medical education programs are assessed. In Foucault's terms, these standards have a 'normalising role' in that they set out expectations of what individual doctors and their institutions need to attain in terms of their competence and identity to ensure their role and standing as doctors and membership of the broader medical profession.

Peer review teams engage in rigorous examination and observation of the quality of programs using multimodal methods, including panel discussions and questions, observation of sites and practice and review of written submissions, products, processes and .other relevant artefacts. In Foucault's terms, these are powerful control mechanisms to ensure the quality of the medical professions.

Part 4: tracing accreditation changes and implications for doctor identity and competence

As its accreditation standards have developed over 30 years, the AMC has articulated a number of key foundational building blocks which have been central to the identity and competence of individual doctors and the broader institutions in which they work. The AMC's thinking has responded to and been shaped by that of other educational institutions and drawn on the key foundational blocks already in use in medical schools in Australia. The key foundational areas of medical practice reinforced through AMC accreditation standards are set out in the following section.

Doctors – technical know-how and science

Science is the dominant discourse of the 19th and 20th centuries. Based on rigorous methods of inquiry, it has served medicine well. Through the emphasis in medical practice on the principles of the scientific method, and its foundations on a broad base of evidence of what works, doctors have consolidated their position within society.

The AMC standards include key requirements for doctors concerning science and scholarship as shown in Box 10.1.

BOX 10.1

Science and Scholarship: the medical graduate as scientist and scholar.

On entry to professional practice, Australian and New Zealand graduates are able to:

1.1 Demonstrate an understanding of established and evolving biological, clinical, epidemiological, social and behavioural sciences.

1.2 Apply core medical and scientific knowledge to individual patients, populations and health systems.

1.3 Describe the aetiology, pathology, clinical features, natural history and prognosis of common and important presentations at all stages of life.

1.4 Access, critically appraise, interpret and apply evidence from the medical and scientific literature.

1.5 Apply knowledge of common scientific methods to formulate relevant research questions and select applicable study designs.

1.6 Demonstrate a commitment to excellence, evidence-based practice and the generation of new scientific knowledge.

This domain focuses on drawing on the scientific method and evidence-based practice to consolidate clinical practices and research and in this way shows a commitment to quality improvement and innovation.

Equally, the doctor's scientific understandings are imbued within a technical base of clinical know-how, skill and practices. See Box 10.2.

BOX 10.2

Clinical Practice: the medical graduate as practitioner.

On entry to professional practice, Australian and New Zealand graduates are able to:

2.1 Demonstrate by listening, sharing and responding, the ability to communicate clearly, sensitively and effectively with patients, their family/caregivers, doctors and other health professionals.

2.2 Elicit an accurate, organised and problem-focused medical history, including family and social occupational and lifestyle features, from the patient, and other sources.

2.3 Perform a full and accurate physical examination, including a mental state examination, or a problem-focused examination as indicated.

2.4 Integrate and interpret findings from the history and examination, to arrive at an initial assessment, including a relevant differential diagnosis. Discriminate between possible differential diagnoses, justify the decisions taken and describe the processes for evaluating these.

2.5 Select and justify common investigations, with regard to the pathological basis of disease, utility, safety and cost-effectiveness, and interpret their results.

2.6 Select and perform safely a range of common procedural skills.

2.7 Make clinical judgements and decisions based on the available evidence. Identify and justify relevant management options alone or in conjunction with colleagues, according to level of training and experience.

2.8 Elicit patients' questions and their views, concerns and preferences, promote rapport and ensure patients' full understanding of their problem(s). Involve patients in decision-making and planning their treatment, including communicating risk and benefits of management options.

Standards for Assessment and Accreditation of Primary Medical Programs by the Australian Medical Council (2012, p 2)

2.9 Provide information to patients, and family/caregivers where relevant, to enable them to make a fully informed choice among various diagnostic, therapeutic and management options.

2.10 Integrate prevention, early detection, health maintenance and chronic condition management where relevant into clinical practice.

(Continued)

2.11 Prescribe medications safely, effectively and economically using objective evidence. Safely administer other therapeutic agents, including fluid, electrolytes, blood products and selected inhalational agents.

2.12 Recognise and assess deteriorating and critically unwell patients who require immediate care. Perform common emergency and life support procedures, including caring for the unconscious patient and performing CPR.

2.13 Describe the principles of care for patients at the end of their lives, avoiding unnecessary investigations or treatment and ensuring physical comfort, including pain relief, psychosocial support and other components of palliative care.

2.14 Place the needs and safety of patients at the centre of the care process. Demonstrate safety skills, including infection control, graded assertiveness, adverse event reporting and effective clinical handover.

2.15 Retrieve, interpret and record information effectively in clinical data systems (both paper and electronic).

These technical skills focus on how doctors need to communicate with their patients and make judgements about their care. This also includes understanding the prevention, early detection and progression of disease as well as understanding how to act in cases of emergencies. Critical to care are the principles of patient-centred care and ability to manage patients and health information accurately and professionally.

It is within the realm of clinical know-how that medical practice intertwines with professionalism. It is within this interconnection between science, technical know-how, professionalism and considerations of the broader community, in which medical practice is embedded, that doctors are confronted with some of the most challenging aspects of medicine. This comes to the core of what it is to be a doctor and to defining competence. It involves the consideration of questions of life and death, the boundaries between the rational and the spiritual, health and well-being. This is often referred to within medical practice as their 'craft', which includes aspects of art and science.

Doctors and their craft – art and science

Technical know-how and science do not explain astounding examples of how doctors craft an identity as selfless healers who risk their own health and, through competence gained through practice, manage health emergency outbreaks. The identity of doctor as healer can also be seen in what may appear to the outsider as less heroic examples where doctors respond empathically to the stories of the ill and needy and give them hope and ways to go on.

The AMC standards reinforce the importance of art and professionalism, so-called non-technical skills such as communication and self-care and qualities such as compassion and humanity, which extend well beyond scientific ways of knowing. See Box 10.3.

BOX 10.3

Professionalism and Leadership: the medical graduate as a professional and leader.

On entry to professional practice, Australian and New Zealand graduates are able to:

3.1 Provide care to all patients according to 'the codes of conduct for medical practitioners in Australia and New Zealand'.

3.2 Demonstrate professional values, including commitment to high-quality clinical standards, compassion, empathy and respect for all patients. Demonstrate the qualities of integrity, honesty, leadership and partnership to patients, the profession and society.

3.3 Describe the principles and practice of professionalism and leadership in healthcare.

3.4 Explain the main principles of ethical practice and apply these to learning scenarios in clinical practice. Communicate effectively about ethical issues with patients, family and other healthcare professionals.

3.5 Demonstrate awareness of factors that affect doctors' health and well-being, including fatigue, stress management and infection control, to mitigate health risks of professional practice. Recognise their own health needs, when to consult and follow advice of a health professional and identify risks posed to patients by their own health.

3.6 Identify the boundaries that define professional and therapeutic relationships and demonstrate respect for these in clinical practice.

3.7 Demonstrate awareness of and explain the options available when personal values or beliefs may influence patient care, including the obligation to refer to another practitioner.

3.8 Describe and respect the roles and expertise of other healthcare professionals, and demonstrate the ability to learn and work effectively as a member of an interprofessional team or other professional groups.

3.9 Self-evaluate their own professional practice; demonstrate lifelong learning behaviours and fundamental skills in educating colleagues. Recognise the limits of their own expertise and involve other professionals as needed to contribute to patient care.

3.10 Describe and apply the fundamental legal responsibilities of health professionals especially those relating to ability to complete relevant certificates and documents, informed consent, duty of care to patients and colleagues, privacy, confidentiality, mandatory reporting and notification. Demonstrate awareness of financial and other conflicts of interest.

Key to professional perspectives of doctor practice is the need to demonstrate a value-based approach to care. This domain acknowledges that personal beliefs and values may not always align with practice. It points to how doctors need to work in line with professional codes and work as part of an interprofessional team considering the perspectives of other professional groups. Within this domain, we also see the importance of self-evaluation and lifelong learning which includes the concepts in Foucault's terms of 'governance of the self' whereby the standards of control and normalisation are internalised and used by the self as a mechanism to ensure one stays in step with current practice and what counts as the norms of the profession.

Accreditation considers heroic stories of doctor identity and competence coupled with negative stories of doctors within the broader community. Landmark cases of doctor misconduct, media reports of bullying and sexual harassment and a growing consumer movement that wants more than a scientific expert and technical know-how from their medical workforce are part of the complex context which accreditors need to heed as they make determinations about quality. It also provides the evidence against which the path is set for future practices – determinations about that which should be maintained from current practice and what should change. Increasingly, regulators and accreditation bodies such as the AMC must have mechanisms and processes to manage complaints, risk and negative stories in the professions. The refinement of methods for dealing with complaints is integral to managing truth and change within the professions. Complaint management provides the boundaries of a site of contestation, which ultimately confirms what comes to count as truth. Smaller stories of injustice are either taken up for inclusion as part of a larger narrative or rebuked. Through complaints processes, and by constant negotiation and re-negotiation of boundaries of practice, the credence of the status quo or call for sanctions and new ways of being within the professions and broader society are confirmed. In this way, these complaints, risk and negative stories and their management form part of the complex messaging surrounding and shaping doctor identity and competence and ultimately contribute to their status in a truth regime. Accreditation plays a vital role in these determinations.

Doctors and community

Within the domain of 'doctors and community', we see examples of important collaborations between the community and doctors which have changed the way medical practice is conceived and implemented. The dual role of community engagement as a 'process and function' (WHO 2020) is a significant lever in dealing with public health challenges, including 'urbanisation, poverty, migration, and poor environmental management, alongside man-made and natural crises such as disease outbreaks, floods and armed conflict' (WHO 2020). Core to the success of any community engagement activity in health is the recognition that 'people are at the centre of any effort to create better health and that resilient people are the foundation of resilient health systems and communities' (WHO 2020).

In 2000, the AMC established connections with consumer groups and updated its standards to include explicit reference to the need for medical education providers and their members to engage with the community to ensure that medical programs meet the needs of the communities they serve.

Central to the expectations of the AMC are standards for doctors, which focus on their role within the broader community (Box 10.4).

BOX 10.4

Health and Society: the medical graduate as health advocate.

On entry to professional practice, Australian and New Zealand graduates are able to:

4.1 Accept responsibility to protect and advance the health and well-being of individuals, communities and populations.

4.2 Explain factors that contribute to the health, illness, disease and success of treatment of populations, including issues relating to health inequities and inequalities, diversity of cultural, spiritual and community values and socio-economic and physical environment factors.

4.3 Communicate effectively in wider roles, including health advocacy, teaching, assessing and appraising.

4.4 Understand and describe the factors that contribute to the health and well-being of Aboriginal and Torres Strait Islander peoples and/or Māori, including history, spirituality and relationship to land, diversity of cultures and communities, epidemiology, social and political determinants of health and health experiences. Demonstrate effective and culturally competent communication and care for Aboriginal and Torres Strait Islander peoples and/or Māori.

4.5 Explain and evaluate common population health screening and prevention approaches, including the use of technology for surveillance and monitoring of the health status of populations. Explain environmental and lifestyle health risks and advocate for healthy lifestyle choices.

4.6 Describe a systems approach to improving the quality and safety of healthcare.

4.7 Understand and describe the roles and relationships between health agencies and services, and explain the principles of efficient and equitable allocation of finite resources, to meet individual, community and national health needs.

4.8 Describe the attributes of the national systems of healthcare, including those that pertain to the healthcare of Aboriginal and Torres Strait Islander peoples and/or Maori.

4.9 Demonstrate an understanding of global health issues and determinants of health and disease, including their relevance to healthcare delivery in Australia and New Zealand and the broader Western Pacific region.

This domain also considers health broadly in the context of global health issues and encourages system-based perspectives on healthcare.

An important decision within the AMC accreditation standards has been to recognise the place of Indigenous Health and to acknowledge the shared rights and expectations of Indigenous and non-Indigenous Australia as well as their different histories and experiences.

In 2004, the Committee of Deans of Australians Medical Schools implemented an *Indigenous health curriculum framework*, a set of guidelines for success in designing and delivering an Indigenous health curriculum in medical programs. The AMC endorsed the framework and, in 2006, introduced revised accreditation standards that required medical programs to include Indigenous health curriculum content and to consider the processes, settings and resources necessary for successful education in this area. This is the only time that the Australian and New Zealand deans of medicine have agreed to a national set of curriculum guidelines and the only time the AMC has reflected such guidelines in the standards.

In the accreditation standards, the AMC privileged the position of Indigenous Health. The revised standards stated, 'Australia has special responsibilities to Aboriginal and Torres Strait Islander people, and New Zealand to Māori, and these responsibilities should be reflected throughout the medical education process'.

The implication of this change has been to ensure that medical students learn about Indigenous people, their history and health and have experience in providing care to Indigenous people. The AMC has since introduced similar standards for other later phases of medical education and training. In 2009, it developed the first national code of conduct for the medical profession in Australia, which acknowledged Australia's culturally diversity, including the culture of Australia's Indigenous people, the need for culturally safe and sensitive practice and the role of the doctor as health advocate. The code stated, '... the Indigenous people of Australia bear the burden of gross social, cultural and health inequity. Good medical practice involves using your expertise and influence to protect and advance the health and well-being of individual patients, communities and populations'.

The focus on doctors and community reflects the constant pull between priorities – doctors as knowers and experts who have the power to self-regulate their profession and define their practices, coupled with the voices of a community, which calls for re-evaluations of expectations and the boundaries of doctors' role in society. Internationally, landmark cases in the United Kingdom such as the children's heart surgery at the Bristol Royal Infirmary (1984–1995) and the 1986 doctors' strike in Canada to protest against a government ban on extra-billing have shaped an international refocus on community needs in the medical profession. These landmark cases resulted in medical organisations and regulators leading work with the broader community to develop a number of frameworks that set out community expectations of doctors. CanMEDS from Canada has been particularly influential worldwide and is summarised in Figure 10.1.

First introduced in the 1990s, the CanMEDS framework, developed by the Royal College of Physicians and Surgeons of Canada, was an important shift in official accounts of doctor identify and competence in that it emphasised not only the role of doctors as the medical expert but also other roles generally considered to be part of the 'hidden curriculum': professional, communicator, collaborator, leader, health advocate and scholar. For the first time, officially, doctors were explicitly taught in these previously unspoken roles and this move has shaped medical education programs worldwide.

In the Australian context, the AMC played a key role in raising awareness of the CanMEDS frameworks with key stakeholders of health, seeing it as a way of engaging in a broader debate in Australia and New Zealand about what is at the core of being a competent doctor. From its earliest accreditation standards for

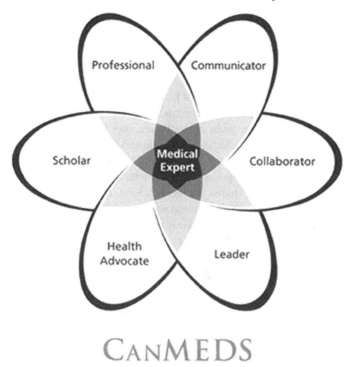

CANMEDS

Figure 10.1 CanMEDS.

Source: Copyright © 2015 The Royal College of Physicians and Surgeons of Canada. http://www. royalcollege.ca/rcsite/canmeds/canmeds-framework-e. Reproduced with permission.

specialist medical programs (2000), the AMC required education providers to explain how they had considered community need in developing the educational goals of their training program and related these goals to the role of the medical specialty in the community. Many Australian and New Zealand medical education providers have adopted a CanMEDS focus to their training standards. Such frameworks demonstrate a shift in the official account of doctors from privileging technical know-how and sciences, including their roles in society and the health community.

Part 5: accreditation standards – on the horizon

In this final section, we draw out implications of 21st-century challenges to the identity and competence of doctors for medical education innovation and the strategy of medical program accreditation bodies. We conclude this chapter with observations on proposed future directions for medical education innovation and accreditation strategies to better prepare doctors and the broader medical profession to navigate anticipated change and disruption to their ways of being and competence.

Recently, at the AMC, we have engaged in a comprehensive horizon scanning strategy-building initiative, which has identified three major areas of external focus impacting doctor identity and competence: changing practices, community need and cultural safety. We anticipate further disruption and opportunities on the horizon within these broad domains, and COVID-19 was just emerging as this was being written. We see some evidence of how such disruptions are being addressed within current medical education programs, particularly in the area of Indigenous Health. There are also some areas of significant gaps particularly with respect to preparedness within medical education training and continuing professional development for the impacts of machine learning and artificial intelligence (AI) on the medical workforce and the adoption of new models of care centred on the principles of patient-centred care and shared decision-making. Equally, the impact of man-made environmental change is a concern which needs to be more clearly articulated within AMC accreditation standards and integrated more fully into medical education programs to ensure that doctors commit to sustainable health practices.

Doctors and disruptive change – future

We see further disruption and opportunities on the horizon, which will require further development of these standards and will shape the entire medical continuum, including intern training.

- **Community needs and shared decision-making**: *Significant shifts occur in community expectations concerning health as individuals and the community seeks more responsibility in healthcare decision-making.*

The broader health community and specific community groups advocate for individuals having an increased role in their own healthcare and decision-making. In this context, the very concept of the patient as passive recipient of care is shifting to one whereby they are an equal partner, with specific rights, and an active role in judgements and decisions about their healthcare. In such situations, the doctor's role of duty of care for patients can collide with the patient and their families' autonomy. What are the boundaries between the doctor's professional knowledge and that of the patient's and their families' decisions? How is the doctor to navigate the space and decisions around what is best in terms of maintaining the balance between quality of life and longevity?

In Australia, a significant community concern with regards to health is the variation in access and health outcomes based on location. Those in rural and outer-metropolitan areas have 'shorter lives, higher levels of disease, and injury and poorer access to and use of health services compared with people living in metropolitan areas' (Australian Institute of Health and Welfare 2020). The provision of accessible high-quality care for Australians is an ongoing challenge for all stakeholders in the healthcare system, including accreditation authorities and healthcare providers. Key questions for doctors are how can we work towards improved equity in health provision across our country? And what are some improved models of education at the point of initial training and lifelong learning to ensure that doctors understand

and experience providing healthcare to underserviced communities and can contribute to diminishing the divide between rural and metropolitan service provision?

Furthermore, the boundaries of what we consider to be 'community' are complex. In a global world with low-, medium- and high-income countries, the health of one community can impact on others. Worthy of consideration is the role of doctors as global citizens and their responsibilities in addressing the public health challenges of urbanisation, poverty and man-made environmental problems alluded to earlier in this chapter. A core question here for doctors is how does their practice contribute to the 'public good?' (WHO 2020). This resonates with the frameworks such as CanMEDS, which challenge doctors to roles as advocates.

Central to delivering on a closer alignment between medical practices and community needs is a refocusing of care on population health, equitable access and human rights. This means shifting investment and prestige at the individual practitioner and system level on secondary and tertiary specialised services towards equity-promoting general and primary care. It also means that practitioners and the organisations and systems in which they work move beyond focusing on the day-to-day routine of operational and implementation concerns. At an individual practitioner and system level, doctors and medical services need to shift to models of embedding learning and predictive capabilities into their practices so they are better able to learn from mistakes, innovate and improve their management of health crises and emergencies (Sheikh et al. 2020).

- **Culturally safe practice and care:** *Doctors (and other practitioners) are called on to critically reflect on health practitioner knowledge, skills, attitudes, practising behaviours and power differentials in delivering safe, accessible and responsive healthcare free of racism.*

While a focus on Indigenous health remains, in February 2020, Australia's national regulators and accreditation authorities for health professions, including the AMC, have endorsed a broader cultural safety strategy. The strategy focuses on achieving patient safety for Aboriginal and Torres Strait Islander peoples as the norm. It sets actions and target dates for aligned definitions, terminology and standards across health professions, frameworks for Aboriginal and Torres Strait Islanders to notify the regulator of health profession practice standards when they have concerns about patient safety, and collecting data to inform change.

Achieving the agreed outcomes will require significant communication, education and evaluation, with individual doctors and institutions. This will further challenge the AMC in its standard setting, examination and thought leadership roles.

- **Interprofessionalism and boundaries of shared practice:** *Doctors are called on to rethink the boundaries of their professional practice and, within the context of people-centred care, find better more collaborative ways of working with peer professional groups in the interest of better patient care.*

The need for better collaboration and reduction of tribalism is an ongoing challenge in health, which needs urgent attention within the health sector globally.

In the context of an ageing population worldwide, many patients have co-morbidities and complex healthcare needs requiring management by various health workers across the sector. To achieve outcomes focused, integrated, people-centred care, it is important to address cultural and system barriers, which have inhibited improved collaboration between the professions. Central to achievement of this goal is also to shift from thinking of medicine and health in isolation towards a model whereby it is seen to be integrally linked with other professions and services, including law, social services and employment. The strengthening of accreditation standards and exploration of better ways to integrate interprofessional learning across the curriculum of vocational training and lifelong learning is an important area of future development for the AMC.

- **Machine learning and AI:** *Doctors are called on to plan for a world where machines can learn and health challenges and systems are increasingly complex.*

Further disruptions are the result of technology enhancement rendered through machine learning and the promises of AI. Technology advancements over the next decade will significantly change the nature of work with the advent of AI-augmented decision-making and support across all professions and fields, including health. This has significant implications for the focus of skills development of health professionals to ensure their employability in a world where machines can learn and have access to huge data sets on which decision-making about care can be made, which will outstrip the accuracy and speed of that a human can make based on their professional knowledge base. The use of AI-augmented decision-making and support will bring to the fore new ethical dilemmas for resolution in health and require of the health workforce a focus on what they add to health by way of humanising care beyond what a machine can achieve more efficiently and cost-effectively. A starting point is improvements to real-time health data through leveraging advancements in information technology aligned with global standards in data integration, personalised care and privacy (Sheikh et al. 2020). We anticipate that these changes will impact significantly on the health workforce and change the nature of the work of doctors presenting new ethical dilemmas which will need careful consideration in the future.

Best practice in adaptive system change in complex systems such as healthcare stress that it is imperative that stakeholders consider disruption strategically and work collaboratively to seek to remove and address current perceived inefficiencies and problems in the current system as well as to work with potential new players in the sector to help create future health provision. The AMC is committed to working with key stakeholders across the system to determine digital capabilities to support doctors to navigate technological changes impacting their practices.

- **Environment issues:** *Doctors are called on to develop more sustainable practices related to healthcare to ensure that the environmental footprint of their work is minimised and kept in balance.*

As we have written our book chapter for this publication, bushfires have ravaged our land on a scale unprecedented in history. Estimates are that over one billion animals have died as a result of the fires, more than 10 million ha of land have been burnt, over 6500 buildings have been destroyed and 34 people lost their lives.

While the current government has called for 'Australians to hold the line and battle the blazes, as they have always done', the populous has united with a different voice and interpretation of events. The scale of the environmental and economic impact carries weight for national and international peoples in all walks of life to take action to address and minimise the impacts of climate devastation.

For doctors, key questions include how in the short term can doctors support the community to manage the mental health challenges of climate destruction and the immediate challenge of disaster management. Equally, and more broadly, is the need to integrate the lens of environmental concerns into health practices to ensure the sustainability of health provision and reduce the footprint of waste.

These changes have consequences for what it means to be a competent doctor and are shaking the very foundations of doctor identity.

Conclusion

In this chapter, we have argued that accreditation standards are a strong lever for changes across the medical profession and have shaped doctor identity and competence over time. We have traced the impact of three particular shifts drawing on the thinking tool of genealogy, as proposed by the French philosopher Foucault. These changes include shifts from scientific ways of knowing to community engagement and recognition in Australia of the importance of addressing the improved health needs of its Indigenous populations. We conclude this article with the recognition that there are further challenges on the horizon which will further shape doctor identity and competence, including technology, consumer activism, interprofessionalism and the yet far from resolved challenges in health experience by our Indigenous populations and environmental and climate change. We anticipate further revisions to AMC accreditation standards in the future to act as a catalyst for change and improvements in these important areas.

References

Australian Institute of Health and Welfare. (2020). www.aihw.gov.au.

Australian Medical Council. (2012). *Standards for assessment and accreditation of primary medical programs.*

Eraut, M. (2004). Informal learning in the workplace. *Studies in Continuing Education*, 26(2), 247–273. https://doi.org/10.1080/158037042000225245.

Ericsson, K. A. (2006). The influence of experience and deliberate practice on the development of superior expert performance. In K. A. Ericsson, N. Charness, P. J. Feltovich and R. R. Hoffman (Eds.), *The Cambridge handbook of expertise and expert performance* (pp. 683–703). Cambridge: Cambridge University Press.

Foucault, M. and Gordon, C. (1980). *Power/knowledge: Selected interviews and other writings* (pp. 1972–1977). New York: Pantheon Books.

Latour, B. (1991). Technology is science made durable. In Law, J (Ed.), *Sociology of monsters: Essays on power, technology and domination*

Sheikh, K., Agyepong, I., Jhalani, M., Ammar, W., Hafeez, A., Pyakuryal, S., et al. (2020). Learning Health Systems: An empowering agenda for low-income and middle income countries. *The Lancet*, 395(102223), 476–477.

Stephenson, J. (1999). *Capability and quality in higher education*. Psychology Press.

The Royal College of Physicians and Surgeons, Canada. (2015). *CanMEDS*. Canada.

Wenger, E. (1998). *Communities of practice: Learning, meaning and identity Cambridge*. Cambridge UK: University Press.

WHO. (2020). *Community engagement for quality integrated, people-centred and resilient health services*. WHO. www.who.int.

11 The measurement of leadership qualities as an aspect of nursing identity

Colin McNeill

Chapter overview

This chapter discusses enhancing assessment of the personal values and attributes underpinning professional identity, leadership and teamworking in a health service facing serious challenges. With a focus on nursing it describes a prototype of an insightful psychometric tool[1] that can be used to select for, identify and develop leadership values and attributes in students at schools of nursing and open a pipeline developing leadership talent.

There exists a great deal of respect and admiration for professionals in the health service and the work they do. But the organisation and its culture face challenge by way of service limitations and effects that are damaging its reputation for professional care and treatment of patients. We describe some major limitations and effects, and the role-enhanced leadership and modified values might play in pushing back against them. More specifically, we wish to describe and demonstrate a psychometric process by which the personal values and professional identity required of a new leadership in an improving service might be measured, selected for and developed in the most effective way.

We make some assumptions. What professional identity and personal identity is, about nursing values that currently exist, that leadership who have mastered application of the right values is essential and that nursing values have a direct effect on quality of care and treatment outcomes.

Assumption one: what professional identity is

There are many approaches to understanding the concept of 'identity'. I want to be clear about our use of the concept. Identity Structure Analysis (ISA), the theoretical basis for our values-based psychometric, draws together and elaborates on several long-established approaches to understanding the development and maintenance of a mature sense of personal and group identity. Concepts derived from these approaches, such as 'ideal self', 'identity variants' [from defensive high self-regard (DHSR) to identity crisis], 'construal', 'self-esteem', 'rating of others', 'identification with others', are defined and integrated. Ambiguities are clarified and definitions made explicit as algorithms. The ISA approach to identity has been described as 'taking a significant pace towards a genuinely scientific psychology' and a work of 'demonstrable and unique value to those who are faced with the upsets and miseries of our complicated form of life'.

ISA assumes, for example, that a person's identity is grounded in childhood and locality, in language used, in subsequent experiences, of life and of other people (parents, friends, peers, role models and so on) and in identifications with and transactions with others. The sense of self is the central core of identity considered in personal terms as 'personal identity' and in group membership terms as 'social identity'. Professional identity of nurses and nursing leaders is the social identity of interest here.

Central to the significance of the 'present moment and situation' for a person's behaviour is the person's construal of self and the others present by means of individualised personal constructs (attitudes, values, beliefs) that help them, subconsciously and consciously, to anticipate the likely thoughts, actions and feelings of self and others and manage relationships. Appraisal is closely associated with construal but takes into account emotive responses evoked by the impact of construal of the situation on a person's sense of well-being and identity.

How does the person's perception of a social situation and the people in it make them feel and how will this affect behaviour? Experience of self, work and life generally leads to a sense of personal and professional identity that can differ from situation to situation. Situations in which one finds oneself evoke values, feelings and responses that are remembered and related to context. This helps make sense of future similar situations but can lead to discomfort and uncertainty as well as familiarity and confidence, or indeed to the emergence of a leadership or 'followership' style of behaviour in response.

Professional identity as a nurse with professional values would be built upon an inherent, coherent, caring, value and belief system underpinning personal identity and should emerge fully fledged from the education process and experience as a registered nurse. It should inform and constrain behaviour as a nurse in the workplace from one situation to another, following others or taking control as sound management of each situation requires.

Assumption two: the best leaders master use of professional nursing values

Our intention is to assess and discuss measurement of the professional and personal values of potential leaders in nursing and we do this later, but we should first be clear about the function values performed in mastery of the leadership role. Leaders should have and seek to maintain the highest professional standards of behaviour since they tend to determine the morality or ethics of the workplace.

Morality, where it derives from the Code of Conduct for Nurses and Midwifery that is external to the individual, must be internalised by the professional as personal professional values informed by work experience – and unprofessional conduct, breaches of the Code of Conduct, can be punished by the profession via a disciplinary process to underpin professional standards. But no set of principles can cover all situations and a nurse's own perspective and inherent personal values, as well as personality and character, will play an important part in decision-making and behaviour.

Morality is thus, to a greater or lesser extent, internal and part of an individual's personal code of conduct, their ideals and the values, the mindset they use to appraise and respond to everyday situations. Note, however, that values often range from deeply committed, core values through everyday values to habitually conflicted ones.

Personal values are the beliefs for which a person has an enduring preference. Ideas help (or hinder) the individual when making judgements about important decisions and more generally making sense of life. They are principles and standards of personal behaviour influenced by character, family, background, culture, religion, community, personal life history and so on. It is clearly an advantage when professional and personal values are well aligned. This is one very good reason for an effective values-based recruitment process.

Assumption three: professional values underpin quality of care and treatment

For the removal of doubt, there is a strong correlation between the abstract concepts espoused as professional values and actual performance at work. There is empirical evidence that personal and professional values do impact behaviour in the workplace, care outcomes and the public image of the health service. The value literature suggests that people attach great importance to their values as behavioural guides and see them as central to self-identity (see Feather, 1990; Rokeach, 1973; Schwartz, 1992; Seligman and Katz, 1996). Values modulate behaviour. Behaviour as leadership style affects performance, including job satisfaction and retention (Abdelhafiz et al., 2016).

In a recent wide-ranging and authoritative review, Sharon Arieli and her research team integrated theories and empirical studies aiming to portray the role of personal values in shaping the choices and behaviour in work settings (Arieli et al., 2019). They concluded that values play a key role in many aspects of organisations: they are associated with occupational choices at the very beginning of the career and predict specific behaviours and decisions. Their broadness and stability make values a predictor of organisational behaviour over time and across contexts.

And other studies in organisational psychology by, for example, Milton Rokeach, Roy Suddaby, Humphrey Bourne and Mark Jenkins and Lilac Sagiv argue that values and beliefs are a predisposition to action and play a central role in guiding organisations, that they exist at multiple levels, defining what is considered right, worthy and desirable for employees, teams and organisations and that 'meaning, values and culture' should be 'brought back in' (Rokeach, 2008; Suddaby et al., 2010; Bourne and Jenkins, 2013; Sagiv et al., 2011).

The contribution of values can be modulated by complexity of the work, personal circumstances, pressures of the moment, unusually challenging decisions, personal relationships and so on, and these factors are being researched but 'people often think of themselves and their actions in terms of abstract values and moral principles ... and often try to live up to their core values'.

So, we can assume that leaders who create and successfully manage the right professional and cultural values for a positive work environment will improve quality of care and outcomes. And the attempt to do so is, 'in the case of inadvertent patient harm and avoidable deaths in a national health service, a moral imperative' (West, 2019).

We will now look at several limitations and challenges to quality of care and treatment. They argue for a rethink of some professional values by the National Health Service, as well as the professional identity of leadership, while also suggesting the sort of change needed. Later we will look at how cultural and personal values can be measured more effectively and changes in mindset of leaders can be quantified.

Leadership factors limiting delivery of a fully professional service

Leadership's personal and professional values are particularly relevant where teamwork is concerned. A review of research on teamwork in healthcare delivery settings provided evidence of the critical role leadership and culture plays in shaping teamwork and collaboration in practice (Rosen et al., 2018). Also see next West's evidence and trenchant comments on the need to improve teamworking in the Nation Health Service (NHS) (West, 2019).

Through a patient safety lens, learning from error through review and reflection is a critical organizational capacity requiring staff to be comfortable recognising, reporting and discussing challenging situations. Nembhard and Edmondson (2006) investigated the effects of leader inclusiveness (i.e., the words or deeds of leaders that may support others' contributions) on the relationship between status and psychological safety in teams. Results indicated that leader inclusiveness helped to overcome some of the negative effects (i.e., low psychological safety) associated with relative status in health-care teams, for example willingness to challenge a higher status team member.

Leadership that encourages good teamworking attitudes and values and creates really effective teams with clear objectives and regular reviews of performance is critical for creating a safe environment for individuals while enabling teams to learn from their mistakes and address West's moral challenge to the National Health Service in the United Kingdom to 'prevent the 5,000 avoidable patient deaths annually'.

Success would also reduce the chronic levels of stress that is associated with poor teamworking, causing damage to the health and well-being of too large a proportion of nurses and also reduce errors that can harm patient care and cause injury and patient mortality West (2019). These are key matters affecting staff well-being and retention.

Acknowledgement by leadership in the profession of the current limitations to mastery of what is professional in care and treatment of patients is important to success in redressing them. Research into such challenges would certainly benefit from a valid and reliable process for assessing professional morality in the service by way of the nursing and leadership values of individual nurses.

These challenges were highlighted recently in an article on the UK's National Health Service, citing evidence from 15 years of data from the NHS Staff Survey – 'data from a quarter of a million people per year'. The author describes a crisis and makes clear the need for better leadership and teamworking if staff are to be retained and the large number of avoidable patient deaths reduced (5000 annually) (West, 2019).

Similar problems are faced by Health and Social Care in the United States. Recent research comprehensively surveyed and synthesised what is known about teams, their structure and context, competencies, improvement strategies and the impact on care delivery outcomes. The authors provide an outline description of the sort of complex issues faced in the United States (and the United Kingdom) that is worth repeating. 'A single visit requires collaboration among a multidisciplinary group of clinicians, administrative staff, patients, and their loved ones. Multiple visits often occur across different clinicians working in different organizations. Ineffective care coordination and the underlying suboptimal teamwork processes are a public health issue. Health-care delivery systems exemplify complex organizations operating under high stakes in dynamic policy and regulatory environments. The coordination and delivery of safe, high-quality care demands reliable teamwork and collaboration within, as well as across, organizational, disciplinary, technical, and cultural boundaries' (Rosen et al., 2018).

Staff attempting to meet the challenge of delivering an effective health service aligned with professional values are finding it hard going. In the NHS, there are 103,000 vacancies, close to 40,000 of them nursing vacancies and high levels of sickness and turnover compared to the rest of industry. 'Lots of people are leaving the NHS for various reasons at every level … chronic levels of stress are associated with errors that can harm patient care and, in the acute sector it's associated with, for higher levels of patient mortality'. (West, 2019).

West provides empirical evidence that 96% of staff in the NHS say they work in teams and about 40% work in 'real teams' – those with clear objectives that meet regularly to review their performance. We also know, he says, that the more people work in what we would call 'pseudo teams' the higher the level of stress, injuries and patient mortality. 'We estimate', he says, 'that if we could increase the percentage of staff in "real teams" in the acute sector in hospitals from 40 percent to just 65 percent that would be associated … with the prevention of 5,000 avoidable patient deaths annually'. We must expand and build the quality of teamworking within the NHS.

Leadership plays a key role in team effectiveness (Rosen et al., 2018) and leadership style affects performance, including job satisfaction and retention (Abdelhafiz et al., 2016). Usama Saleh concluded in a qualitative study of 35 nurses working in different specialisms in a Saudi Arabian medical centre that 'The leadership style employed by nurse managers has a major impact on nurses' satisfaction, turnover, and the quality of patient care they deliver' (Saleh, 2018).

There are unique challenges facing the nursing profession and a need for a quality of nursing leadership at every level that is up to the meeting them – leadership to build quality work environments, enhance teamworking, implement new models of care and bring health and well-being to an exhausted and stretched nursing workforce. Leaders with the right value sets will have to be recruited, selected educated and trained if job satisfaction for nurses and healthy work environments underpinning retention are to be achieved.

The uniqueness of the challenge

The limiting factors as referred previously provide a complex and difficult challenge to the leadership of the NHS and the nursing profession as a whole. Like the innovative and foundational work on military teams or aviation crews in past decades, health-care provides a uniquely challenging setting for team researchers to develop and test theories of team effectiveness.

NHS teams are under stress for resources, fragmented duties adversely affect communication and emergencies can create life or death time pressures. Such a pressured environment is a breeding ground for misunderstandings and mistakes. Consequently, it is crucially important to resolve the deference issue (willingness to challenge, willingness to seek the cause of major mistakes and willingness to encourage this to happen). Matthew Syed talks of 'cognitive dissonance', the term Festinger coined to describe the inner tension we feel when things go wrong and self-esteem is threatened. Too often in the NHS, the response is not acceptance and reflection to prevent recurrence but denial and reframing to avoid blame (Syed, 2015, p. 80–81; Festinger, 1957).

So, findings about team leadership in extreme environments and the need for retraining of 'already leaders' to be followers when appropriate may be relevant in nursing. 'Many astronaut candidates enter the corps with experience and skills in leadership; however, the leadership role is shared during a long-duration mission, even if a formal mission commander has been assigned' (Burke et al., 2018). 'Thus, new astronauts with typical leadership skills at selection may need training on aspects of followership and shared leadership in concert with team orientation' (Landon et al., 2018).

Susan McDaniel undertook a scholarly inquiry into the contribution of research on teamwork and collaboration to psychology and healthcare. A special research issue, guest edited with Eduardo Salas, concluded, 'Then we turn to health care, which today is dominated by teamwork …we are still trying to understand how best to train, reinforce, and evaluate team-based skills'.

'And so, we hope this special issue motivates better, longitudinal, methodologically robust, and relevant research. Teams and effective teamwork matter in our airplanes, hospitals, and work environments; in our national security; in space exploration; in the generation of knowledge; and in our economy. Teamwork and collaboration matter, and although we have learned much— more is needed!'

They are focussing on the methods and processes that make collaborations more efficient and successful. 'Interdisciplinary teams are the way to make that happen' and improvement in 'Leadership training [that] targets a team leader's knowledge, skills and abilities' have been shown to be supportive of effective team processes (McDaniel and Salas, 2018; Salas et al., 2018).

The abovementioned issues present as a broad spectrum of serious and urgent matters requiring a reframing of the delivery of care in resource-strapped health services, in particular learning from the investigation of preventable medical error – see, for example, Starmer et al. (2014) and Rodziewicz and Hipskind (2019). These complex matters will surely challenge leadership.

I think it is generally well known and accepted in the United Kingdom that the NHS has some limitations and challenges. West's data analysis and Rosen's research (Rodziewicz and Hipskind, 2019) describe the stark reality for the NHS and major health services elsewhere and highlight the need for more effective leadership at every level. Leaders are required who have mastered professional values and have productive attitudes to relationships particularly teamworking. At a corporate level, leaders who can deliver funding and resources for 'on-the-job' training in leadership and teamworking and aare required who can n enhance recruitment and education to provide future leaders of the right calibre.

The answer to these challenges begins with recruitment, selection and education and the opening of a pipeline to a growing pool of leaders with the right values and beliefs and a range of different styles. Such a process would benefit from a psychometric to provide valid and reliable description and measurement of values and personal attributes for use in selection and education as would research to help understand more fully the science of teamworking in the complex environment of the NHS.

The scoring, assessment and development of leadership values and attributes

It is important to the success of such a project to have a valid and reliable measure of values and attributes. Recent research has established that NM is both valid and reliable test for assessing nursing values (McNeill et al., 2019). Leadership qualities can be inferred from the assessment of nursing values by NML.

We assume in our theoretical base (McNeill et al., 2019, p. 1) that professional identity may be expressed as a set of professional values that come together as a professional mindset. And that a nurse's behaviour will be guided and constrained in any caring role by such a professional belief system. The mature professional mindset will emerge out of inherent values and beliefs as these are modulated and enhanced by the education process and experience as a registered nurse.

A nurse leader will, we presume, excel in the sensible and effective application of professional nursing values to the requirements, uncertainties and challenges of the real world of nursing care and treatment. A potential leader will start from a better place if they have strongly core values and attributes such as willingness to make decisions when competent to do so and a natural capacity to influence the behaviour of others.

Professional identity can be scored and assessed effectively and consistently using a given set of professional values. Profiles of scores on values and attributes will vary from unique individual to unique individual. As we shall see later, potential natural leaders can be distinguished from potential natural followers by the values and attributes they aspire to and use to make sense of life.

A pipeline of recruitment, education and on-the-job training built upon such a valid and reliable assessment of applicants and students would provide the health service with a fresh stream of nurse leadership equipped with the values and attributes necessary to push back against the limitations and challenges we have described while maintaining the best existing qualities of the nursing profession.

Design of a suitable test of leadership values

Background

After a systematic review of policy and research reports Cummings et al. (2010) stated, 'Numerous policy and research reports call for leadership to build quality work environments, implement new models of care, and bring health and well-being to an exhausted and stretched nursing workforce ... Our results document evidence of various forms of leadership and their differential effects on the nursing workforce and work environments. Efforts by organizations and individuals to encourage and develop transformational and relational leadership are needed to enhance nurse satisfaction, recruitment, retention, and healthy work environments, particularly in this current and worsening nursing shortage'.

We gathered further evidence from the literature of serious challenges and limitations faced by the health service, and it has been expressed above (p. 4–7).

Recent theoretical and empirical developments in the leadership literature are currently receiving attention in terms of research, theory and practice. 'We began by examining authentic leadership ...'. (Avolio et al., 2008). 'There are many identified styles of nursing leadership ... Servant ... Transformational ... Democratic ... Authoritarian ... Laissez-faire ...' (Frandsen, 2014). 'Development of student leadership capacity and efficacy is critical to the nursing profession' (Waite et al., 2014) who also made the point that authentic leadership is a popular leadership theory and that an authentic leadership course has been very well received by Fellowship students.

Authentic leadership is an approach to leadership that emphasises building the leader's legitimacy through honest relationships with followers who value their input and are built on an ethical foundation. Generally, authentic leaders are positive people with truthful self-concepts who promote openness. By building trust and generating enthusiastic support from their subordinates, authentic leaders can improve individual and team performance (Gardner et al., 2011; Waite et al., 2014). Authentic leaders are genuine with people and have a real interest in their health and welfare.

The study

The objective of the study was to demonstrate how an applicant's leadership qualities might be better understood using ISA and an instrument such as NM. The NM instrument was modified to measure leadership qualities (see Tables 11.1 and 11.2) and named NML. The specific aim was to show how one might answer the question 'To what extent does this applicant embody 'authentic leadership' qualities?'

The question of leadership in the profession can be a vexing one. In order to better understand the question and inform the use of NM in its assessment, we expanded the desktop literature search to include leadership generally.

We acknowledge from the literature that leadership is not a unitary concept but exists to various degrees and in various kinds in different individuals, workplaces and situations. Also, as a broad generalisation, that the 'great leaders' are 'born not made'.

The design focus fell on one aspect of leadership in nursing practice, caring for people (as opposed, for example, to resource or financial management) and on one style authentic leadership (as opposed to, for example, transformational or democratic). We used the concept of 'Authentic Leadership', familiar to leadership theorists, as the concept around which to design the NML psychometric (Avolio et al., 2008; Waite et al., 2014).

Nursing values were reworked into themes related to authentic leadership and NM scores on values were used to calculate theme scores, summed as scores on leadership (see Tables 11.1 and 11.2).

Table 11.1 Qualities of the authentic leader

Qualities of an Authentic Leader	
CONF	Confidence
COMM	Commitment
DMC	Decision-making capability
CIO	Capacity to inspire others
H&I	Honesty and integrity
GCS	Good communication skills
EMP	Empathy
ICT	Innovation and creative thinking
ACC	Accountability

Table 11.2 Leadership qualities and nursing values

Nursing Values[a]	C No.	CONF	COMM	DMC	CIO	H&I	GCS	EMP	ICT	ACC
				Leadership Qualities						
Rights	1			1		1				1
Safety	2			2		2				2
Discomfort	3	3	3	3	3	3	3			
Teamwork	4			4				4		4
Influence	5	5		5	5		5	5		5
Learning	6	6	6	6	6				6	6
Listening	7	7		7			7	7		
Honesty	8	8			8	8	8			8
Coping	9	9	9	9	9				9	9
Challenging	10	10	10	10	10	10				10
Deciding	11	11	11	11	11				11	11
Responsibility	12	12		12					12	12
Carefulness	13		13			13				13
Communication	14	14			14		14	14		
Getting on	15	15			15		15	15		
Reliability	16		16	16		16	16			16
Independence	17	17		17		17			17	
Awareness	18			18	18		18	18	18	18
Reflectivity	19			19				19	19	19
Selflessness	20	20	20		20	20		20		

[a] A full description of the value choices made can be found at Paragraph 2.2.1 of the Replication Study (Traynor et al., 2019).

Since the 20 nursing values we have been using with NM mapped well to nine 'authentic leadership' attributes, we were able to design a pilot instrument to assess and score our sample of applicants on qualities associated with authentic leadership.

The assumption which could be made here is that to become a great authentic leader, you should have all the qualities set out in Table 11.1. And if you lack any one of them, then you might struggle to make a mark as a leader. The reality of course is somewhat different being more a matter of strong features and limitations, degree and kind, time and place.

To the extent to which you show commitment, empathy, honesty and integrity and accountability, you will set a good example which others will follow. The quality of your communication skills and decision-making capabilities will also play a vital role in effective leadership. Lastly, innovation and creative thinking (ICT) and the capacity to deal effectively and well with discomforting and difficult decisions will help you stand out as an authentic leader.

We will consider our findings using NM shortly and, in these terms, but first let us say something about the leadership measure we devised. This is not a fully developed instrument. It has been designed to demonstrate how better quantitative data on leadership might be acquired, beginning with the applicant to nursing and following through longitudinally. We have used qualities associated with one form of leadership, but the instrument might have addressed any other form of leadership by simply changing the values to match the form of leadership being studied.

A backdrop to our consideration of leadership qualities is that we have a measure of personal nursing values from which to infer leadership characteristics. In doing so, it seems reasonable to suppose that successful nurses, those that have the required nursing values to the required standard, will, to a greater or lesser extent, have authentic leadership qualities. Effective nursing means taking control in a caring way.

Nursing values tell you quite a lot about leadership qualities, but not everything, since personality, character, personal identity, personal circumstances and skills are among other factors affecting performance. Our task here is to focus on nursing values and leadership, although ISA analytics permit a closer look at personal identity and circumstances if required.

Rank ordering applicants using the NML psychometric is one way of distinguishing those better endowed with the qualities of authentic leadership from the less well endowed, but each applicant has different strengths and limitations in their leadership profile and is a unique leadership asset. Any process of professional development should carefully weight each talent and consider what might be done to nurture it. This uniqueness reflects the real world of leadership and identity instruments like NML can be of great assistance with staff development.

Data analysis

The epistemological position we adopt is essentially constructionist. That is, a person develops a unique sense of self and perspective by way of personal experience of self-in-the-world (see ISA meta-theory. The criteria we adopted to address validity and reliability provide the NM test with qualitative and quantitative rigour, are based accordingly on this philosophical position and methodology and are described in considerable detail elsewhere (McNeill et al., 2019 and at paragraph 2.7.3 Replication Study; Traynor et al., 2019).

The units of measurement remain the reliable and valid S-scores on nursing values. The validity of deriving the L-scores from these valid and reliable S-scores is grounded in expertise, experience and common sense. Work is required to reaffirm it. This is acceptable here since our aim is to demonstrate the viability of the NML process as a test of leadership qualities and is not to establish its validity and reliability.

The instrument worked well, profiling and rank ordering the sample of applicants by score on leadership qualities. Psychometric test standards were met (see the 'Statistical properties' section). Two successful applicants were described in terms of their leadership qualities, highlighting their strengths and limitations and illustrating the use of the test in offering insight into leadership potential and leadership style (see the 'Applicant SUI 148' and 'Applicant SUI 226' sections).

NM identity analytics, inherent functionality not previously used in the context of nursing, facilitated identification of nursing characteristics that enhanced or adversely affected leadership performance demonstrating how leadership skills might be more fully appraised and development encouraged.

The outcome demonstrated how a well-designed NM-style Leadership instrument could provide quantitative and qualitative research data on leadership in nursing that is not currently available.

The findings

Nurse Match as a measure of the qualities of an 'authentic leader' (objective 1)

NML proved to be effective as a process for rank ordering applicants on leadership qualities as part of a selection process and as a practical tool for the more detailed appraisal of individuals who score well on it (see the 'Applicant SUI 148' and 'Applicant SUI 226' sections). Statistical analysis of the data supported the expectation that a test like NML would meet international test standards were it to be subject to a proper developmental process.

Statistical properties

The scoring process conforms to internationally accepted standards for a psychometric test, including internal reliability (Cronbach's alpha 0.9753) (see Table 11.3).

The distribution of the overall scores (mean L^{TOT} scores) is normal (see Figure 11.1). Anderson–Darling statistic was used to appraise normality

Table 11.3 Descriptive statistics for mean 'Authentic Leadership' (L^{TOT}) score

	Statistic (N = 228)	Comment
AD test	0.386	Normal Dist.
p-Value[a]	0.388	Alpha = 0.05
St Dev.	13.40	
Mean	51.63	Close to median
Median	51.35	Close to mean
Skewness	0.09	Symmetrical
Skew SE	0.16	
Kurtosis	−0.10	Low 'tailiness'
Kurt SE	0.32	
Cronbach's alpha	0.9753	VG reliability

[a] The null hypothesis (H_0) for the Anderson–Darling (AD) test is that the distribution is normal. Here there is no reason to reject the null hypothesis p-value >0.05.

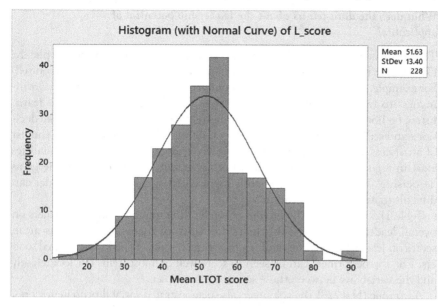

Figure 11.1 Descriptive statistics for mean 'Authentic Leadership' (L^{TOT}).

(AD = 0.386: p-value = 0.388 with alpha = 0.05). All nine-item scores are normally distributed (AD statistic and p-values are reported in Appendix B at Table BA of the research report).

Table 11.4 illustrates the substantive difference between the measure of values and the measure of leadership – each participant was scored on both measures (N = 228). The substantive difference is reflected in the mean scores, i.e. 47.82 for values and 51.46 for authentic leadership. The 'unit of measurement' is the same in both cases. It is the S-score on each of the 20 values. A t-test indicated a real difference between the measures, and this was significant, p-value 0.003 (alpha = 0.05). The effect size was small (Cohen's d = 0.28) and correlation was high (r = 0.998).

Table 11.4 Suitability S^{TOT} and Leadership L^{TOT} test scores: high correlation but real difference

Mean S^{TOT}	Mean L^{TOT}	Comment
47.82	51.46	Substantive difference
	Statistic: L-score cf. S-score	
t-Test (crit. t = 1.96)	−2.97	Real difference
p-Value	0.003	(Alpha = 0.05) significant difference
Cohen's d =	0.28	Small effect size
Correlation (r)	0.998	Extremely high

What does the data tell us about the leadership potential of applicants?

The instrument assesses 9 authentic leadership qualities of an applicant (Table 11.1) by making certain assumptions about what attributes are required. For example, the leadership quality of confidence will be demonstrated by a willingness to take on unpleasant tasks, being able to influence others, to learn, listen, be honest, cope with resource limitations, take responsibility, make decisions and still get on with others and remain self-less: see Table 11.2 for the list of attributes and values concerned for each leadership quality. All 9 qualities exist in a good leader, to a greater or lesser extent, and interact to emerge as 'leadership'. If one is absent or poorly represented, a reputation as a leader can difficult to establish or maintain.

Table 11.5 sets out (a) the profiles of some of the top individual performers on overall leadership qualities, (b) the performance of the whole sample as mean scores on leadership qualities and (c), in contrast, some of the lowest ranked scorers. The top performers can be seen to score well on most items but look closely and the variability between these scores is plain to see.

As a group (N = 228), the volunteers also demonstrated variability on item scores, strongest on good communication skills (GCS) and empathy (EMP) and noticeably weaker on ICT. The lowest ranking applicants generally did not score well on items; nevertheless, individual variability between item scores is readily apparent. It was also apparent that individuals of similar rank would often differ considerably in their strength on a leadership quality.

The high level of correlation between nursing values and leadership qualities (see Table 11.4) makes sense since our nine leadership values are those of the

Table 11.5 High and low and mean output scores on nine elements of leadership

SUI	CONF	COMM	DMC	CIO	H&I	GCS	EMP	ICT	ACC	L_score	R/O
169	69.09	84.76	83.78	74.29	84.63	70.27	88.32	71.31	68.32	77.20	5
148	72.87	75.95	75.37	77.62	75.06	85.30	84.09	66.48	73.13	76.21	6
226	68.07	79.56	81.83	70.00	76.59	77.79	92.31	65.30	72.51	75.99	7
125	71.52	72.07	75.45	75.17	71.42	86.02	86.72	66.49	75.05	75.54	8
8	73.47	81.59	75.73	72.75	72.06	75.88	81.86	72.22	71.85	75.27	9
MEAN	49.57	54.47	50.58	53.70	49.47	58.30	58.36	43.21	47.03	51.63	Mean
4	32.34	20.05	32.85	33.44	13.74	36.09	52.21	28.44	25.09	30.47	217
184	30.76	25.51	31.86	26.79	38.29	24.65	36.11	29.12	28.67	30.19	218
98	35.10	23.71	25.24	31.13	26.31	44.55	44.80	19.35	13.58	29.31	219
74	24.87	30.95	23.50	35.02	22.73	38.60	40.36	13.79	29.85	28.85	220
10	31.13	18.40	32.53	23.97	32.86	31.29	20.60	28.19	31.98	27.88	221

'authentic leader' whose sense of identity is grounded in having the right professional values and ethical thinking and applying them to colleagues as well as patients.

The mean score on the leadership items is used to rank order applicants but, since a leader is unlikely to show the same strength across all qualities, even high-ranking profiles should be examined for limitations in one or more elements. Any limitations or suspected limitations can be examined more closely, and an explanation sought using the additional analytics provided by the Ipseus (NM) software as shown next.

The applicants we are most interested in here are those who have scored well on nursing values using NM and have been offered a place on a course. We can now do an assessment of the potential of these applicants (now students) as leaders.

Selection involves a broader assessment that is provided here by a psychometric test, and not all the applicants who scored well on nursing values were offered a nursing course. In fact, only two of those listed in Table 11.5 were offered a course, SUI 148 and SUI 226. We will use these two examples to demonstrate the potential of NM in the assessment of leadership potential.

Applicant SUI 148

The defining leadership qualities of this applicant are *empathy* and *good communication:* see Figures 11.1 (L^{TOT} = 84.09 and 85.30) and 11.2. That is, the student can be characterised as giving considerable importance and emotional significance to influencing people's behaviour, doing unpleasant tasks, listening, communicating effectively, being reliable, honest and unselfish, being aware of what is going on, being reflective rather than responsive and just plain getting on with people. See Table 11.2 for all the values underpinning these two qualities, the scores on which will vary a little.

See Figure 11.3 for the clustering of scores on her core nursing values: a representation of her mindset or value and belief system, setting importance of a value (sp) against its emotional significance (ES).

Other main drivers of respect for a leader are present as good scores on accountability, honesty and integrity. They underpin her authentic leadership credentials. Confidence is an essential quality and is present. The capacity to inspire others features strongly, (L^{TOT} = 77.62) emerging just short of empathy and good communication. Strong scores on decision-making and commitment complete a strong hand of leadership qualities, except perhaps for innovative and creative thinking, one quality that is less impressive. These qualities are summarised in Figure 11.2.

In order to pin down the reason for the lower score on innovative and creative thinking (ICT), (L^{TOT} = 66.48), with a view to enhancing that quality, we can go back into Table 11.2 and look under ICT where we find that the value constructs that constitute ICT are coping (with lack of resources), decision-making, experiential learning, independence, awareness and reflectivity.

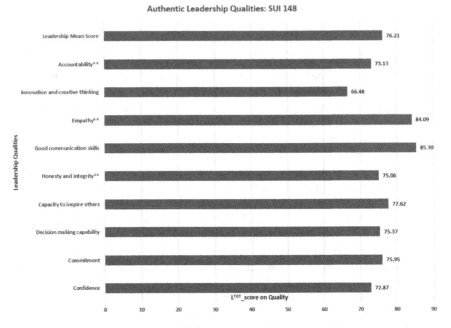

Figure 11.2 Leadership qualities of SUI 148, a successful applicant.

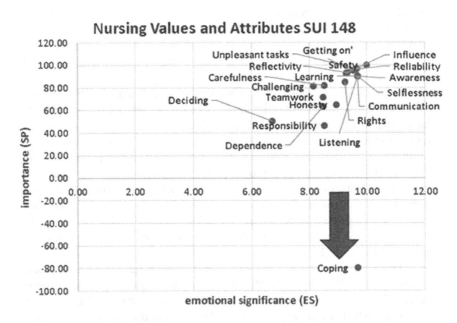

Figure 11.3 Core nursing values showing concern about coping with pressure on resources.

When we use the 'hidden' analytical resources of NM, we find a probable cause for the lower score on innovative and creative thinking. One of the constituent value constructs 'Coping' (construct 9 in Table 11.2) is highly conflicted (sp $\geq$ −79.98: threshold to low importance is sp $\leq$ +35.99) and emotional significance is high (ES = 9.67: threshold to high is 9.89).

This bipolar value dimension sets out two alternative points of view one of which a respondent should choose. When describing 'model nurse' this would present as 'A model nurse thinks … resource constraints at work are no excuse for lack of kindness and sympathy/pressures on resources can leave less room for kindness and sympathy'. The professional response is the first alternative. It is a nursing value to aspire to. The applicant prefers the alternative point of view and it has strong emotional significance for her. She believes very strongly that pressure on resources can leave less room for kindness and sympathy. This attitude is unprofessional since it becomes an excuse for not aspiring to be kind and sympathetic and results in conflicted thinking about quality of care, and so conflicted behaviour.

The negativity (dissonance) around this construct is very high. See Figure 11.3 for a clear picture of the impact of coping on her value and belief system. For her, the very low importance of the aspiration to cope well with resource limitations (follow the arrow) is due to its very low usefulness to her in making sense of life in the workplace and its very high 'emotional significance' is due to the large amount of negative feeling associated with it.

In short, this student believes that pressure on resources can leave less room for kindness and sympathy. She sees difficulty coping with this situation and feels strongly about it.

Given the cluster of strong core values (top right corner) that underpins the applicant's nursing identity, it would be a pity to let this genuine concern fester to possibly undermine her convictions about professional nursing and her leadership potential – which is evident in her flagging of this concern.

Her *identity variant* is 'Balanced' so that she has a coherent sense of work identity and a moderately high sense of self-esteem. She is the sort of person who normally copes well and sensibly with personal differences and difficulties at work. However, one has to consider the possible effect of this coping issue on her morale and resilience and any future leadership role she might have and what might be done during her education to help her see the need for clear aspirations in this regard.

Applicant SUI 226

This student presents with a very strong leadership score on empathy and strong scores on 'commitment' and 'decision-making capability' (DMC) (see Figure 11.4). Good scores on communication skills, honesty and integrity and, to a lesser extent, accountability fully complement those leadership virtues but scores on capacity to inspire others, confidence and innovative and creative thinking are not so impressive.

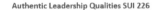

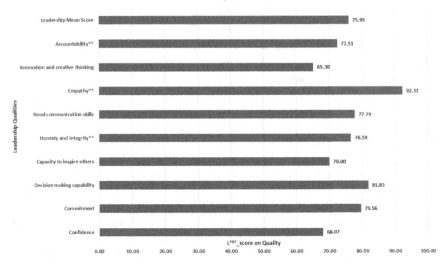

Figure 11.4 Leadership qualities of SUI 226, a successful applicant.

NM analytics can help explore the factors in play here and consider what, if anything, might be done to enhance the less impressive leadership qualities or at least raise awareness about them to allow their effective management. Before we look at these three qualities, it is necessary to deal with (a) a concern about the nursing value deciding (construct 11) that is linked to DMC and (b) the defensive identity variant DHSR both flagged by NM.

Despite scoring well on the leadership quality DMC the student appears to have difficulty with decision-making in nursing. One of the factors contributing to DMC is the nursing value 'Deciding' – construct 11 – which presents as '*prefer to make the decisions within my area of competence*/in a shared area of competence I sometimes prefer the other person to take decisions'. Analytics shows that the student aspires to the left-hand discourse (in italics) but this choice is associated with substantial emotional discomfort since it is conflicted (sp = –31.70: the threshold to low sp = +52.37.) being associated with substantially greater dissonance than consonance.

The effect can be clearly seen in Figure 11.5 at bottom right (follow the arrow). For some reason, the student is discomforted when acknowledging the importance of making decisions within their area of competence. 'Negative Importance' can mean 'double talk', saying one thing and meaning another. Perhaps she would really prefer some other competent person to make the decisions. In any case, this is a vexing matter for her (emotional significance = 10, maximum) and it would be useful to clarify what is going on here for developmental reasons. As we will see in a moment this student has a somewhat defensive type of identity and this may be relevant.

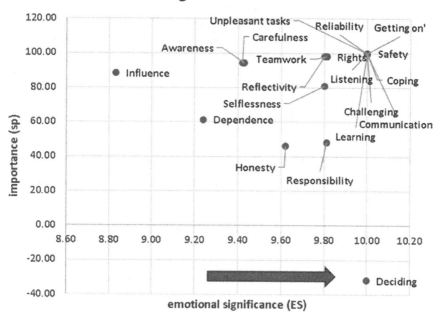

Figure 11.5 Nine immutable core nursing values and conflicted decision-making (deciding).

Analytics indicates that the nature of the student's personal identity is an important factor in her leadership style (identity variant is DHSR). Her appraisal of her success in pursuing her aspirations (self-evaluation) is quite high and identity diffusion is low indicating a very precise and somewhat inflexible sense of what it is to be a nurse. This is a defensive state of mind which does not accept difference as normal and tends to see things in black and white terms – see Figure 11.5, top right, cluster of nine nursing values (all have 'importance' 100: 'emotional significance' 10).

DHSR, this tendency to rigid and immutable expression of personal values and beliefs, might on the face of it be the source of dissonance or doubt associated with making decisions within her area of competence, 'Deciding' (see above). The interaction between deciding and DHSR, could be creating dissonance, which is not resolved over time by adjusting behaviour, so reducing the student's perception of her confidence, her capacity to inspire others, and her innovative and creative thinking. In any event, the negative L-score on deciding (value construct 11) will have reduced her L^{TOT} score on all three leadership qualities.

The L^{TOT} scores on confidence and the capacity to inspire others will also have been reduced somewhat by the student's 'unprofessional' take on nursing value construct 08 (honesty) where she had to choose between 'it is better to be open and honest in everything you do/*sometimes it is wiser to manage the truth in the best interests of all concerned*. She indicates a preference to managing the truth when the professional preference is to aspire to be open and honest'.

One could go on, but the point has been made. This student would probably benefit from an opportunity to reflect on this aspect of her leadership profile. Whether this is done tangentially in a shared lecture experience addressing these considerations as matters of educational importance or face to face as staff development is a matter for tutorial staff.

Discussion

Strengths of NM Leadership test

Nurse Match – Leadership version – has all the strengths of the main NM psychometric (see McNeill et al., 2019). The 20 values scored using NM have been allocated selectively to represent leadership qualities. These qualities are difficult to research so that their understanding is constrained by having too little quantitative data. Here we have an approach which uses a person's value and belief system to profile or model their leadership potential in qualitative and quantitative terms that permit us to work on enhancement or at least encouragement of growth in leadership qualities.

Limitations

The limitations of the core NM approach are discussed more fully in Section 4.2 of the Replication Study (Traynor et al., 2019).

Briefly stated they are that valid and reliable self-reports rely on sound motivation, openness, honesty and astute self-awareness which is difficult to ensure. This is managed in part by encouraging quick intuitive responses. 'Social desirability' bias, responding in the way you think is socially desirable, is minimised by the NM scoring process. NM provides a snapshot of values held at one moment in time-taking account of randomly occurring personal factors that influence responses so that some values may vary considerably over time. Some respondents with very high self-regard and very firm preferred views may score exceptionally well when a more balanced and equitable demeanour with a more moderate score may be preferable – a situation best managed at interview.

Suitability in terms of nursing values and attributes can only be part of the process of assessment. There is clearly a need for complementarity in the means of appraisal of nurses and candidates for both developmental and recruitment purposes.

There are also limitations associated specifically with NM Leadership. When using NM analytics, a certain amount of specialist knowledge and experience in the use of the analytics is required. An element of synthesis and subjectivity is involved in interpretation of the data about individual applicants or students. This means, initially at least, that the use of ISA analytics will be limited to research on leadership in nursing for which this specialist knowledge is available.

On the other hand, this could be an advantage since it would enable idiographic work with those acknowledged as 'the best leaders' in the field to generate some fresh insight into what makes for successful leadership.

Finally, the choice of values used to represent leadership qualities has not been subjected to the degree of developmental testing that it otherwise would and that is acceptable here only because the test is merely being used for demonstration purposes.

Summary and recommendations

Recognised issues within the organisation

Issues such as underfunding, low staffing levels, high levels of sickness, poor levels of staff retention make headlines and provide a ready explanation for failures of treatment and care. A closer look at the facts, however, points to a defensive culture, inappropriate deference, defects in quality of leadership and team working as important factors. Cultural attitudes and values underpin issues such as the following and they can be addressed directly.

a *Update professional codes* of practice to deal firmly, fairly and constructively with defensiveness and denial by staff in the face of allegations of poor treatment outcomes, care or attitudes.

b *Resolve the deference issue*: Encourage 'shared leadership' and 'followership' in the education of nurses and doctors. Introduce as a team concept, task-dependent 'leaders and followers', in which leaders can be followers and followers can be leaders determined by task role. The team being familiar with who does what.

c *Improve teamworking practice*: Poor teamwork equals stress, ill-health and poor retention while good teamwork equals satisfactory and satisfying outcomes.

 1 Promote effective teamworking early in the education process treating belief in and capacity for good teamworking as a key aspect of professional identity.

 2 Educate on best practice when working in a team; teamworking attitudes and values, setting clear objectives, generating safety, learning from mistakes.

 3 Teach 'review and reflect' on team outcomes and shared responsibility.

d *Educate for leadership*: 'Nurses at the point of registration need to be equipped with the necessary leadership skills' Marian Traynor has described in some detail a leadership module in the nursing curriculum at a school of nursing (Traynor, 2018).

e *Measure leadership potential* and provide feedback: Assess student's take on nursing values as their professional belief system emerges to assess their leadership potential. Provide a feedback process within the module to encourage development.

Recognising and reframing

The first step in promoting more effective leadership in the nursing profession is acknowledgement by leaders of the limitations to their understanding and mastery of what is professional in care and treatment of patients: acceptance that there are some well-recognised deficiencies in practice and a willingness to address them.

Professional values underpin professional performance at work, care outcomes and public image of a health service. The service in the United Kingdom is highly respected, admired, by the general public which is why people are so disillusioned when things go wrong. In recent years, there have been a large number of avoidable patient deaths annually (circa, 5000). Doing something about this has become a moral imperative.

We have considered which values require review and will round off the chapter by considering how values might be reframed in this context and improve performance.

Doing it

Such reframing of culture standards and leadership to be fit for purpose is needed to build better quality work environments, enhance teamworking, implement new models of care and bring health and well-being to an exhausted and stretched nursing workforce. Leaders with the right standards and aspirations, caring and talented, will have to be recruited, selected, educated and trained if best quality care, job satisfaction for nurses and healthy work environments underpinning retention are to be achieved.

Ideally, cultural identity should change gradually through a process of review of outcome and reflection on experience once enough time has elapsed. There are, today, some strong voices speaking out about change and where it is needed. Probably the last thing the health service needs is a comprehensive review. But it does need to improve outcomes for patients and reduce avoidable harm in a sustainable way.

How might this be managed? One mechanism that has been suggested is the seeding of the profession with a pipeline of new nurses with an enhanced set of professional values whose leadership potential has been appraised, encouraged and developed.

This will require a commitment to gradual and sustainable revision of professional standards via a process of conception, application, review and reflection – ideally by the combined efforts of academics and experienced practitioners. Implementation should begin by attracting and selecting applicants with the right inherent values and leadership potential.

It would be important to ensure awareness by existing staff of such a programme of change, what well-recognised issues are being addressing and what benefits the changes are expected to bring about, that is encourage participation of practitioners and seek their buy-in to the process of change.

Educating for change

Reframed value concepts as they emerge could be drip-fed by schools of nursing into the curriculum where professional identity, leadership or teamworking is being addressed.

A valid and reliable psychometric test like NML should be used to measure (score) and monitor development of professional identity and leadership potential during the education process in the manner we have described (pp. 13–18 previously) and beyond that with specialist practitioners and nurse educators if the will was there.

The education process, i.e. the course syllabus should be reworked to take account of these issues. Bring in lecturers from other disciplines as necessary. The aim of the education process being to establish a pipeline into the profession of nurses imbued with up-to-date values and leadership attributes (see Traynor, 2018 for an exposition).

Using a custom-built leadership psychometric

I demonstrated in this chapter (pp. 13–18) how a psychometric (NML) built using a revised value set could improve this process of developing professional standards and professional leadership in nursing staff at a time of great need by providing a valid measure of the personal significance of professional nursing values for behaviour, that is by making key processes more effective and transparent – processes such as recruitment and selection, education, staff assessment, staff development and the provision of better quantitative and qualitative research data on leadership in nursing.

Resolving the enigma of professional identity

The narrative here has been about a very useful new 'Match' tool for conceptualising and measuring the personal and professional identity of individuals who are or might become leaders of organisations and teams. The prototype tool used to demonstrate the use of 'Match' in a health service in crisis is NML. It offers for each employee, self's view of self and self's view of nurses, leadership and teamwork in terms of professional nursing values.

The Match class of psychometric is most effective in appraising a person's professional values and beliefs as core or conflicted drivers of behaviour and in scoring the match with an organisation's expressed values. It becomes most useful when it is necessary to rework an organisation's standards or its leadership culture in the face of an existing crisis or need to enhance organisational performance in some way.

When the health service recovers from the COVID-19 pandemic, there may be a prospect of further change to improve working conditions and efficacy of treatment and care to reward the health service for the self-sacrifice shown. One can expect, hope for, fresh financial resources to address key issues like staffing levels but inherent issues of concern remain about treatment and care of some patients, stress on and retention of staff, too much poor teamworking, uneven quality of leadership and, underpinning this, too much resistance to constructive change, denial and defensiveness in the face of avoidable harm done. The issues are interwoven, complex and intractable and will have to be simplified if a measure of success is to be achieved.

Our narrative has been about a very real crisis in an organisation and the challenges of resolving it by way of cultural change in behaviour. I have demonstrated how NML using a simple scoring system can check the extent of the buy-in by staff to the change in leadership and teamwork values facilitating the process of change – and how that work can be done transparently, systematically and effectively via a valid and reliable measure of leadership values, to professional test standards.

Note

1. Nurse Match (NM) Leadership (NML) is a psychometric derivative of the established NM psychometric tool that successfully completed a pilot use with applicants run by a research team at Queen's University School of Nursing in collaboration with Identity Exploration Ltd: contact Dr Marian Traynor (M.Traynor@qub.ac.uk).

References

Abdelhafiz, I.M., Alloubani, A.M.D., & Almatari, M. (2016) 'Impact of leadership styles adopted by head nurses on job satisfaction: A comparative study between governmental and private hospitals in Jordan', Journal of Nursing Management, 24(3). doi: 10.1111/jonm.12333.

Arieli, S., Sagiv, L., & Roccas, S. (2019) 'Values at work: The impact of personal values in organisations', Applied Psychology. doi: 10.1111/apps.12181.

Avolio, B.J., Walumbwa, F.O., & Weber, T.J., (2008) 'Leadership: Current theories, research, and future directions', Annual Review of Psychology, 60(1), 421–449. Available at: https://doi.org/10.1146/annurev.psych.60.110707.163621.

Bourne, H., & Jenkins, M. (2013) 'Organizational values: A dynamic perspective'. Organization Studies, 34(4), 495–514. https://doi.org/10.1177/0170840612467155

Burke, C.S., Shuffler, M.L., & Wiese, C.W. (2018) 'Examining the behavioral and structural characteristics of team leadership in extreme environments', Journal of Organizational Behavior. doi: 10.1002/job.2290.

Cummings, G.G. et al. (2010) 'Leadership styles and outcome patterns for the nursing workforce and work environment: A systematic review', International Journal of Nursing Studies. doi: 10.1016/j.ijnurstu.2009.08.006.

Feather, N.T. (1990) 'Bridging the gap between values and actions: Recent applications of the expectancy-value model', In E. T. H. R. M. Sorrentino (Ed.), Handbook of motivation and cognition: Foundations of social behavior, Vol. 2 (pp. 151–192). New York: Guilford Press.

Festinger, L. (1957) 'An introduction to the theory of dissonance', A Theory of Cognitive Dissonance. doi: 10.1037/10318-001.

Frandsen, B., 2014. Nursing leadership: Management & leadership styles. London: AANAC Extras.

Gardner, W.L. et al., 2011. 'Authentic leadership: A review of the literature and research agenda', The Leadership Quarterly, 22, 1120–1145.

Landon, L.B., Slack, K.J., & Barrett, J.D. (2018) 'Teamwork and collaboration in long-duration space missions: Going to extremes', American Psychologist. doi: 10.1037/amp0000260.

McDaniel, S.H., & Salas, E. (2018) 'The science of teamwork: Introduction to the special issue', American Psychologist, 73(4), 305–307. http://dx.doi.org/10.1037/amp0000337

McNeill, C. et al. (2019) 'Developing nurse match: A selection tool for evoking and scoring an applicant's nursing values and attributes', Nursing Open. Wiley-Blackwell Publishing Ltd, 6(1), pp. 59–71. doi: 10.1002/nop2.183.

Nembhard, I.M., & Edmondson, A.C. (2006) 'Making it safe: The effects of leader inclusiveness and professional status on psychological safety and improvement efforts in health care teams', Journal of Organizational Behavior, 27, 941–966. http://dx.doi.org/10.1002/job.413

Rodziewicz, T.L., & Hipskind, J.E. (2019) Medical error prevention. London: StatPearls.

Rokeach, M. (1973) Rokeach values survey. In The nature of human values. New York: Simon and Shuster.

Rokeach, M. (2008) Understanding human values. New York: Simon and Schuster.

Rosen, M.A. et al. (2018) 'Teamwork in healthcare: Key discoveries enabling safer, high-quality care', American Psychological Association, 73(4), 433–450.

Sagiv, L., Schwartz, S.H., & Arieli, S. (2011) Personal values, national culture and organizations: Insights applying the Schwartz value framework. In: N. N. Ashkanasy, C. Wilderom, & M. F. Peterson (Eds.), The handbook of organizational culture and climate (pp. 515–537). Newbury Park, CA: Sage.

Salas, E., Reyes, D.L., & McDaniel, S.H. (2018) 'The science of teamwork: Progress, reflections, and the road ahead', American Psychologist, 73(4), 593.

Saleh, U. et al. (2018) 'The impact of nurse managers' leadership styles on ward staff', British Journal of Nursing, 27(4). doi: 10.12968/bjon.2018.27.4.197.

Schwartz, S.H. (1992) 'Universals in the content and structure of values: Theoretical advances and empirical tests in 20 countries', Advances in Experimental Social Psychology, 25(C), 1–65. doi: 10.1016/S0065-2601(08)60281-6.

Seligman, C., & Katz, A.N. (1996) The dynamics of value systems. In The psychology of values: The Ontario symposium, Vol. 8 (pp. 53–75). London: Erlbaum.

Starmer, A.J. et al. (2014) 'Changes in medical errors after implementation of a handoff program', New England Journal of Medicine. doi: 10.1056/NEJMsa1405556.

Suddaby, R., Elsbach, K.D., Greenwood, R., Meyer, J.W., & Zilber, T.B. (2010) 'Organizations and their institutional environments – bringing meaning, values, and culture back in: Introduction to the special research forum', Academy of Management Journal, 53(6), 1234–1240. https://doi.org/10.2139/ssrn.2266086.

Syed, M. (2015) Wrongful convictions. London: John Murray. Available at: www.johnmurray.co.uk.

Traynor, M. (Queen's U. S. of N. and M.) (2018) Developing a leadership programme for nursing students. Belfast. Available at: m.traynor@qub.ac.uk.

Traynor et al. (2019) Burdett Trust for Nursing Final Report "What Matters to Patients?": Identifying Applicants to Nursing who have the Personal Values Required to Build a Skilled and Competent Workforce and Lead the Nursing Profession in Northern

Ireland'. Executive Summary A. Belfast. Available at: https://www.qub.ac.uk/schools/SchoolofNursingandMidwifery/FileStore/Filetoupload,945100,en.pdf.'

Waite, R. et al., 2014. 'The embodiment of authentic leadership', Journal of Professional Nursing.

West, M.A. (2019) 'It doesn't have to be this way', The Psychologist, August, pp. 30–33. Available at: www.thepsychologist.org.uk.Landon, L. B., Slack, K. J. and Barrett, J. D. (2018) 'Teamwork and collaboration in long-duration space missions: Going to extremes', American Psychologist. doi: 10.1037/amp0000260.

12 Are we admitting the right students?

Seeking the "best fit" with institutional values and professional identity development and professionalism in US medical school admission processes

Joel Lanphear, Marie C. Matte, Chris Austin, Lyman Mower and John Clements

For any student, the process of becoming a competent health professional involves learning about oneself, the profession, the content and processes of patient care, and the milieu in which one will practice. It also involves the development of one's professional identity.

The context of medical practice in the United States and Canada has changed as a result of a number of influences. Among them, but not limited to, are the increasing cost of health care, lack of primary care physicians in less populated areas, lack of or few minority students and practitioners, increased preventable health problems related to diet and lifestyle, the development of team approaches to health care, and the positive and negative impact of social media.

Some medical schools and institutions have developed new courses, implemented entire new curricula, and modified their mission statements in an effort to address the changing environment. Other medical schools, particularly those whose mission statements and curricula are focused specifically on addressing the issues listed previously are asking "are we admitting the right students?" Is there a way to change our admissions and selection processes to identify and measure the candidates most likely to fit the mission of the school and to maximize the development of their professional identity? This chapter describes how some North American Medical Schools have addressed the issue. In addition, this chapter addresses how one new North American Medical School has included consideration of the meaning, measurement, and mastery of professional identity formation in its admissions processes.

Introduction

Internationally, the components of many medical school admission processes include some form of standardized examination. The best known of these in North America is the Medical College Admissions Test (MCAT). The MCAT is used to evaluate a then applicant's knowledge of natural, behavioral, and social science concepts and principles, as well as problem solving and critical thinking skills that are required in medical school. The MCAT has four sections assessing the following subjects:

1 Chemical and Physical Foundations of Biological Systems
2 Critical Analysis and Reasoning Skills
3 Biological and Biochemical Foundations of Living Systems
4 Psychological, Social and Biological Foundations of Behavior

The results of the MCAT are reported to the student and institutions to which they apply (1). Other standard parts of the application process include letters of recommendation from faculty or a panel from the undergraduate institution, undergraduate grades, personal statement by the applicant as to their motivation for becoming a physician, and some form of "face-to-face" interview. Finally, based on the criteria of the institution, an Admissions Committee constituted from the faculty and administration meets to select the final candidates for admission. This chapter deals with the admissions process and new models of the "interview" focusing on the broader or more holistic aspects of admission. The purpose of which is an attempt to identify the "best fit" for institutional mission and health-care needs of the population served.

The interview process: tradition and history

The purposes most often cited in the research by Goho and Blackman for using an interview in the admissions process are to "predict success in medical school, measure noncognitive/humanistic skills, clarify information in the written application and provide a public relations service" (1). They state that selecting applicants that would become good physicians was another intended goal of the interview.

Historically, interviews for medical school have been conducted either by one interviewer or a panel/group of interviewers and a set of standard questions for all applicants. In an effort to obtain greater reliability and validity than offered by the individual interviewer model, applicants are often interviewed by three separate interviewers at different times. Another approach is the group or panel method often employed using a panel of three, with set questions asked in turn by each panelist. Edwards et al. classify interviews as structured, semi-structured, and unstructured indicating that as structure increases and so does the reliability and validity of the interview (2). As noted by Kreiter and Axelson, research on the types of traditional admissions interview has shown that interrater reliability (reproducibility) is very low with the implications for validity very questionable. They conclude, based on a meta-analysis of 20 interview studies on admissions in four countries, that the interviews weakly predicted both academic success and performance in the clinical environment (2).

Concern for the reliability and validity of the admissions interview process, given its wide use in medical schools, has led to a number of studies (3). As early as 1990, Edwards et al. conducted meta-analyses of interviews that were structured, semi-structured and unstructured. The 17 structured interview studies for nonmedical applicants ranging from sales positions to police officers, had the highest predictive validity (.63) and interrater reliability of .82. However, as noted by Edwards et al., most of the employment and medical admissions studies they reviewed were semi-structured at best. In reviewing these studies, the reliability coefficients ranged from .23 to .99 and validity coefficients from −.17 to .61. The authors concluded that by adding tasks to the structured interview based on job analysis and standardizing questions, both reliability and validity could be increased (4). This view is supported in other health professions including pharmaceutical education by Joyner et al (5). As Kreiter and Axelson point out, assuring validity and reliability in the process of medical school admission interviews has suffered from the failure to develop outcome measures not only for success in medical school, but for the more difficult question of determining what constitutes a "successful physician" (2).

Admissions issues beyond reliability and validity

As important as these concepts of reliability and validity are to the selection process, there are additional factors that are believed to contribute toward creating the successful physician and in the broader context to better meeting the healthcare needs of society as a whole. These factors include the development of professional identity. In many countries including the United States, Canada, and beyond, minority populations are underrepresented in the medical schools that prepare the physician workforce. The Association of American medical Colleges (2016) reported that African Americans represented 8% of total applicants followed by multiple race (7%) and Hispanic or Latino (6%). Graduation rates for the same time periods and groups generally reflected application levels (5). The population of the United States reported in the 2010 census data indicated that White citizens represented 72.4 of the population followed by 16.3 Hispanic, 13% Black, 5% Asian, 2% mixed and 1% native American (6). In examining the US physician population in 2017, it is clear that disparities exist between physicians by racial and ethnic group. White physicians constitute 70% of the work force followed by 21% Asian, 6% Hispanic or Latino, and 6% Black, while the remaining categories are other, pacific islander, and multiple ethnicity groups (7). Thus, these ethnic disparities between physician workforce, medical school matriculants, and graduation data have challenged the admissions process of some medical schools to create admission processes that address these inequities. These approaches are addressed in a later portion of this chapter.

As early as 2001 Dr. Jordan Cohen, the President of the Association of American Medical Colleges admonished US medical schools for current admissions processes that did not place adequate emphasis on what he termed the "personal characteristics of applicants." In many ways, this was yet another call for the development of outcome measures against which applicants can be assessed (8).

Koenig et al. reported on the work of the Association of American Medical Schools (AAMC) Innovative Lab Working Group (ILWG) multiyear project to identify personal competencies of medical school applicants most likely contribute positively to the medical school and practice community (9). The study, as described by the authors, identified nine personal competencies as important for entering students. They were ethical responsibility to self and others, reliability and dependability, service orientation, social skills, capacity for improvement, resilience and adaptability, cultural competence, oral communication, and teamwork (8). The authors noted that consensus about personal characteristics among varying constituencies is difficult at best and identifying and/or developing the tools to measure them is also a challenge. Their strong recommendation to medical schools was clear that without including measures of personal characteristics in their admissions process that changing the composition of future matriculating classes was not likely to change. In carefully addressing personal characteristics of applicants, it may be just be possible to begin addressing some of the inequities noted earlier.

Much has been written about the role of the healthcare team in medical practice primarily as a method to reduce adverse results of patient outcomes and to systematize what has been described as fragmented care (10). Yet, a common concern of medical students is "they expect us to function in a healthcare team, but don't teach us how in medical school." In 2017, Nelson et al. completed a review of the literature on interprofessional team training the purposes of which include many that are similar to the personal attributes identified by the ILWG. Among these are communication skills, adaptability, hat teamwork, and reflection and reassessment. They conclude that although interprofessional education has been a priority in medical schools that there remain gaps in this training and that the best practices for interprofessional education are yet to be identified (11). The very lock step nature of the most if not all professional curricula creates a significant barrier to even scheduling of interprofessional experiences across colleges and schools (12). From the purpose of identifying the best students to fit the mission of any medical school, the question remains, "if medicine is a team sport, and if we expect graduates to function in healthcare teams, then can we develop methods to assess their potential for this on admission?"

The literature has demonstrated the critical importance of professional identity formation and professionalism in medical education. In the United States and Canada, concerns about professionalism in residents (i.e. house officers) rank among the highest reasons for remedial training programs for these positions (12, 13). There is reason to believe that professionalism issues in residency training may have resulted from a lack of proper training and education during the first 4 years of medical school (14). It is beyond the scope of this chapter to present a complete review of the literature on identity formation in the context of the human socialization process. However, as Cruess et al. have noted, students enter medical school with a personal identity already formed and will develop an identity as a medical student, resident and eventually as a physician (15).

Stuart Lane has provided a helpful view of the relationship between professional identity formation and professionalism noting that the former is developed at the individual level and the latter constructed at and by the level of community and medical profession interaction (15). It appears that there is a relationship between the ability of physicians to reflect and their ability to adequately perform clinical reasoning tasks, so critical to functioning as a physician (16). Physicians routinely encounter and are challenged to critically assess information within their own values, beliefs and context, and those of their patients, and this, in turn, impacts the physician–patient relationship, clinical reasoning, and decision-making (17). For this reason, medical schools and accrediting bodies have moved to insure that self-reflection, professional identity formation, and professionalism are included in their curricula (18). Cruess et al. suggest that admissions criteria be reviewed from the perspective of identity formation in the context of a medical professional (15). In the light of this, the College of Medicine at Central Michigan University (CMU) developed a number of Multiple Mini Interview (MMI) stations designed to assess the extent to which applicants reflected the mission of the college, their potential to self-reflect and for becoming a competent medical professional. These are addressed late in the chapter.

Perhaps the most significant development in medical professions admissions arose from the research of Eva et al. (19). As previously described, interrater reliability in the traditional admissions interview varied widely based on the way interviews were administered. That is, structured interviews tend to yield higher reliability and validity, and it was suggested that these could be inflated by interviewers having information about the applicant and/or nonverbal communication between interviewers (20). In addition, Turnbull (1996) had shown that while interrater reliability in oral examinations was high that generalizability across a number of sessions was low, thus reducing overall rest reliability (21). Finally, the authors suggested that the context within which a candidate is asked to perform cognitive functions is more important than individual traits. Thus, the generalizability of the results of one interview is questionable. To test these questions, the researchers created the MMI similar to the 10-station concept of the Objective Structured Clinical Examination. Results from this study and others that followed demonstrated the advantage of multiple insight into the candidates abilities, a dilution of the effects of chance and examiner bias, structured stations so that all candidates answer the same question, and perhaps most importantly the ability to create scenarios designed to identify applicants that better fit the mission statement of the institution (20).

In 2007, the AAMC created Holistic Review Project that initially designed to create tools to assist medical schools in creating and sustaining diversity (21). It soon took on a broader focus as a catalyst for examining how to conduct the admissions process differently (AAMC, 2013). The AAMC holistic review approach uses the Experiences–Attributes–Metrics (E–A–M) Model (22). Metrics include grade point averages (GPAs), MCAT scores, and grade trends indicating that scholarship forms an important baseline. However, the inclusion of grade trends allows for consideration of grade improvement in all years of study. The attributes circle of the diagram includes 21 separate categories which contribute importantly to the holistic concept. Finally, the outer circle focuses on four major experience categories and eight subtopics. These form the basis of holistic review, and it should be noted that institutions are free to emphasize those that best fit their missions. The core concepts of holistic review are as follows:

1 Promotion of numerous aspects of diversity essential to excellence.
2 Selection criteria includes experiences and attributes as well as academic performance.
3 Consideration by Schools of each applicant's potential contribution to the school and field of medicine with flexibility to balance a class to meet institutional goals.
4 Consideration of race and ethnicity in making admission-related decisions only when aligned with the mission and goals of the institution and within a broad range of other factors such as personal attributes, experiential factors, demographics, and other considerations (23).

A case study in admissions process reform

In 2010, a new medical school was created in Mount Pleasant Michigan at CMU. The Mission statement was:

> The Central Michigan University College of Medicine educates diverse students and trains culturally competent physicians to provide comprehensive healthcare and services to underserved populations in Michigan and beyond. Our faculty, staff and graduates advance health and wellness through exceptional medical education, innovative research, quality patient care and strategic collaborations to improve the health and well-being of individuals and communities (24).

From the perspective of a new medical school with this mission, the MMI model coupled with the Holistic Admission Approach provided real promise for creating an admissions process to identify a "best fit" of applicants with the school's mission. Thus, prior to recruitment of the inaugural class, CMU decided to adopt the holistic admissions process to aid in the development of this process. The college participated in one of AAMC's holistic admissions training programs. This multiday event was attended by key individuals who would be heavily involved in the recruitment of the inaugural class. The workshop provided a basic framework for creating a holistic admissions process, and the college was tasked for refining the various components of screening and selection that aligned with mission of the college. In all subsequent admissions processes, a training workshop was held for all participants to ensure that each fully understood their role and tasks in the process (25).

The components/participants of the entire admissions process were:

1　Admission staffs review to assure applications were complete
2　Initial screening by faculty of electronic submission of application
3　On-sight MMI process
4　Admission committee's decision
5　Offer of admission made to applicant

Once staff had determined that the applicant met the basic application require-ments, two individual faculty reviewers rated each candidate on their individual application essay, and their answers to a series of eight questions focused on the college mission. The reviewers rated the applicant using a rubric that included academic metrics, academic attributes, personal attributes, experiences, and dis-tance traveled. Each is reflective of the AAMC's A-E-M model.

During the first admissions cycle, the primary goal in the process of screening applicants was to eliminate screener bias in relation to an applicant's academic metrics. The solution was to "blind" our secondary application screeners from both the MCAT scores and overall GPA metrics of any applicant they reviewed. The Secondary Application screeners comprised College of Medicine faculty and staff, with the largest percentage of screeners being faculty. It was also important for any faculty member who served on the admissions committee to participate in the screening process. The idea behind not blinding the coursework and grades associated with the coursework was so that screeners could use academic rigor and grade trends as part of their overall evaluation. It became evident during the post cycle review process for the secondary application screening process that our screeners having the ability to see applicants' grades, even though they were not privy to the overall GPA, still introduced bias into the screening process.

The next cycle and each subsequent cycle, the academic record was removed from the view of our secondary screeners. It was decided that while academic history and course rigor is an important element in the decision process, it was best that the admissions committee use this information to ultimately determine if the academic qualifications of our applicants were acceptable for an offer of admission.

While several changes and variations to the process have been introduced over the years, the goal has always been to appropriately measure the prepa-ration and readiness of the applicant for success in medical school and to assure their fit with our mission. In this context, success includes the ability to self-reflect and develop a professional identity. The main components of the secondary review process have always measured the experiences and narrative components of an application. During our first cycle, one individual provided an overall rating of an applicant's entire application using the AAMC Strength of Evidence scoring system. Subsequently two screener reviews for each applicant were required and used the combined screener scores to create a ranked order list for potential interview selection. In subsequent years, the screening process was changed to include input from as many as five individuals, each reviewing smaller components of an individual application. This included two narrative reviews, two experience reviews, and one academic review—the academic review *is completed* exclusively by the admissions office. Introducing additional individual screeners to the review of an applicant provided a more comprehensive review. The idea behind this reference was that by adding more input, the feedback/review of the applicant is more comprehensive and helped to address any interrater reliability among our secondary screeners. Training of reviewers, by the Admissions Office staff, clearly defined goals for the process, and constant attention to the reliability is aligned with the potential for improvement of the overall success of the process.

At CMU, the holistic admissions process is used to help identify applicants who have the personal attributes and characteristics that align with the mission, have demonstrated proper preparation for medical school evidenced through pre-professional experiences, and have shown that they are academically prepared for the rigors of medical school. The commitment to this goal has allowed the college to design an admissions process that provides unique insight into our applicants and allows us to select applicants best suited to meet our mission.

As described earlier, the MMI has been shown to improve reliability across a number of data points through the use multiple interview stations with set questions for each examiner. Typically, an MMI station includes a scenario posted on the outside of the interview room, an examiner with a score sheet and a defined time of 3 minutes for the applicant to respond. A typical scenario is as follows: "A close friend in your year 1 medical school class tells you that his mother has just been diagnosed with breast cancer. He feels overwhelmed by his studies and is considering dropping out of medical school to spend more time with his mother."

You have just met with your friend. Please talk about this conversation now with the interviewer. The applicant is scored using a 10-point scale on their communication skills, strength of arguments, and empathy displayed. In addition to the individual encounters, there is always that involves two or more applicants that required teamwork since that is an important aspect of the future or medical practice.

Also, as discussed earlier, self-reflection and professional identity formation are important abilities for successful practitioners. This some MMI stations were designed to assess this potential in applicants as follows: these stations include the following:

Life's purpose: Take the next 2 minutes to consider your life's purpose. What is your purpose and how does CMED fit into it?

Leadership and followership: Medical school applicants are often asked to reflect on their leadership experiences. Both an understanding of leadership principles and practical leadership experiences are undoubtedly important for future physicians. Followers, however, are the necessary condition for leaders to exist. There is no leader, after all, without followers.

What makes a good follower in a group or team? How do you know when you should lead or follow? What are the duties of leaders and followers? Discuss these questions with the assessor.

> *Skill development:* What skills or abilities do you think are most important for new medical students? Do you currently have these skills? What skill or expertise do you feel like you are still missing?
>
> *Health care mission:* Take the next 2 minutes to consider your healthcare mission.

What is this mission and what role will the College of Medicine play in helping you fulfill it?

> *Being a rural physician:* A major focus of the CMU College of Medicine is to provide physicians to meet the needs of the underserved areas of Michigan, with an emphasis on the rural areas of the central and northern parts of the state. What challenges do think physicians in these regions face? What qualities do you think they need to be successful?
>
> *Physician excellence:* Other than attaining medical knowledge and clinical skills, what do you think you will need to work on in order to be an excellent physician and meet CMED's mission and values?

Several changes have been introduced to interview scoring over the prior cycles. These changes have been made in order to introduce greater range into the data, aiding the admissions committee in making meaningful distinctions between applicants. In the first application cycle for CMU, in 2013, interviewers rated candidates on a 1–10 scale and had an opportunity to provide comments and other narrative feedback. Interviewers were also asked to note a conflict of interest, should it arise.

Changes came in subsequent cycles that refined these results in an attempt to link them even more closely to outcomes the college was seeking. In the 2014 cycle, interviewers were asked to answer a yes/no question about an applicant: "Would you want this applicant as your physician?" The addition of this query was driven by a desire to link assessor feedback with the values of the College. Assessors were trained to answer yes if the candidate exhibited characteristics consistent with the mission, vision, and values of CMU and know if they found evidence to the contrary. The answer to this question was meant to be addressed in the comments. This question remained a part of the interview process for 5 years, unchanged. It was updated in the 2020 cycle to ask instead if there is "compelling information" about this applicant to share. As noted above, teamwork was always the focus of one station and these have also evolved over time.

The first three application cycles at CMU featured one (1) teamwork-focused station in the MMI. In this station, two candidates were paired to work on a task, together, while observed by an assessor. The candidates had to work in tandem to complete a puzzle or accomplish some objective. Examples of the tasks included determining the correct order for a sequence of images to building a house of cards. The college recognized teamwork as an important characteristic for medical students. The teamwork stations, however, were not successful in assessing teamwork as a competency to the extent desired.

The challenges were the limited time and the limited complexity of the activity of the activity. An MMI station lasted 7 minutes. This constraint limited the scope of the activity that could be presented to the candidates. Hence, in the application cycles from 2013 to 2016, candidates were presented with a brief collaborative activity. In the overwhelming majority of cases, candidates completed the activity and did so in a way consistent with the personal characteristics sought by the admissions process. Candidates were only very infrequently frustrated with one another or otherwise challenged to work through a more difficult set of circumstances. In many respects, the teamwork stations failed to identify anything beyond eliminating a very small group of extreme responses.

To increase the challenge and gain additional insight into candidates and their teamwork capabilities, the admissions team added a large group activity to the interview day in 2017. This activity involved a group of 12 candidates and took 1 hour to complete. This was facilitated by separating it from the MMI stations of the interview, rather than working a group activity, somewhat artificially, into the rotation of MMI stations.

The introduction of the large group activity addressed the two challenges present in prior attempts to capture meaningful information relative to candidates and their teamwork capabilities. The greater length of time allowed for the introduction of a complex task and a deeper look into the merits and deficiencies of individual ways of contributing. Perhaps the most important result of devoting more time to these activities was the emergence of individual leadership and followership styles among the candidates. Group roles emerged and it became much easier to understand the ways in which individuals were either supporting or detracting from the objective of the team. As such, it became easier to score the performance of individual candidates and their measure their individual contributions. This facilitated the selection of candidates that appeared to maximally have skill in advancing group objectives. It also facilitated the rejection of candidates that clearly struggled to contribute or otherwise detracted from the objective at hand. Candidates who were easily frustrated, spoke over and interrupted others or were otherwise disruptive and typically less suitable for selection.

The large group activity also addressed the limitations of the original teamwork station as part of the MMI. However, there are other challenges to taking a group of 12 and assessing the performance of all members. With an inadequate number of trained assessors, it may be difficult to keep track of the behaviors and contributions of each candidate. Also, medical students are expected to work in groups of many sizes and contribute to teams that are configured in a variety of ways. Given this, the admissions team modified the interview day again to incorporate additional group activities, focused on smaller teams.

In the 2018 cycle, CMU added small group team activities to the interview. The interview format consisted of an MMI with six stations, four small group team activities, and 1-hour-long large group activity, which worked the same way as in the 2017 cycle. The small group activities took about twice as long as a regular MMI station, or about 14 minutes. This additional time allowed for the group to participate in a more complex task. And because the group was small, only three candidates, it was easy for the assessor to understand the contributions of each individual participant.

One additional advantage of these small group activities is that a variety of skills could be tested, rather than just the one tested through the large group activity. Candidates were asked to work together to solve problems, contribute equally to a discussion, reach consensus on a course of action, or other activities that challenged different dimensions of teamwork, communication, and interpersonal skills.

In total, these approaches to group activities, both in larger and smaller formats, allowed the admissions team to meaningfully assess candidates in terms of the preprofessional competencies for medical students as identified not only by the AAMC but as they relate to the practice of medicine.

It has been 5 years since the initial class of students were admitted to the College of Medicine. All Graduates are now in residency training in a number of locations in the United States. The final act of this play will take a good deal of time to conclude but the sign for creating graduates that will meet the school's mission is positive. Tracking studies are underway to determine the extent to which graduates select primary care specialties for graduate training and where they chose to locate to practice.

Summary

In this chapter, we have addressed some of the historical forces that have impacted the admissions process in US and Canadian Medical Schools and how organizations and institutions have begun to change to develop new approaches to improve the admissions process. The creation of more diverse medical school classes and enriching those classes with a broader range of individual experiences, interests, and perspectives is destined to create a richer experience for all students. And, in the end our hope is for physicians who are self-reflective and are committed to carrying out the mission of the school as compassionate, technically competent practitioners who improve the health and well-being of the individuals and communities they serve.

In summary, to select the "right" students, the authors recommend the following:

1. Assure that the process of applicant selection is reliable and valid across all reviewers by training them in the specific applicant characteristics that are being sought.
2. Assure that the characteristics of the selected applicants are a "best fit" for the mission of the institution.

3 The applicant pool and the selected applicants must reflect the patient population to be served.

4 Recognize that academic performance, while important to success in medical school, is only one dimension of any applicant—assess applicants on other variables that will contribute to successful professional identity formation.

5 Have the courage to change admission approaches to meet the changing nature of medical practice in the context of a changing world environment.

References

(1) Retrieved from https://students-residents. Aamc.org/applying-medical-school// taking mcat-exam/about-mcat-exam.

(2) Edwards, Janine C., Johnson, Eugene K., and John B. Molidor. The Interview in the Admission Process. *Academic Medicine* 1990: 65 (3); 167–177.

(3) Kreiter, Clarence D., and Rick D. Axelson. A Perspective on Medical School Admission Research and Practice over the Last 24 Years. *Teaching and Learning in Medicine* 2013: 25 (S1); S50–S56.

(4) Goho, James, and Ashley Blackman. The Effectiveness of Academic Admission Interviews: an Exploratory Meta-Analysis. *Medical Teacher* 2006: 28; 335–340.

(5) Joyner, Pamela U., Cox, Wendy C., White-Harris Carla, and Susan J. Blalock. The Structured Interview and Interviewer Training in the Admissions Process. *American Journal of Pharmaceutical Education* 2007: 71 (5); 83–88.

(6) Retrieved from https://aamcdiversityfactsandfigures2016.org/report-section/secion-3/.

(7) Retrieved from https://statisticalatlas.com/united-states/race-and-ethnicity/ 2010.

(8) Cohen, J. Facing the Future. President's Address Delivered at: Annual Meeting of the Association of American Medical Colleges; November 4, 2001, Washington, DC.

(9) Retrieved from https://datausa.io/profile/soc/291060/ 2019.

(10) Koenig, Thomas W., Parrish, Samuel K., Terregino, Carol A., Williams, Joy P., Dunleavy, Dana M., and Joseph Volsch. Core Personal Competencies Important to Entering Students' Success in 92 Medical School: What are They and How Could They Be Assessed Early in the Admissions Process? *Academic Medicine* 2013: 88; 603–613.

(11) Kohn, L.T., Corrigan, J.M., and M.S. Donaldson, Eds. To Err is Human: Building a Safer Health Care System. 2017 Retrieved from http//www.ncbi.nlm.gov/ pubmed/25077248.

(12) Nelson, Sioban, White Catriona F., Hodges, Brian D., and Maria Tassone. Interprofessional Team Training at the Prelicensure Level: A Review of the Literature. Academic Medicine licensure Level: A Review of the Literature. *Academic Medicine* 2017: 92; 709–716.

(13) Regan, Linda, Hexom, Bradon, Nazario, Steven, Chinai, Sneha A., Visconti, Anette, and Christine Sullivan. Remediation Methods for Milestones Related to Interpersonal and Communication Skills and Professionalism. *Journal of Graduate Medical Education* February 2016: 8 (1).

(14) Svystun, O., and S. Ross. Difficulties in Residency: An Examination of Clinical Rotations and Competencies Where Family Medicine Residents Most Often Struggle. *Family Medicine* 2018: 50 (8); 613–616

(15) Cruesss, Richarde L., Cruess, Sylvia R., Boudreau, J. Donald, Snell, Linda, and Yvonne Steinert. A Schematic Representation of the Professional Identity Formation and Socialization of Medical Students. *Academic Medicine* 2015: 90 (6).

(16) Stewart, Lane. Professionalism and Professional Identity: What Are They and What Are They to You? Retrieved from https://www.amsj.org/archive/6924.\; 1–4

(17) Coulehan, J., and P. Williams. Conflicting Professional Values in Medical Education. *Cambridge Quarterly of Healthcare Ethics* 2013: 12; 7–20.

(18) Hargreaves, Ken. Reflection in Medical Education. *Journal of University Teaching and Learning Practice* 2016: 13 (2). Available at http://ro.uow. edu.au/jutlp/vol 13/iss2/6.

(19) Eva, Kevin W., Rosenfeld, Jack, Reiter, Harold I., and Geoffrey R. Norman. An Admissions OSCE: The Multiple Mini-Interview. *Medical Education* 2004: 38; 314–326.

(20) O'sullivan, Helen, Van Mook, Walther, Fewtrell, Ray, and Val Mass. Integrating Professionalism into the Curriculum: AMEE Guide No. 61. *Medical Teacher* 34 (2); e64–e77.

(21) Turnbull, J., Dannoff, D., and G.R. Norman. Content Specificity and Oral Examinations. *Medical Education* 1996: 30; 56–59.

(22) Eva 2004

(23) Retrieved from https://www.aamc.org.initiatives/holistic review/2019.

(24) Retrieved from https://www.aamc.org/services/member-capacitybuilding/holistic-review. 2019.

(25) Retrieved from https://www.cmich.edu/colleges/med/Education/MD/Admissions/pages/default/aspx. 2019.

13 Identity structure analysis as a means to explore social worker professional identity

Marta B. Erdos, Rebeka Javor and Balázs Ákos Vass

Introduction

A previous paper discussed the issue of professionalization as a society-level determinant of the position of an occupational group and professional identity (B. Erdos & Gomory, in this volume). In the current chapter, we focus on social workers' identity constituents, identity development processes and conflicted areas. A great number of publications discuss the recent crisis of social work. Signs and symptoms of the crisis are closely related to social workers' professional identity, especially the shift from close client–helper interactions towards controlling, administrative roles (Asquith, Clark & Waterhouse, 2005; Webb, 2017b; Hobbs & Evans, 2017; Navrátil & Bajer, 2018; Szabó, 2017; Szoboszlai, 2014). How does one become a professional social worker in this debated and unstable context for the area in Hungary? What are the core professional values, attitudes and visions of a social worker? How are these identity constituents shaped in the direct practice of the profession – and by the anomic societal context? How is professional identity maintained and reconstructed? In what ways do social workers serve as role models for their clients in their psychosocial development?

In the first part of the chapter, we explore the key components of social worker professional identity by reviewing the professional literature, and by conducting a qualitative content analysis on practitioner and student interviews. The study involves a more specific exploration of the concept of threatened identity, concentrating on the role of negative public perceptions, on the impact of working in liminal/marginal settings, and on possible significance of professionals' own traumatic experiences.

Qualitative analysis, in addition to yielding an insight into the area, serves as an input for identity structure analysis (ISA) (Weinreich & Saunderson, 2004; Weinreich, 2010a) and for building its associated measuring tool, Ipseus, designed for the complex study of identity.

ISA is an exceptional method to analyse the dynamics of professional, personal and societal values, and one's identifications and conflicted areas in order to assist selection processes and practitioners' continuing professional development (CPD). Further, if we know more about social worker practitioners' identities, then this knowledge may serve as a basis for supporting identity development of students in social work. In the second part of the chapter, we summarize our experiences concerning the development of the instrument to measure social worker professional identity and analyse the key findings of our project.

Professional and personal identities

Professional identity – a decisive factor of career success – can be defined as *'one's professional self-concept based on attributes, beliefs, values, motives and experiences'* by which people *'define themselves in specialized, skill- and education-based occupations'* (Slay & Smith, 2010:1,3). Hogard determines identity as *the totality of values, attitudes, memories, convictions, aspirations, and reflections that are unique to an individual* (Hogard, 2014:1). One's or a group's professional values as identity elements are determined by the professional area and the immediate work environment.

Personal identity is articulated in one's narrative (life story) and is reflected in the evaluations of relevant entities that make up the totality of self-construals (Weinreich, 2004). Professional identity elements are predominantly shaped by a special rhetoric associated with a profession, by the organizational culture of the given institution, and by one's own specific work experiences. Accessible role models, feedback from supervisors, clients and colleagues on work performance and periods of career transition play a key role in the formation of professional identity (Slay & Smith, 2010). It is a continuous, career-long process of interpretation and customization to ever-changing work environments (Webb, 2017a, 2017b).

With the change of traditional workplace structures, such as the introduction of flexible forms of employment, and with major changes in the most wanted competencies with new emphasis on personal and interpersonal skills as collaboration, creativity, critical thinking and communication skills, professional identities have become more intertwined with personal identities than before. This statement is even more relevant in the area of helping professions. Social workers, just like counsellors, *'bring the instrument of themselves into the therapeutic setting.'* (Black & Weinreich, 2014:339) Professional identities include personal domains, one's own life experiences and reflections that are not necessarily related to the domain of work, but more to one's private life, as acknowledged in the Global Standards (2012), a key policy document for social work: ...*recognition of the relationship between personal life experiences and personal value systems and social work practice.* The inherent paradox of the profession is that helpers' own selves are considered to serve as an instrument to conduce constructive change in a process involving very personal elements, though the process itself normally takes place in a highly institutionalized context.

Who is a social worker in Hungary today?

A common feature of contemporary careers is shifting boundaries (Slay & Smith, 2010) and the associated fights for professional monopolies. The boundaries of social work have been rather vague in the international arena (What is and what is not social work?). As for social worker identities, we face some difficulties due to the contextual nature of the profession. First, there are diverse traditions of social work as a profession in the different countries. From time to time, the question whether there is a distinct professional identity or not arises (Fargion, 2008; Payne, 2014; Global Definition of Social Work, 2014).

> Such a document should reflect some consensus around key issues, roles and purposes of social work. However, given the profession's historically fragmented strands; the contemporary debates around social work's intraprofessional identity; its identity vis-à-vis other categories of personnel in the welfare sector such as development workers, child care workers, probation officers, community workers and youth workers (where such categories of personnel are differentiated from social work); and the enormous diversities across nations and regions, there was some scepticism about the possibility of identifying any such 'universal'. The suggestion was that such a document must be sufficiently flexible to be applicable to any context. Such flexibility should allow for interpretations of locally specific social work education and practice, and take into account each country's or region's socio-political, cultural, economic and historical contexts while adhering to international standards.
>
> (Global Definition of Social Work, 2014)

Some authors highlight the centrality of social problems (Navrátil & Bajer, 2018; Szöllősi, 2012) when determining the area of social work. However, a narrow focus on social problems might result in disempowerment, scapegoating and stigmatization, which is quite contrary to the mission of the profession (Saleebey, 2006).

Payne (2014) – referring to Asquith, Clark and Waterhouse (2005) – distinguished between five service philosophies that influence social workers' professional attitudes:

- Welfarism (social democratic paternalism)
- Professionalism, highlighting expertise and authority
- Consumerism, regarding service users as consumers
- Managerialism with strong economic concerns and
- Participationism (equality of service providers and service users in the helping process)

The 2014 global definition on social work explicitly defines the core issues of the profession, though admitting local variations:

> Social work is a practice-based profession and an academic discipline that promotes social change and development, social cohesion, and the empowerment and liberation of people. Principles of social justice, human rights, collective responsibility and respect for diversities are central to social work. Underpinned by theories of social work, social sciences,

humanities and indigenous knowledge, social work engages people and structures to address life challenges and enhance wellbeing. The above definition may be amplified at national and/or regional levels....The social work profession's core mandates include promoting social change, social development, social cohesion, and the empowerment and liberation of people.

The definition relies mainly on participationism and professionalism that are also acknowledged in the key documents on social work in Hungary (e.g. A szociális munka etikai kódexe/Code of Ethics, 2016). Paternalistic traditions and the deep impact of sudden political shifts in the country from the very beginnings have hindered the implementation of these guidelines. In a study conducted in 2001, social workers considered neither their participation in professional organizations nor the role of professional education and CPD important (Fónai, Patyán & Szoboszlai, 2001), what contradicts both participationism and professionalism as service philosophies.

There seems to be one common conclusion of the debate on social workers' professional identity internationally and in the domestic literature, namely that this is a *matter of concern* (Webb, 2017b; Hobbs & Evans, 2017; Szoboszlai, 2014; Pataki, 2013; Vass s.d.; Budai, 2004). Motivated by the wish to minimize spendings on social care, decision makers do not necessarily regard social workers' professional identity as a resource, rather, they may expect some self-sacrificing attitude to life, and some skills to control and educate clients of social work. The academic sector has long recognized that social workers' identity is a matter of deep concern indeed, and perhaps a matter of worries, as this career is less and less attractive for prospective students.

Shortly after the social transition in Hungary in 1989, almost any professionals could pass as a social worker in any settings, and the number of qualified professionals in the field was insignificant (Kozma, 1994). The differences among social workers with an academic degree (ISCED 6-8), social assistants with a secondary education (ISCED 4) social carers (ISCED 2-4) and 'social workers' with practically any type of academic degree (e.g. education or sociology) were merged in the statistics (Horváth & Lévai, 1996a, b). According to Nagy, *social workers are those who do social work* (Nagy, 2003:28). In the public discourse, 'social professionals' are not understood as professionals with a *relevant* academic degree, but practically all the employees (including carers) in the social sector (Bugarszki, 2014).

The previous said explain why the estimated number of social workers changes between 5000 and 100,000 (Talyigás and Hegyesi, 2014; Bass and Márton, 2005). Farkas (2005) commented on the data of the National Statistical Bureau and stated that approximately 70,000 persons were employed in the social sector, with 35,000 social workers/carers. A total of 7000 had a degree in an academic field, whereas only 3500 had a degree in social work, social pedagogy and social policy. The number of qualified professionals – based on higher education statistics – was around 12,000 (Farkas, 2005); or, according to a more recent estimate, taking into consideration the brief temporary expansion in higher education, 20,000 (Szoboszlai, 2014). The rate of retention found in the previous study (about 30%, Farkas, 2005) is very low indeed and is a salient indicator of the lasting crisis of the profession. A ministerial decree (1/2000 [I.7.]) determines who may be employed as a social worker, that is, who is entitled to deliver social services. For example, in homeless care, any degree is accepted – the only requirement is a minimum of ISCED 6 level and 50% of skilled workforce. Similarly, a chief manager in a residential home providing social care can be a lawyer, an economist or a theologian. The lack of competent workforce and the huge administrative workload in many areas have resulted in a negative spiral on both training and retention. Recently, short courses have been introduced to compensate for the lack of workforce and make one a social professional.

Today, after three decades of the rebirth of the profession, it is not easy to answer even the simplest question: Who is a social worker? Institutions of higher education would insist that a social worker has a degree in social work and, accordingly, is employed as a social worker. Many other professionals whose qualifications and job titles are different in Hungary would be regarded as social workers in an international context: social pedagogues as school social workers/child protection workers, community coordinators as cultural social workers/community workers, mental health counsellors as clinical social workers, probation officers as criminal justice social workers and 'child protection nurses' as health social workers. In the countries where the professionalization of social work is more advanced, there is a common social worker knowledge base and a licensure process for all these professionals. This is not so in Hungary. The chaos concerning the question '*Who is a social worker in Hungary?*' has its deep negative impact on professionals' identity, including other-ascribed components of identity.

Researchers on the theme face difficulties in sampling but may also have the opportunity to ask new types of questions and compare the different groups. If the differences between social and non-social professionals are not particularly high, then we can argue for the relevance of practice-based training; if there are major differences, then we should argue for the necessity of Higher Education Institution (HEI)-based, more traditional forms of professional education.

Authenticity, roles and role conflicts

Webb (2017a) addresses the issue of sentimental politics of authenticity, that is, a social worker should represent the values and carry out the mission of social work. *'a residual tension remains among some social workers on how to integrate the objective scientific observer with the empathic counselor and passionate action-oriented reformer ….'* (Maschi et al., 2012:27). Due to a relatively low level of several major domains in professionalization, and high-level government influence on social affairs, the Hungarian public may perceive social workers in a more polarized manner: as charity workers, simple souls, our everyday heroes piously befriending the needy (Kormányos, 2015) or – the other extreme – inflexible and courageous resistance fighters. Misrepresentations ('socialist', that is, state socialist or 'communist' workers) are widespread among the elderly; and the image of the control worker is also present in the media. Negative or missing public perceptions contribute to the crisis of social work (Asquith, Clark & Waterhouse, 2005; Webb, 2017b; Navrátil & Bajer, 2018). All these inconsistent misrepresentations are very far from the image of a genuine professional.

In 2011, Pataki in her analysis, relying on Seithe's typology (2010), differentiates between the following role models:

- The patient helper: Provides support and care, often at the expense of own needs (possibly: compulsive helper/Lefever, 2007/).
- The conservative professional: Believes in the glorious past and would refuse the significance of external forces that shape the professional field.
- The tricky helper: Tricks help one to cope with seemingly hopeless situations.
- The indifferent professional: A manager who considers attempts at societal criticism ridiculous and would not cherish any ideals.
- Harmonizers: Introducing market relations into the area of social services.
- Modernizers: Reshaping social work through ethical and theoretical considerations.

The role of a social worker includes the role of a defender, counsellor, case worker, partner, risk assessor, care manager and social control agent. This list is without doubt not exhaustive. It rather hints at the conflict potential of these roles (Navrátil & Bajer, 2018:2). For Szoboszlai *a social worker is a rebel, an innovator, a collaborator – and above all, a helper*

(Szoboszlai, 2014:88)

A peculiar feature of in-group ideations is highlighting practice, often at the expense of continuing education and practice-based research activities. A true social worker in Hungary is primarily 'practical'. This is in accordance with public views and with the opinions formed by other disciplines, but not with international standards. University lecturers who teach social workers are expected to be 'practical' too, that is, to follow praxis even if it is ineffective, what is more, is potentially harmful. For example, a well-built counselling process demands adequate time frame, a proper physical and psychological space, and full attention on part of the social worker. Part-time students sometimes warn the lecturer that they might have an average of only 10–15 minutes for a family – every second or third week. This is regarded neither counselling nor social work by the lecturer but is identified as social work in the institutional context that struggles with the lack of finances and, consequently, lack of workforce. The problem is that therapies are (very *practically*) not available for clients of social work, and social workers' generally poor reflective competencies will result only in crafts professionalism, when case management is understood only as a series of specific and automatic actions and reactions (Szabó, 2017).

Empirical investigations concerning social workers' professional identity

In the domestic professional literature, identity issues of Hungarian social workers are frequently theorized but rarely researched. Targeted, complex and national-level empirical studies on social worker identities are missing. Studies are available on some related themes, as social workers' value system (Pilinszki et al., 2004), perceptions on professional career (Fónai, Patyán & Szoboszlai, 2001), and on the moral and societal crisis of the profession (Bugarszki, 2014; Németh, 2014; Szoboszlai, 2014). Though the risks of burnout are also a frequent theme in the social professional literature, systematic studies are accessible only on teachers and health professionals (Mihálka, 2015).

In 2001, Fónai, Patyán and Szoboszlai in their research design did not differentiate between qualified social workers and other professionals who were employed as social workers: an idea that highlights practical experiences and legal requirements concerning employment over professional education. In their early study, they asked social workers to evaluate different hypothetical solutions to professional problems. The cases involved ethical dilemmas: workable, but not to-rule solutions, openly unethical behaviour and going beyond one's professional competencies. The results showed that social work was surprisingly professionalized in terms of professional roles, and social workers had a distinct sense of mission. The vast majority of the participants respected the rules and competency boundaries and were characterized by strong client-centred approaches.

Pilinszki et al. (2004) conducted a study among Hungarian social workers by utilizing Rokeach Value Survey and compared values of the Hungarian population with those of the social workers. Authors found significant differences for terminal values with higher evaluations of self-respect, inner harmony and sense of accomplishment among the social workers, while they considered pleasure (the Hungarian equivalent also translates as welfare), comfortable life and a world of beauty less important. As for the instrumental values, social workers favoured broad-mindedness, creativity, capability and logic but appreciated cleanliness, love and politeness less than the respondents in the representative national sample (Pilinszki et al., 2004). Authors concluded that social workers appreciate consumer society values less than the Hungarian public.

In a study on 84 individuals utilizing Woo's Professional Identity Scale Counselling and a concurrent metaphor-analysis, no significant differences were found between students of social work and social worker practitioners as for their professional identities (Ruzsa & Homoki, 2015).

Aczél (2016) has studied the role of gender differences in the career path of male and female social workers and found that men's stories are about heroic struggles, while women's stories are primarily concerned with ethic of care.

Interpretations on threatened identity. Social workers as wounded healers

In a number of countries, including Hungary, social work equals to semi-professionalism or quasi-professionalism in the eyes of the public; and the position of social work among the other academic disciplines is (or, in the luckier cases, previously was) highly debated (Fargion, 2008; Szoboszlai, 2014; Navrátil & Bajer, 2018). The high rate of paraprofessionals in Central and East-European countries reflects a relative failure in the accomplishment of the professional project, that is, competition for public recognition and economic and political influence (Navrátil & Bajer, 2018).

Weak monopolies are only one side of the coin. Slay and Smith (2010) in their analysis on a seemingly distant theme (the identity of Black journalists) claim that though professional roles are normally associated with prestige and autonomy, an accompanying and interfering stigmatized cultural identity would result in the repeated experiences of an 'outsider', and in questioning prestigious occupational rhetoric. A stigmatized identity is a reduced, one-dimensional image of the self, when *too little truth is told about us* (Slay & Smith, 2010:13). Carrying the social stigma as a professional is partly due to close connections with underprivileged or vulnerable populations (Hobbs & Evans, 2017).

The concept of liminality is a useful theoretical tool to explain social workers' stigmatized positions. Liminality is an in-between, insecure and unpredictable state, a necessary phase, a space of possible in the traditional rites of passages, in which persons move from one social status towards another while obtaining new knowledge on own roles and identities (van Gennep, 1960; Turner, 1982). Liminality involves a temporary dissociation from ordinary social structures by definition. Under certain conditions – in dictatorships, and also in globalized contexts without locally meaningful frames of reference – a permanent but non-realistic liminal structure is built when entire societies are captured in absurd, upside down societal relations (Szakolczai, 2015). This was the case in Hungary during the years of open and the subsequent soft forms of dictatorship. For the majority of the population, frozen liminality is quite an uneasy but very familiar social context.

In such a societal context – and naturally not only in Hungary – more and more groups and communities are deprived of their chances of reintegration into society. They become marginalized and stigmatized. Social workers normally work with these vulnerable groups and communities, that is, they have direct contact with people in liminal or marginal positions. '*Overt stigmatisation of social workers can occur when social workers are marginalised by their association with the vulnerable client groups they work with*'(Hobbs & Evans, 2017:20). Negative, false or missing media portrayals of social workers engrave the problem. In some countries, a negative image is often a consequence of the 'control work' done in the frameworks of child protection system, that is, removing the at-risk child from the family (Hobbs and Evans, 2017).

The idea of threatened identity (Weinreich, 2004) is a useful conceptual tool to explain this dimension of social worker identities. According to Weinreich's (2004:68) definition, '*one's social identity is threatened when other people view oneself as a member of a social group in ways that are grossly discrepant from one's own view of self as member of that group*'. One possible reaction to this identity state is establishing a defensive position by either ignoring or overreacting the threat. Results of an empirical investigation support the first option, i.e., ignoring the threat, and at the same time, refusing some of the dominant society values (Pilinszki et al., 2004). Possible reactions to existing or perceived threats often prevent the representatives of the profession to enter into balanced discussions with decision makers, rather, they would fight (*freedom fighters*) in most of the cases, what actually may diminish the chances of representing both the clients and the professional groups themselves. Diffusion, on the other hand, would result in incorporating the threat into own, conflicted image of the professional self, which results in confusion and uncertainty. Demoralization is a learned helplessness attitude which makes the person apathetic and results in low self-evaluation (Weinreich, 2004). Hobbs and Evans conclude that Australian social workers' self-stigma is much stronger than negative public judgments. Self-stigmatization takes place through identification processes with the 'aggressor's' views. Strong self-stigmatization, as a finding, is embarrassing: '*Social workers commit to a lifetime of work empowering others and promoting equal rights for all people. It is ironic then, that as a profession, social work still needs to fight for recognition, acceptance and a sense of belonging within the professional realm*' (Hobbs & Evans, 2017:30). There are two main alternatives for a professional with stigmatized identity. Adaptation takes place through role model identification, provisional selves experimentation and evaluation of these experiments, based on an internal value system and external validation. Redefinition includes reconstructing the stigma. Stigma is inherently a Janus-faced phenomenon with its strong negative and positive connotations.

We can conclude that social workers' professional identity is a threatened identity: partly because of the Flexner-syndrome (*is social work a profession at all?*), which, more than after a century, continues to determine the positions in interprofessional collaboration. Social workers report high power differences in interprofessional settings, especially in health social work. In interdisciplinary teams, stigmatization may be subtle and is manifested in doubting social workers' competencies. In a relatively early study in Hungary, social worker practitioners were asked to rank other professionals for collaboration potentials. They ranked social pedagogues first; then members of the local council's social committee; judges, nurses, teachers, sociologists, psychologists, politicians, policemen, lawyers, ministers, social politicians, journalists, doctors and supervisors (understood here as clinical supervisors) (Fónai, Patyán, & Szoboszlai, 2001). Very probably, the results would be different today. The role of the local council has significantly diminished due to domestic centralization tendencies; parallel, the high prestige of social politicians is on the decrease. Inviting and financially supporting the churches to intervene in the area of social problems might have changed the position of ministers as well. It is worth noting that in this study, clinical supervisors were seen more as an enemy than a professional resource, which is a threat for identity development, continuing professional education and a risk for burnout.

In order to redefine one's professional identity, and to maintain and develop such an identity, further, to think of own self more independently of the values of the dominant culture, the professional needs community resources – an alternative value system and alternative discursive resources that are social and professional in-group resources. They should reach a developmental level that is beyond technical rationalism. Social workers either conform themselves to the public image and accept the stigma or accept *and* reinterpret the stigma and become reflexive professionals (Jones & Joss, 1995; Schön, 1983).

Self-reflection is regarded as a means to protect one against burnout:

> The development of the critically self-reflective practitioner, who is able to practice within the value perspective of the social work profession, and shares responsibility with the employer for their well being and professional development, including the avoidance of 'burn-out'.
> (Global Standards, 2012, 4.2.2 Domain of the Social Work Professional)

In a study conducted in the United States on mental health problems occurring among social worker practitioners, two astonishing results emerged. First, more than 40% of the social workers reported mental health problems before starting their career – not a problem in itself, as wounded healers as experts of experience may become most effective reflective professionals. They know very well how important it is to maintain hope and be patient in the process of transition, and they also know that substantial change in one's life is a possibility. However, more than 52% reported such problems *after* commencing their professional practice, with 28% experiencing the problems at the time of data collection (Straussner, Senreich & Steen, 2018). One plausible explanation could be that these professionals simply have more insight on their problems, and this explains the increased rate in comparison with the general population – but this is definitely not in accordance with professional requirements. Webb (2017b) refers to a study by Grant and Kinman who report that *'social workers regard it as "unprofessional" to admit that traumatic cases affected them emotionally and that not mixing your personal life with work is considered as truly "being professional"'* (Webb, 2017b:7). This attitude, if extended to own emotional wounds, is quite risky, as helpers will probably project their own unresolved problems onto clients.

Strength-based, solution-focussed methods in social work empower clients to cope with stresses in life and maintain hope even in seemingly hopeless situations (Saleebey, 2006). In order to apply these methods in a competent manner and in a number of different work environments, social workers must develop certain skills and attitudes, such as empathy, self-reflection, resilience and empowerment via experiential learning. This may begin in a formal learning environment, but the majority of the helpers are also 'wounded healers'. A preceding trauma or lasting deprivation in their lives motivates them in their career choice and leads them to enter formal training. The trauma can (and in a helper's role, should) be solved in profound and constructive life-transformation processes. Formal training adds underpinning theories to social workers' own stories of redemption (McAdams, 2006), facilitating congruent and empathetic responses to clients, as well as the further development of self-reflective skills and a motivation to continuously practising the care of self.

By contrast, practising 'control work', a distancing and mechanical way of 'helping' may be the outcome of an extremely demanding work environment, which increases the risks of burnout. Another possible explanation for such preferences for control work does not lie in the context but in the person. Unsuccessful coping with own traumatic experiences and emotional abuse may result in rigid identification with authority figures and a disposition for exercising control over their clients (Fekete, 2000). In this sense, control work is a culturally supported outcome of Schmidbauer's Helfer Syndrome.

Results of the qualitative interviews

A substantial literature review is an important prerequisite for designing a specific instrument for ISA. Additional qualitative interviews assist the researchers to focus more on significant themes and domains, and design the instrument to match respondents' discursive patterns or the 'speech codes' governing their worldviews. One of the strength in ISA investigations is that the wording of the instrument makes respondents 'feel at home' while answering the particular items. Interviews do not only serve as some raw material for further analyses but also facilitate the in-depth explorations on sensitive issues.

We used three different sets of interview data: 13 interviews on social workers' career paths; 8 interviews on social workers' required competencies and professional development (conducted with six social workers, a teacher and a medical doctor in leadership/mentoring positions in social institutions) and an additional group of 6 interviews on social worker student attrition, probably representing the very first crisis of the professional (Tinto, 1987). See Table 13.1.

The interviews do not reflect gender rates among social professionals for a number of reasons. First, due to the low prestige of the profession, student dropout is higher among male students than among female ones; second, because of strong cultural traditions, there are more men than women in prestigious leadership positions. Gender rate among social workers in Hungary is an estimated 1:5, with much more women than men working in the area (Pilinszki et al., 2004).

Social worker interviewees represented a great variety of the professional areas (family support, homeless care, addiction treatment centre, hospice care, centre for persons with learning disabilities, school social work and community development in state, NGO, and church-based institutions). Interview questions

Table 13.1 Interviews

Interview type	Male	Female	Age range
1. Career path	4	9	30–64 (average 45)
2. Competencies and professional development (C1-8)	4	4	32–62 (average 48)
3. Student dropout (D1-6)	3	3	21–60 (average 31)

differed according to the goals of the three different types of interviews. The method was a thematic analysis, including some narrative aspects in types 1 and 3 interviews.

Career path interviews

Career path interviews bore some resemblance to what McAdams (2006) identified as 'stories of redemption', in which bad things turn to good in one's life. In these stories, people have an early experience on some family resource or 'blessings' (either a sign of a special talent or enjoying distinguished care and attention) and develop an early sensitivity to social and human problems. Narratives are characterized by a clear and stable personal philosophy and persons' readiness to serve their communities.

Eight respondents could identify a key childhood experience (a trauma, lasting deprivation or some relevant experience such as a visit in a segregated area) as a motivation for career choice. Five of them referred to early sensitivity to social issues. The presence of a role model in their lives was decisive both before career choice and on commencing their studies. Main sources of job satisfaction were engagement in client–helper interactions, and the related sense of competence, opportunities for self-actualization, acknowledgements on part of the workplace and working in a good team. Main problems concerning the social worker career were an extreme workload, stresses and conflicts, management problems, difficult clients, very low reimbursement and low levels of public recognition. Their aspirations included security and stability of employment, and opportunities for continuing professional education and recreation. As for the future of the profession, they asserted that – due to worsening social conditions – the need for social workers is on the increase, but the profession is currently in a crisis in Hungary (Vass, s.d.).

Social workers' competencies

Interviews on social workers' required competencies reflected the main focus of the profession – person-in-environment. Respondents related the issue of social change

- to the need for programme evaluation and adequate feedback on professional experiences, as a possible focus of social work research;
- to the representation of client interests and profession's interests; and
- to the distorted public image on social workers' professional activities.

They prioritized knowledge on the following:

- Social networks
- Psychosocial counselling skills (especially family counselling)
- The system of social care and administration
- And skills to motivate clients

Personal aptitude equals to the following:

- Openness (including a non-judgmental attitude)
- Empathy
- Congruence
- Commitment and perseverance
- Creativity
- Self-reflectivity
- And a practical approach to problems

According to the interviewees, the development of these identity components largely depends on own motivations and experiences (including working through early traumas). Supervision has a main role in professionals' lifelong development. Knowledge on professional boundaries and frameworks are relevant in interprofessional collaboration, balancing between professional and private lives, professional autonomy and facilitating adequate client participation in the helping process. Failures are partly due to systemic problems, such as the overall weak positions of social workers in the Hungarian society; and to interpersonal/personal issues as collusion, co-dependency or compulsive help. Professional identity development themes as motivations, aspirations and own experiences were frequent in the interviews.

C1, in addition to being a social worker and an addiction counsellor, is an expert by experience who uses his own personal experiences on addiction and recovery as a powerful professional resource. As a competent helper and mentor, he has substantial experiences on the problems of professionals who are reluctant to work through their own traumatic experiences. He emphasizes the importance of lifelong development of the professional, and the importance of self-reflective capacities:

> I think a social worker who has some life experiences is a more effective helper. I would not only highlight the years of drinking but experiences on recovery, especially the misleads of recovery. Social professional careers are usually chosen by people who previously obtained personal experiences on social problems, and this is very true for alcoholics. [1]Many social workers' career choices are motivated by the wish to help problem families that they themselves were raised in – but they have not worked through their own experiences. (…) I think that there are often dysfunctional motivations in the career choice of social workers…when someone wants to transfer one's own helplessness into helping others, and compensate for the shortcomings originating from own unprocessed experiences by helping others. This should be controlled in the selection process – or more exactly, it can be developed in one's professional education (…) A family can be dysfunctional in many different ways (…) and you cannot be a helper if you are stuck in your own life. There are two ways to cope with that: one is to recognize own barriers and exceed them, and this is how I am enabled to work in many more areas

of social work. As long as I am stuck with a problem I should not work in that particular area. If I am in the midst of a personal divorce crisis I will be not able to help my clients manage their divorce. This is my temporary limitation or inadequacy.

C2 is a social worker in a hospice providing palliative care. Her motivations were grounded by her own experiences, which made her realize the personal impacts of some of the harms of general (non-hospice) health care systems.

> I often visited my father, almost every day. When I could see that he was about to leave this world, I was just standing at his bedside, entrapped in my sadness. For some reason, I left the hospital room for some minutes. A nurse came to me and ordered me not to cry in my father's presence and not to tell him about any negative things as it was not allowed there. I felt very angry, I could feel I would explode because I was not allowed to express my own feelings towards my father (…) there was the emotion, my anger that made me do something about this case. This is when I decided that I would work in the hospice, that I must change the relationship of a dying person with their loved ones, to make it different from my own experiences.[2]

C4 is a teacher, head of a school who worked long decades to promote the educational chances of Roma children living in segregated city areas. She has always considered the employment of qualified school social workers a priority, what was rather unusual in the majority of the schools:

> …a social worker may be involved in many different roles. They can fill an administrative post and do paperwork (…) but you, as HEIs should provide a list of competencies together with the degree, on their particular strengths and weaknesses. (…) many courses should be introduced on personality development…you can learn how to be in the background…how to communicate in a non-controlling, non-judgmental, non-demanding way, or how to encourage the clients to speak up for themselves. Students can acquire knowledge, no problem with that, but these are skills and attitudes… this is a dramatic role. You have to commit yourself, be definite about it. They have to work on their own personalities to make a determined and competent woman of Mommy's good little girl. A person who knows exactly why she is there, what she wants, who she works with, and is courageous, while at the same time knows that it is not her who should dominate the situation.

Student interviews on dropout

Due to the lack of information on social work among the public, deficits in public recognition and an overall low prestige of the profession, social work career is not attractive. Many social worker students who commit themselves to the profession have some own experiences on traumatization or lasting deprivation, and this is a very strong motivation. Some students – mostly non-traditional students lacking many of the resources to pursue university-level studies – see it as a chance for social mobility (Pusztai, 2013). Others, who have not made up their minds yet on a prospective career, want to postpone the decision (psychosocial moratorium). Members of the latter two groups have a higher risk for dropout.

The narrative of these students is as follows: on application, the student is rather ambivalent concerning the profession; the decision is often 'by chance'. When reaching a turning point or personal crisis in life (e.g. end of a romantic relationship or facing financial problems), the idea that they should leave the study programme emerges. The social network is not supportive either – from open refusal to indifference concerning the person's ambitions. Sometimes the family considers obtaining a degree as a 'family mission' that the student has to accomplish, irrespective of students' personal motivations and own choices. The decision on dropout is often underpinned by perceived shortcomings of the study programme, lecturers' 'unfriendly' attitudes, and 'useless' or 'non-practical' subjects. These are used as rationalizations for the decision. Some students come back and continue; they acquire life experiences and reconstruct their own motivations. They are open for new knowledge, and their choice of career is now recognized as own commitment.

D1, a Roma woman in her early twenties from a segregated village had a family mission to become a first-generation professional. Her boyfriend, however, wanted to live with her and she gave up her studies to earn some money for their independent living as a couple. This seems a priority in D1's life over her studies. In the next excerpt, she refers to a common misconception: social workers in Hungary are often mistaken for workers for public utility, a workfare approach to support the needy and lead them back to the labour market:

> When I go home (to the original family) they keep asking me about my exams. I cannot explain to them that currently I work, and I am not interested in my studies any more… as it is very important to them…more important than to me. (…) My grandpa keeps telling everyone that I will be a lawyer, he does not understand what social work is, that it is not some unskilled work for public utility, like sweeping the streets in those horrible orange jackets for some miserable social benefits.

D6, a man in his late 30s, is currently employed as a social worker. After more than 10 years, he returned to finish his studies, as this is the precondition for obtaining a leadership post in his workplace, where he is acknowledged as a competent and committed team member. He recollects his experiences on dropout as a crisis (Tinto, 1987) or a liminal experience of a rite of passage (van Gennep, 1960), leading to mature professional motivations and identity:

> I lost my scholarship. I had just registered for one or two courses that I did not attend. And there came the bill…and I said to myself that okay, that

was it. I went to the UK to work, and when I got home there was the mail on my dismissal from the university…it hurt. Previously I had never been dismissed from anywhere: I could not forgive myself. (…) I went back to the UK to make ends meet. There was the economic crisis and I had a Swiss francs loan…you know. A nadir point in my life (…) In the UK I worked as a recycling sorter at a city dump and earned four times as much as here at home as a qualified professional. No responsibility. Big money. (…) Then I came home and went back to my previous workplace. I took shifts to earn some more money and decided to pick up loose threads.

Measuring identity with ISA/Ipseus

As a conclusion of the international and domestic literature review, measuring social workers' identity seems necessary in a number of areas, especially in educational and workplace settings. Explorations on identity seem notably useful in:

- Education programme development (designing study programmes and pre–post evaluation)
- CPD programmes design and evaluation
- Workplace selection, with special regard to the varied and contextual nature of social work
- Detecting workplace conflict resources
- Identifying 'temporary limitations' in times of major transitions in the professional's life
- Refining national and international standards, policies and practices
- Identifying conflicts in interprofessional collaboration
- Conducting scientific studies, including the comparison of student and practitioner identities; time series evaluations during one's career as a social worker; studying gender differences, comparisons between the different areas and sectors of praxis; comparisons in the global context

The use of ISA, and its linked measure, Ipseus, facilitates well-grounded explorations on social workers' professional identities by disclosing personal and interpersonal dynamics related to one's or a given group's values, identifications, reflections and crisis/conflict zones. The fundamental principle of ISA is the following: *A person's appraisal of the social world and its significance is an expression of his or her identity* (Weinreich, 2004: xix). Our identity largely depends on the integration of our experiences on the social situations we are involved in, and it governs our current behaviour and future aspirations. ISA is a constructionist theory, a unique and a creative synthesis on mainly but not exclusively Kelly's (1955) personal construct theory, Erikson's (1968) psychosocial development theory, Festinger's (1957) cognitive dissonance theory, Mead's (1934, cit. Weinreich, 2004) symbolic interactionism, Berne's (1968) transaction analysis and Harré's (1998) discursive self-theory. ISA conceives identity as the totality of our constructs on ourselves, where there is a continuity with our concepts on experiences and future aspirations (Weinreich, 2004). Our constructs are determined by our appraisals on the social network of significant others, and also by macro-level cultural perspectives.

An ISA instrument (Ipseus) contains domains, represented by entities, and themes, represented by bipolar constructs. Entities include one's own self in different temporal perspectives, in a number of situations or as seen by others (exploratory selves and metaperspectives), as well as some significant others. Constructs are ideas that have proven relevant in the qualitative studies grounding the contents for an Ipseus social work instrument. The person is asked to appraise the discourses that are made up of the entities and the bipolar constructs. One of the strength of the instrument is that it is sensitive to cultural-discursive traditions of the target group, using own central themes, language and metaphors (Weinreich, 2010a; McNeill et al., 2018). During the appraisal, a nine-point scale is provided where extremes −4 and +4 correspond to two polarities, and 0 is neutral. Respondents are asked to appraise each entity in the instrument, using the scale on all the given bipolar values. For example, 'My boss…treats clients as equal partners in the helping process/is patronizing and controls the clients' The numbers are represented by deepening colours, that is the person will not be influenced by common connotations on negative (−) or positive (+) values or low/high numbers. Considering that identity is a personal issue, ISA is both internally and externally standardized, that is, also relative to the person's and own group's/own culture's evaluations.

Our instrument was based on a substantial review on the professional literature, on the results of the interviews and on repeated discussions with practitioners. We also introduced an initial pilot with five respondents (whose appraisals were excluded from the final sample) to detect any problems concerning the domains (entities), themes (constructs) and wording. As a result, we removed one theme that openly referred to unethical behaviour and was possibly offensive and simplified sentence structures. The instrument used with 59 respondents was based on the following domains and themes:

1   Balancing between the personal/psychosocial and the social/societal (Darvas and Hegyesi, 2003): the significance of individual or social change.
2   Dilemmas of social work as an academic discipline: contrasting traditional scientific vs. highly personalized interventions (Fargion, 2008); the role of professional education and social work research.
3   The impact of preferences for technical rationality in the dominant culture. Craft professionalism or reflective professionals characterized by autonomy (Jones and Joss, 1995; Fargion, 2008).
4   Social justice vs. conformity.
5   Distance between professional definitions, public perceptions and political requirements (Navrátil & Bajer, 2018).
6   Social workers' understandings on empowerment/control work, including client autonomy, the possibility of life transformations in clients' lives and attitudes of the compulsive helper.
7   Wounded helpers vs. helpers' perfectness.

8   The role of personal ideologies.
9   Empathy vs. objective, distancing attitudes.
10 Eudaimonic/spiritual vs. hedonistic values (in comparison with consumer society values).
11 Collaborations: the lonely hero vs. team player.

The themes were included in 21 corresponding constructs as shown in Table 13.2.

Table 13.2 Constructs

	Label left	:	*Label right*
01	Client as equal		Patronizing and control
02	Continuing education		Finished education
03	Flexible about rules		Rigid about rules
04	Favours self-reflection		Refuses self-reflection
05	Deserving clients only		A chance for everyone
06	Part of clients' lives		Client autonomy
07	Interpersonal relations		Societal problems
08	Refuses research		Research in practice
09	Externally formed frameworks		Own responsibility for frameworks
10	Respect boundaries		Help at all price
11	Natural skills and practice		A degree in social work
12	Free from own problems		Wounded helper
13	Perfect solution		Tolerates insecurities
14	Empathetic		Objective
15	Autonomous decisions		Externally controlled
16	Distance from own ideologies		Teaches own ideologies
17	Critical thinking		Never questions guidelines
18	Societal catch-up		Societal changes
19	Faith in clients' capacity		People cannot change
20	Spiritual orientation		Welfare and success
21	Team player		Can count only on oneself

Domains (entities)

Entities (15) included past, current, future, ideal and contra-ideal selves; exploratory selves (Me in private life; Me, when solving a difficult problem); an admired (my professional role model) and a disliked person (disrespected colleague); two metaperspectives (Me as seen by the clients, Me as seen by my closest colleague) and some additional external entities as 'my best friend', 'the state' (in Hungary the government is traditionally termed as 'state'), 'people in Hungary' and 'my boss'. See Table 13.3.

The highly contextual and rapidly changing nature of social work in Hungary and limitations of sampling – a convenience sample that is not representative of the social workers for the reasons detailed earlier – would yield only the formulation of few tentative hypotheses:

1   Both the state (as main employer) and the public are seen as maintaining values opposite to those of social workers.

Table 13.3 Entities

	Label	Classification
01	When decided	Past self
02	Currently I	Current self
03	Private self	Exploratory self
04	Disrespected colleague	Disliked person
05	Solving a difficult...	Exploratory self
06	The government	–
07	My best friend	–
08	My boss	–
09	Professional role model	Admired person
10	People in Hungary	–
11	In 10 years	Future self
12	I as a bad professional	Contra ideal self
13	Clients think I	Metaperspective
14	Close colleague thinks I	Metaperspective
15	Ideally, I	Ideal self

2 Professional education and scientific research are not prioritized among social workers (though participants of the Pécs sample related to a university environment might have been affected by the context of data recording).
3 Conflicted areas include the psychosocial vs. societal level as the focus of interventions; the wounded healer concept; control work vs. empowerment, critical thinking and empathetic vs. distancing/objective attitudes.

Data recording and analysis

Our sample was a convenience sample of social worker practitioners invited into our research by the first and second authors through their own professional networks. The only inclusion criteria were that the respondent should be employed as a social worker. Among our respondents (SWD group), 42 had a degree in social work/social pedagogy/social policy that are considered as equivalents both in the labour market and in higher education (e.g. on admissions to master-level programmes). A total of 15 persons (other degree [OD] group) had some ODs and 2 have not finished their graduate studies yet. All of the respondents volunteered to participate in the study. When it seemed appropriate, we also asked for the permission and support of the manager of the given facility. Data were obtained in two Hungarian towns, in a variety of social services, and with part-time students, at the university. The sample included very diverse employment contexts (homeless shelter, addiction treatment centre, child and family protection services, community/settlement/work, day-care centres/community care for persons with mental disorders/learning disabilities). The majority of the respondents worked for state-run social institutions, with some church-based services and very few NGOs. Ethical approval was obtained from the Ethical Committee on Social

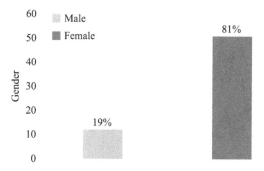

Figure 13.1 Gender rates of respondents.

Research (no. 1/2019) and allows the anonymous, nomothetic use/statistical processing of data, considering part-time students' and field instructors' participation in the sample. Each participant was assigned an individual code for identification. In addition to answering the instrument, we asked the participants about their basic demographic data (age range, gender and focus of employment) and also asked them for a short evaluation on the instrument. We did not record any data concerning respondents' work environment, as this could have identified them. Figure 13.1 shows that gender rates fully correspond to national estimates.

The majority of our respondents have substantial professional and life experiences; about 75% of them were between 31 and 55 years old (Figure 13.2). This is perhaps due to recent decrease in social professional education as young professionals are missing.

Approximately two-thirds of the respondents work in direct client–helper interactions (Figure 13.3).

Data included in Figures 13.4–13.7 suggest that respondents found the themes relevant and the instrument is easy to answer.

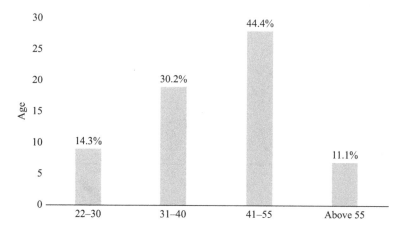

Figure 13.2 Age ranges of the respondents.

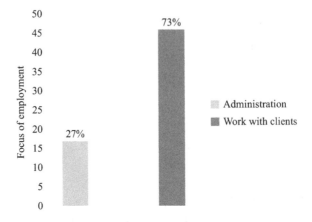

Figure 13.3 Focus of employment.

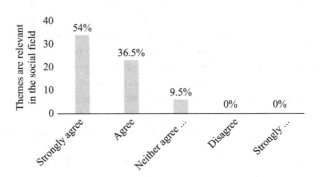

Figure 13.4 Evaluations on the relevance of themes.

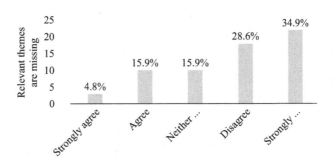

Figure 13.5 Evaluation on possible gaps in the instrument.

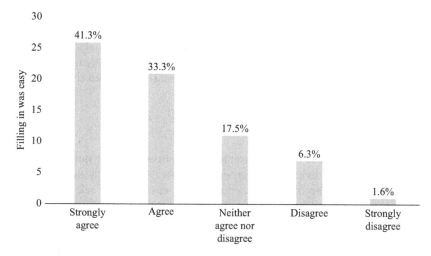

Figure 13.6 Evaluation on design (easy).

Appreciation and gratitude

Respondents could elaborate on the earlier issues by answering open questions (optional), but only two persons commented ('one or two items were difficult to interpret'; 'not all of the entities are relevant for some of the themes and this might be a source of distortion' – perhaps this person did not read the instructions that explicitly explain the role of 0 in rating). Oral feedback was more frequent: *the institution that first was very cautious on collaboration finally lent the necessary laptops to quicken data collection and asked all the colleagues to respond. They said*

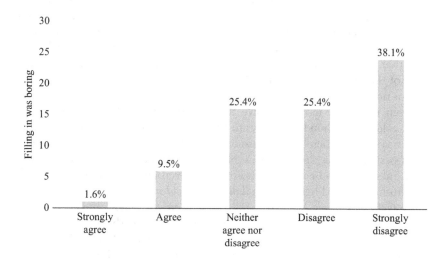

Figure 13.7 Evaluation on design (interesting; inverse statement).

they could hardly wait to read the results; respondents were a bit sceptical but finally all of them liked the instrument; this was very good, and the questions were most interesting. When a researcher asks the members of a silent and relatively marginalized group to share their views, one possible result of the investigation is mutual gratitude. Perhaps, this is the case with any group if the questions that we ask are truly relevant.

Results

Ipseus generates a wide variety of results, which answer a large number of questions concerning individual and group identities. Accordingly, we may focus on individual or group differences, compare the evaluation of relevant entities, including own self-states or the use of bipolar constructs within a given group or between groups. In the current sample, all the 59 individuals are employed in some segments of social work (*social workers are those who do social work* by Nagy, 2003), 15 of them have a university degree but not in social work or a closely related area (that is social work, social pedagogy or social policy) and 2 persons are undergraduates. First, we comment on the results of the total sample and relate our main findings to the wounded healer and threatened identity concept, and then compare the two main groups of social and other graduate professionals.

Self-summary

Self-summary is based on the combination of two key parameters (1) self-evaluation that shows one's endeavours to implement one's identity aspirations and (2) identity diffusion, which is about one's attempts to re-synthesize one's identifications with others (Weinreich, 2010b).

ISA's external standardization [3] provides the researcher with a possibility to compare results across different cultures, groups or persons, while internal standardization is interpreted in the context of local/workplace settings or on the level of the individual. Here, we utilize external standards (represented by black thick lines), that is, analyse social workers' identity states as defined by the parameter ranges of the general population. The rationale behind this decision is twofold: first, it is not particularly helpful for a client to meet a social worker who is defensive, even if not any more defensive than other social workers. Second, social worker values have found their ways to Hungarian practitioners mostly from the Western countries; therefore, the use of external standards of the British sample in this particular case seems a plausible choice. While external standard lines (black lines) seem to be close to those of the given group (blue lines) for identity diffusion (defined here as *overall dispersion and magnitude of one's identification conflicts with others*, Weinreich, 2004:64), there are major differences in the parameter ranges in self-evaluation, significantly extending the zone of moderate self-evaluation at the expense of high evaluation. The latter coincides with the maximum value, what might mean that the group sets very high standards for themselves – a possible source of dissatisfaction.

Table 13.4 Possible identity variants

Self-evaluation	Identity diffusion		
	Low (foreclosed)	Moderate	High
High	Defensive high self-regard	Confident	Diffuse high self-regard
Moderate	Defensive	Indeterminate	Diffusion
Low	Defensive negative	Negative	Crisis

Source: Weinreich (2004, p. 106).

Based on Marcia's original idea on a variety of identity states, ISA differentiates among nine different identity variants, determined by the level of identity diffusion and self-evaluation (see Table 13.4). In the clinical practice, terms as 'defensive' or 'diffuse' are often used as value judgments; ISA is more neutral in this respect and defines these variations as 'vulnerable'. The concepts are to be interpreted as relative to the overall status of the given group (Weinreich, 2004); e.g. one would expect a social worker to be open to others' values, even if these are different from their own priorities.

In Figure 13.8, the position of contra-ideal professional self is in the crisis zone, what seems evident. Past self (when deciding to be a social worker), and the self-solving a difficult problem are in the indeterminate zones. The position of the past self is the second lowest for self-evaluation, what might indicate some relatively difficult experience at the time of the decision for some professionals. Current professional selves, the exploratory self-solving a difficult problem and private selves are very close to each other, probably indicating the relevance of the idea helpers' being *instruments of themselves*, and the predominance of professional challenges. Future selves and ideal selves are in the confident zones. On this group level, the positions of past, current and future selves and that of the ideal self-portraying professionals' highest aspirations show a steady line of development. This is reflected in a complementary statistical analysis on our data. Paired sample T-tests have confirmed the marked differences in the evaluation of past, present and future selves, and, parallel, involvement with present and future selves. Refer to Table 13.5.

If we want an elaborate answer to our question concerning the wounded healer concept and threatened identities, these group-level explorations should be complemented by a summary on the individual cases. The 'wounded helper' concept involves a specific trajectory: initial presence of a vulnerable or negative identity state (past self) that is developing into a more desirable state (indeterminate or confident) which is compatible with the requirements of the profession, detailed in the first part of the chapter. Further, we analysed defensive patterns, the types of vulnerable states (Weinreich, 2004) that are hardly congruent with professional requirements. 'Defensive identities tend to be rigid and unreceptive to alternative perspectives, the vulnerability then being a lack of adaptability and flexibility in changing circumstances' (Weinreich, 2004:67). This is not the identity variant of a social worker, a reflective professional by definition, but that of a control worker with rather fragile self-assuredness. Defensive high self-regard states, though these

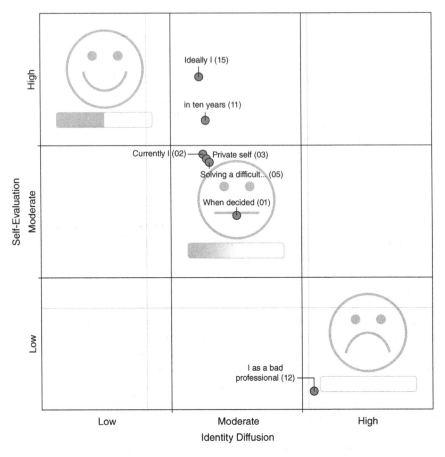

Figure 13.8 Self-summary of the 59 persons employed as social workers.

Table 13.5 Changes in past/current/future self (57 respondents with a university degree)

	t	*df*	*Asymp. Sig. (two tailed)*	*Effect size (Cohen's d)*
Inv_Past – Inv_Current	.277	56	.783 (n.s.)	–
Inv_Current – Inv_Future	−3.101	56	.003[b]	.40
Inv_Past – Inv_Future	−2.061	56	.044[a]	.27
Eval_Past – Eval_Current	−5.881	56	.000[b]	.78
Eval_Current – Eval_Future	−3.852	56	.000[b]	.51
Eval_Past – Eval_Future	−7.164	56	.000[b]	.95

[a] p < .05.

[b] p < .01.

may seem comfortable for the person in an ever-changing environment, were also considered as alien to central values of social work as openness, and acceptance of diversity and change. In our exploration on the individual cases, past self (career choice, 'when deciding…') was selected as baseline, and the positions of current self shaped by today's experiences, future self as expectations and ideal self as aspirations were compared to this baseline. Contra-ideal selves are also included in the table, as these identity states motivate defence.

The number of possible variations is rather high but can be reduced to some basic, relevant patterns determined by dominant identity states and developmental trends (Table 13.6).

Table 13.6 Identity variants of persons employed as social workers with a degree in social work (SWD = 42), some other degree (OD = 15) and social assistants without a degree (ND = 2) currently in part-time education

Respondent	Past self	Current self	Future self	Ideal self	Contra-ideal self	Trajectory
ND_01	Indet.	Conf.	Conf.	Conf.	Neg.	Positive
ND_02	Indet.	Indet.	Indet.	Indet.	Crisis	Stable
OD_01	Def.	Def.	Def.	Def.	Crisis	Foreclosed-stable
OD_02	Indet.	Indet.	Conf.	Conf.	Def. neg	Positive
OD_03	Indet.	Def.	Def.	Def. HSR	Crisis	Foreclosed-positive
OD_04	Def.	Def. HSR	Def. HSR	Def. HSR	Crisis	Foreclosed-positive
OD_05	Diff.	Indet.	Conf.	Conf.	Crisis	Wounded-positive
OD_06	Def. HSR	Def. HSR	Def. HSR	Def. HSR	Crisis	Foreclosed-stable
OD_07	Indet.	Conf.	Diff. HSR	Conf.	Crisis	Varied
OD_08	Indet.	Conf.	Indet.	Conf.	Crisis	Varied
OD_09	Indet.	Def. HSR	Def. HSR	Def. HSR	Crisis	Foreclosed-positive
OD_10	Indet.	Indet.	Conf.	Conf.	Neg.	Positive
OD_11	Neg.	Conf.	Indet.	Conf.	Crisis	Wounded-pessimistic
OD_12	Def. HSR	Def. HSR	Def. HSR	Def. HSR	Neg.	Foreclosed-stable
OD_13	Neg.	Indet.	Conf.	Conf.	Neg.	Wounded-positive
OD_14	Indet.	Conf.	Conf.	Conf.	Neg.	Positive
OD_15	Def.	Def. HSR	Def. HSR	Def. HSR	Crisis	Foreclosed-positive
SWD_01	Indet.	Indet.	Diff. HSR	Diff. HSR	Neg.	Varied
SWD_02	Indet.	Indet.	Conf.	Conf.	Crisis	Positive
SWD_03	Indet.	Indet.	Conf.	Conf.	Crisis	Positive
SWD_04	Conf.	Conf.	Conf.	Conf.	Def. neg	Stable
SWD_05	Neg.	Indet.	Diff.	Conf.	Neg.	Varied
SWD_06	Indet.	Conf.	Conf.	Def. HSR	Neg.	Positive!
SWD_07	Indet.	Indet.	Indet.	Indet.	Neg.	Stable
SWD_08	Crisis	Def. HSR	Def. HSR	Def. HSR	Crisis	Foreclosed-positive
SWD_09	Indet.	Indet.	Indet.	Indet.	Crisis	Stable
SWD_10	Diff.	Diff.	Diff.	Diff. HSR	Neg.	Diffuse
SWD_11	Def.	Def. HSR	Def. HSR	Def. HSR	Crisis	Foreclosed-positive
SWD_12	Crisis	Def. HSR	Conf.	Conf.	Crisis	Wounded-varied
SWD_13	Diff.	Diff.	Diff. HSR	Diff. HSR	Crisis	Diff.-positive
SWD_14	Indet.	Indet.	Conf.	Conf.	Neg.	Positive

(Continued)

Table 13.6 Identity variants of persons employed as social workers with a degree in social work (SWD = 42), some other degree (OD = 15) and social assistants without a degree (ND = 2) currently in part-time education (*Continued*)

Respondent	Past self	Current self	Future self	Ideal self	Contra-ideal self	Trajectory
SWD_15	Indet.	Indet.	Conf.	Conf.	Def. Neg	Positive
SWD_16	Conf.	Conf.	Conf.	Conf.	Crisis	Stable
SWD_17	Diff.	Indet.	Conf.	Conf.	Crisis	Wounded-positive
SWD_18	Indet.	Indet.	Indet.	Conf.	Neg.	Stable
SWD_19	Neg.	Def.	Def. HSR	Def.	Crisis	Foreclosed-positive
SWD_20	Def.	Def. HSR	Def. HSR	Def. HSR	Crisis	Foreclosed-positive
SWD_21	Def.	Def.	Def.	Def.	Crisis	Foreclosed-stable
SWD_22	Neg.	Indet.	Conf.	Conf.	Crisis	Wounded-positive
SWD_23	Conf.	Indet.	Conf.	Conf.	Neg.	Varied
SWD_24	Indet.	Def. HSR	Def.	Def. HSR	Crisis	Foreclosed-positive
SWD_25	Indet.	Def. HSR	Def. HSR	Def. HSR	Crisis	Problematic
SWD_26	Crisis	Indet.	Conf.	Conf.	Crisis	Wounded
SWD_27	Indet.	Conf.	Def. HSR	Def.	Crisis	Varied
SWD_28	Def. HSR	Def.	Def. HSR	Def. HSR	Neg.	Foreclosed-positive
SWD_29	Indet.	Def. HSR	Def. HSR	Def. HSR	Crisis	Foreclosed-positive
SWD_30	Diff.	Indet.	Diff.	Conf.	Crisis	Varied
SWD_31	Diff.	Diff. HSR	Diff. HSR	Conf.	Neg.	Diff.-positive
SWD_32	Def.	Def. HSR	Def. HSR	Def. HSR	Crisis	Problematic
SWD_33	Conf.	Conf.	Conf.	Conf.	Crisis	Stable
SWD_34	Diff.	Diff.	Diff. HSR	Diff. HSR	Neg.	Foreclosed-positive
SWD_35	Indet.	Conf.	Conf.	Conf.	Crisis	Positive
SWD_36	Indet.	Def.	Def.	Def.	Crisis	Foreclosed-stable
SWD_37	Def.	Def.	Def.	Def.	Crisis	Foreclosed-stable
SWD_38	Def. HSR	Def. HSR	Def. HSR	Def. HSR	Def.	Foreclosed-stable
SWD_39	Def.	Def. HSR	Def. HSR	Def. HSR	Neg.	Foreclosed-positive
SWD_40	Indet.	Indet.	Indet.	Indet.	Neg.	Stable
SWD_41	Indet.	Conf.	Conf.	Conf.	Crisis	Positive
SWD_42	Indet.	Indet.	Indet.	Def. HSR	Crisis	Stable!

Foreclosed (positive/stable) identities: One's development/expected/aspired self-development is mostly characterized by defensive states as solutions to earlier professional or personal transformations. Self-evaluations may increase (positive) or do not change (stable). The 22 cases of such defensive identity states and aspirations are interpreted as a response to social workers' threatened identity and – considering that these versions make up more than one-third of the sample – are probably not only individual choices but are the results of some societal or cultural factors.

Positive identity development (11 cases) reveals a pattern that is fully compatible with professional guidelines and is a comfortable identity state for the professional as well.

Stable identity (nine cases) is not characterized by the perception of marked identity development on part of the person, but it is fully compatible with professional requirements and is probably convenient for the person. (In one of the cases, aspirations/ideal self are towards a more defensive position with higher self-evaluation.)

Wounded helper identity development: Some initial vulnerable/negative state evolves into a more positive state which is compatible with professional requirements as well (indeterminate and confident). In one of the seven cases, expectations are less positive than current state (the case is labelled here as wounded-pessimistic); and in another case (wounded-varied), the position of the current self is defensive, but both the expectations and the aspirations are aimed at statuses that are more suitable for a social worker.

Diffuse and varied: The remaining 10 cases were characterized by diffusion and mixed patterns. Diffusion (three cases), understood here as a sign of unusual openness or a chaotic, changing value system and a parallel tolerance towards ambiguities and paradoxes, is not necessarily a problematic position in social work. '*Diffuse identities are likely to be over-receptive to varieties of beliefs and values, potentially reinforcing or adding to the vulnerabilities of existing confusions, uncertainties and vacillations*' (Weinreich, 2004:67). In seven cases, the pattern was varied, not yielding a well-grounded interpretation concerning the wounded healer concept or threatened identity.

The relatively low number of cases with wounded helper identity development, and, parallel, the presence of foreclosed/defensive identities in more than one-third of the sample suggest that our interpretation concerning social worker professional identity as threatened identity is a plausible one. It is worth noting that the most destructive variant in this context (defensive negative) is not present in the sample, only as contra-ideal self, in three cases. Research results are not available on any other group of professional helpers and this is why we cannot tell if the results here are particularly 'good' or 'bad' if compared. In any case, a helper with a defensive position would not serve clients' needs very well in direct interactions.

Entity summary

Figure 13.9 on entity summary is a combination of parameters *ego-involvement* and *evaluation* of the entities; if ego-involvement is relatively high then low-level evaluation is quite problematic for the person. Obviously, this is the case for contra-ideal self. Evaluation is negative, but ego-involvement is moderate with the negative role model (disrespected colleague) and for the entity representing the public (the majority of people in Hungary). Evaluation of the 'state' (government as main employer) is low, almost negative. All these might be a response to identity threats and establish a marginal position (they don't like me, but I don't care too much about it). Ego-involvement is higher with past, current, ideal and future selves, the professional role model, the problem-solving and private life selves; but only the selves representing expectations (future self) and ultimate aspirations (Ideal self) are evaluated higher (would still be situated in the moderate range if we compared to internal standard lines). Similarly, to self-summary, the temporal perspectives depicted in entity summary delineate a progressive narrative (Gergen and Gergen, 1997) where future seems better than present or past states.

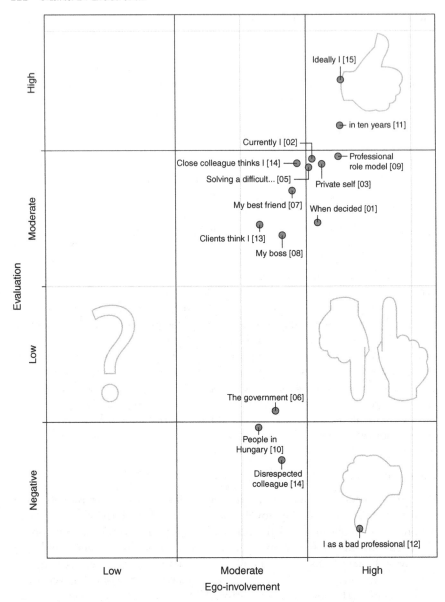

Figure 13.9 Entity summary on the 59 respondents.

Construct summary

Construct summary is a combination of parameters emotional significance (ES) and structural pressure (SP). Preferred poles of the appraisals are determined by ideal self-ratings (for the details, please see Appendix 1 at the end of this chapter, Figure 13.A1). SP is a measure to determine construct stability (compatibilities over incompatibilities of appraisals), differentiating among rigid, core, secondary, conflicted or contradictory patterns. Unlike with self and entity summaries, where comparing the results to a general population pattern seemed plausible (e.g. *defensive as compared to an average person*), here we mostly rely on in-group standards (represented by the blue thin lines) to interpret the results. It is worth to consider though, that part of what would qualify as an emotionally significant core construct with high stability for the wider public (external standards) counts as of moderate ES and less stable for the social worker.[4]

When using internal, group-level standard lines, ranges of both core and secondary constructs are narrower as compared to general population standards, while the conflicted area is extended. Only five of the constructs (client autonomy, client as equal, a chance for everyone, self-reflection and continuing education) have a relatively higher, but still moderate ES; three of these are the central social worker values associated with client–helper interactions and the two latter are related to practitioners' developmental needs. Secondary constructs that are very near to core ones are faith in client's capacity and eudaimonic/spiritual orientation. Other secondary constructs with moderate ES include emphasis on interpersonal relations over societal problems, research in practice, critical thinking, the wounded healer concept, taking own responsibility for frameworks, autonomous decisions, respecting boundaries, tolerating insecurities and being a team player. In the domestic literature, there is a continuing debate on the role of social workers in the treatment of macro-level societal problems, in contrast with their work with individuals in the sphere of interpersonal relations. Our respondents favoured working in the interpersonal domain to managing societal challenges. Conflicted constructs include balancing between objectivity vs. empathy, the promotion of societal changes vs. societal catch-up, distancing from own ideologies (logically related to the issue of objectivity), flexibility vs. strict adherence to rules and a degree in social work – and all of these potential conflict areas have moderate ES. Societal catch-up or 'closed up' is a frequent element in government rhetoric and is in contrast with the promotion of social change, which is a core idea in social work (*facilitate constructive confrontation and change where certain cultural beliefs, values and traditions violate peoples' basic human rights. As culture is socially constructed and dynamic, it is subject to deconstruction and change.* Global Definition of Social Work, 2014).

Altogether, the pattern suggests a distancing attitude on part of the social workers. Figure 13.10 shows construct summary.

Differences between subsamples of respondents with a degree in social work and some other degree

ISA/Ipseus has a built-in facility for determining group level differences, showing preferred poles, summary data on dissonances and consonances, and the resulting SP and ES (Appendix 1, Figure 13.A1). When we have checked the subsamples for possible differences by using Ipseus' majority–minority facility, there seemed to be very little differences between the SWD group's and OD group's preferences.

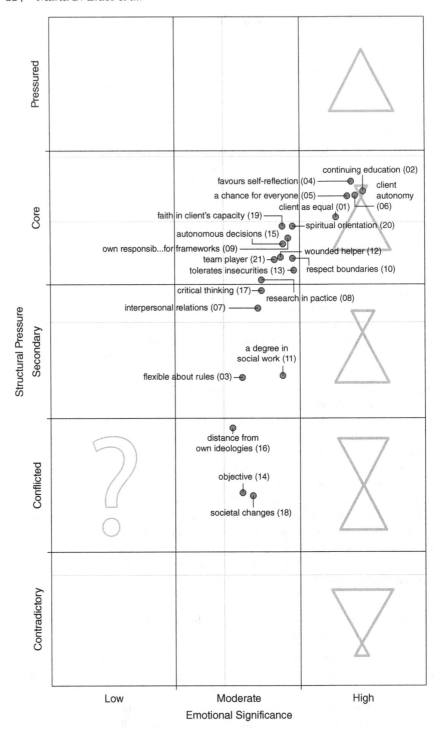

Figure 13.10 Construct summary on the 59 respondents.

Our sample was not balanced as the number of respondents with a degree in social work or equivalent (SWD) was significantly higher than the number of respondents employed as social workers with some OD. In order to compare the subsamples and identify statistically significant differences, if any, we randomly selected 15 persons of the SWD group to compare the results to the group of 15 other professionals, utilizing the excel output files produced by the software. Independent samples T-test was performed to identify possible differences in the evaluation of entities; in construct stability, indicated by SP and in ES. Practically no such differences were found in any of these major dimensions, apart from the evaluation of one of the entities (close colleague Metaperspective). Further significant differences were identified in extensiveness of the responses on two role models (boss and admired person). Dissonance significantly differed in the treatment of societal problems vs. working with interpersonal relations and objectivity over empathy, indicating a possible impact of the formal training that lays great emphasis on both themes. Detailed results of the statistical analyses are provided in Appendix 1, in Tables 13.A1 and 13.A2. Altogether, the number of significant differences between the two groups was very low and related mostly to external entities, what indicates the predominance of practice over formal training.

Discussion

Systematic, national-level studies on the professional identity of social workers have not yet been conducted in Hungary, though there is consent that professional identity is a key resource in the helping field. Identity formation is associated with the recent crisis of the profession brought about by the decline of the welfare state. Further, as Győri stated in 2014, social workers are strongly influenced by the political changes concerning the professional area. All these transformations have continued to have a deep impact on the conceptions, practices and the consolidating value system of the newly reborn profession in Hungary, indicating that the second birth of a profession is not necessarily less demanding than the first one. The quality question of competent and committed workforce in the social field soon turned into a quantity question of ensuring the necessary workforce at all (Varga, 2008). Even so, effective service of the clients of social work and service of the society would definitely demand quality workforce.

Based on our results, the concept of threatened identity and social workers' liminal status seems pertinent to the societal position of the Hungarian social workers. In the eyes of social workers, public perceptions on social issues are quite contrary to the profession's value system. For the social workers, newly introduced, hedonistic consumer society values of welfare and success were less favoured than the search for meaning in life, a spiritual-eudaimonic orientation, and also a constituent of the sense of coherence concept (Antonovsky, 1987). People are usually critical on any government; however, for social workers, the government is the main employer, and this is why negative evaluative connotations are more of a potential source of conflicts. Adherence to rules and guidelines has also proven a conflicted area; no wonder, as these rules and guidelines do not always seem to work well in everyday practice (Németh, 2014) and should be adapted to real-life conditions. This step could ensure that feedback from the practitioners be heard by the decision makers, what would presumably positively influence perceptions on the government on part of the social workers.

On exploring the theme of wounded helpers, we have found that the evaluation of past self (at the point of career choice) is lower than those of current or future selves. A further analysis on the individual cases have revealed that overall developmental patterns are in accordance with professional requirements of social work, and several persons were successful in their efforts to turn initial crises or negative states into future resources. However, defensive attitudes were also present in about one-third of the sample. The idea that previous difficulties in life become a precious professional resource was accepted, but appeared as of secondary importance, what might indicate that the idea is quite well known among the professionals but is not a lived experience for quite a number of social workers.

Evaluating objectivity over empathy, the latter understood as sharing in the states of mind of the other, is a distancing, and at the same time conflicted attitude on part of the respondents, some of whom may confuse *emotionally abstinent* approaches (Kozma, 1996:114) with *emotionally absent* ones. This might refer to burnout (client as object, Fekete, 2000). Considering the overall positive attitude towards clients as reflected in the importance of client participation, autonomy and empowerment, and mostly positive evaluations on current selves and future aspirations, respondents of the sample as a whole do not seem to suffer from burnout and do not seem to be compulsive helpers either. A specific feature of Hungarian social work, a relative lack of counselling skills with marked emphasis on societal facts in the training programmes (B. Erdos & Gomory, in this volume); fears from being 'unprofessionally' involved (Webb, 2017b) and recent tendencies of control work in the area of social work yield a more consistent explanation for these findings. Further, approximately one-third of the respondents were employed in administrative positions and not in direct client–helper interactions. Administrative posts might increase one's preferences for clearly determined settings, with less alternatives and conflicts.

The fact that neither research (together with critical thinking) nor a social work degree are priorities among the respondents establishes a problematic position for the domestic training and research institutions, and also for the experts involved in social services development. These findings echo the statistical data on social worker admissions to HEIs, with students' marked preferences for part-time education on masters' levels,[5] which they often utilize as a form of practice-based continuing education. The results are related to our other findings, disclosing that there were not any significant differences among the persons employed as social workers with a relevant degree (SWD) and some OD. Another possible explanation for the relative lack of differences is the homogenizing nature of social work *practice*: the work environment is perhaps more decisive in forming one's identity than professional training, especially when the primary focus of HEIs is on knowledge and not on a wide variety of competences. The introduction of licensure could stop the recruitment of non-social professionals for social worker positions without providing them with adequate training. At the same time, academic institutions should focus more on the development of identity issues and introduce trainings on counselling, more specifically on empathy, mentalization and self-reflection. Sources for CPD – as trainings, short courses and supervision – would be appreciated by the Hungarian social workers.

The strength of the profession lies in the integration of three key areas: practice, education and research. Practice-based education could be a viable option on undergraduate levels as well, only if salaries were attractive enough for the prospective students in the social sector, and qualified mentors were available. Large-scale introduction of evaluation research with the aim of service development (Ellis, 2013) seems highly problematic in Hungary, as social worker practitioners do not consider social work research an important area.

Based on our general conclusions, we propose some further, more specific improvements in a number of areas, namely:

- Modifications in the training programmes in social work education (working through personal crises states or early wounds; reflective trainings; working closer to practice, but insist on good, evidence-based practices)
- The introduction of a wide variety of CPD programmes for the practitioners, including clinical supervision
- Media campaigns and other measures to change public perceptions on social workers
- Policy/legislation changes concerning prestige, monopolization of the profession and ensuring professional autonomy
- Research on a larger/more representative sample, including identity research and research on 'control work' issues

Our study has some important limitations, mainly due to sample size and sampling procedure. A convenience sample does not represent the entirety of a professional group (which, in this case, is still a fluid concept in the domestic professional literature). The university environment in data collection with approximately one-third of the sample could directly influence respondents' judgments on themes of social work research and education. Some of the possible impacts are less direct: involvement in continuing professional education reduces the risks of burnout (Fekete, 2000) and probably increases the overall level of positive future aspirations.

Our instrument worked quite well, and findings are in accordance with most of what is known about social work today in Hungary. In the light of our findings, however, certain modifications could make the picture even clearer. One of the priorities was to keep the instrument short enough so that respondents would agree to participate in the study even if they have little spare time. Most practitioners found our instrument relevant to the theme and easy to answer. However, the inclusion of further entities could contribute to a more elaborate view on one's identification processes. Adding childhood self, primary carers, a mentor/lecturer in social work, church/NGO organizations as entities would enable us to elaborate on the identity processes concerning career choice, and also on the wounded healer concept; to study the nature of the perceived gap between practice and education and the role of further employers in the social sector.

We often referred to external standards of the British sample, and we had good reasons to do so as social work has its traditions in the western countries, including Great Britain. Hungarian standards are not available yet but might be different from the British ones. The differences that we could identify with the social worker group, where 'high' evaluation is understood as (almost) the maximum, similarly to high ES, taken together with the extended zone of conflicted constructs – another salient feature – might not be a pattern characteristic only of the Hungarian social workers but an overall domestic pattern due to differences in history and culture.

The flexibility of ISA/Ipseus approaches and the rich complexity of the data the software produces are an abundant resource for the researcher. The completion of one project generally opens new study fields. Inter-professional and cross-cultural comparisons and the analysis of different subsamples to identify what is common and what is specific about social worker identities are among the potential future directions.

Notes

1. It is important to note that alcoholic is not a stigma term in 12-step fellowships. Rather, it is associated with sense of belonging and acknowledgment (for more, please see Diane Rae Davis, Golie G. Jansen, Making Meaning of Alcoholics Anonymous for Social Workers: Myths, Metaphors, and Realities, Social Work, Volume 43, Issue 2, March 1998, Pages 169–182, https://doi.org/10.1093/sw/43.2.169)
2. This interview was made by Zoltán Szabadi for his thesis work (2019, University of Pécs) on the role of social workers in hospice care (supervisor: Marta B. Erdos)
3. Comparisons are made with respect to external standards specified on a British sample.
4. Here we do not refer to the specific contents of the given construct but the differences in parameter range between the general population and our sample, which might indicate a difference in overall evaluative attitudes.
5. A BA in Social Work is not a prerequisite for an MA in Social Work; practically any degree in the humanities or social sciences is eligible.

References

A szociális munka etikai kódexe (Code of Ethics) (2016) Szociális Szakmai Szövetség. http://3sz.hu/sites/default/files/Etikai.pdf

Aczél, Zs. (2016) *Egy gender-olvasat a szociális munkáról (Social work in terms of gender)* PhD dissertation, Budapest: ELTE http://edit.elte.hu/xmlui/bitstream/handle/10831/38098/disszert%C3%A1cio_Acz%C3%A9lZs.pdf?sequence=1&isAllowed=y

Antonovsky, A. (1987) *Unraveling the Mystery of Health. How People Manage Stress and Stay Well.* San Francisco, Jossey-Bass Publishers.

Asquith, S., Clark, C., Waterhouse, L., & Education Dept, Scotland (2005) *The Role of the Social Worker in the 21st Century: A Literature Review.* Edinburgh: Scottish Executive Education Department.

Bass, L., Márton, I. (2005) *A szociális munkások helyzete ma. Social workers Today.* Szociális Szakmai Szövetség http://www.3sz.hu/tartalom/szocialis-munka

Berne, E. (1968) *Games People Play. The Psychology of Human Relationships.* Andre Deutch Ltd., London.

Black, S., Weinreich, P. (2004) An exploration of counselling identity in counsellors who deal with trauma. Weinreich, P. & Saunderson, W. (Eds.) (2004). *Analysing Identity: Cross-Cultural, Societal and Clinical Contexts.* London & New York: Routledge. 339–360.

Budai, I. (2004) "...szakmai identitásában megerősödve lépjen ki a gyakorlatba..." "(...begin practice with strengthened professional identities...") *Esély*, 1, 61–79.

Bugarszki, Zs. (2014) A magyarországi szociális munka válsága. (The crisis of social work in Hungary) *Esély*, 3, 64–73.

Darvas, Á. & Hegyesi, G. (2003) Hungary. In: Weiss, I., Gal, J. & Dixon, J (ed.) *Professional Ideologies and Preferences in Social Work: A Global Study.* Westport: Praeger Publishers, 125–141.

Ellis, R. (2013). Policy, evaluation and practice. *Szociális Szemle*, 6 (1–2), 7–9.

Erikson, E.H. (1968). *Identity: Youth and Crisis.* New York: Norton.

Fargion, S. (2008). Reflections on social work's identity. International themes in Italian practitioners' representation of social work. *International Social Work*, 51 (2), 206–219.

Farkas A. (2005). *A szociális szakma szerepe ma Magyarországon. (The role of social work today in Hungary.)* Szociális Szakmai Szövetség http://www.3sz.hu/tartalom/szocialis-munka

Fekete, S. (2000): Segítő foglalkozások kockázatai – Helfer szindróma és burnout jelenség. (Risks of the helping professions – Helfer syndrome and burnout) In: Kelemen G. (szerk.) *Tele-dialógus.* Pro Pannonia. Pécs. 179–191.

Festinger, L. (1957). *A Theory of Cognitive Dissonance.* California: Stanford University Press.

Fónai, M., Patyán, L., Szoboszlai, K. (2001) Szociális munkások pályaképének néhány eleme. (Some element of social workers' careers) *Esély*, 6, 89–109.

Gergen, K. & Gergen, M. (1997). Narratives of the Self. *Memory, Identity, Community: The Idea of Narrative in the Human Sciences.* 161–184.

Global Definition of Social Work (2014) IASSW. https://www.iassw-aiets.org/global-definition-of-social-work-review-of-the-global-definition/

Global Standards (2012) https://www.ifsw.org/global-standards/

Győri P. (2014). Néhány szubjektív gondolat a szociális szakmáról.(*Some subjective thoughts on the social profession.*) *Esély*, 3, 74–78.

Harré, R. (1998). *The Singular Self. An Introduction to the Psychology of Personhood.* Sage, London.

Hobbs, E., Evans, N. (2017) Social work perceptions and identity: How social workers perceive public and professional attitudes towards their vocation and discipline. *Aotearoa New Zealand Social Work*, 29 (4), 19–31.

Hogard, E. (2014). Evaluating the identity of program recipients using an identity exploration instrument. *Canadian Journal of Program Evaluation*, 29 (1), 1–35. doi: 10.3138/cjpe.29.1.1

Horváth, A., Lévai. K.(1996a) Szociális munkások (I. rész).(Social workers. Part I.) *Esély*, 4, 71–87.

Horváth, A., Lévai. K.(1996b) Szociális munkások (II. rész). (Social workers. Part II.) *Esély*, 6, 33–56.

Jones, S. & Joss, R. (1995). Models of professionalism. In: Yelloly, M. & Henkel, M. (eds.): *Learning and Teaching in Social Work. Towards Reflective Practice.* London and Bristol, Pennsylvania: Jessica Kingsley Publishers, 15–33.

Kelly, G. (1955) *The Psychology of Personal Constructs.* Norton, New York.

Kormányos, K. (2015) A szociális szakma és a társadalmi környezet – gondolatok egy vita kapcsán. (The social profession and its societal environment – thoughts on a debate.) *Párbeszéd,* 2.

Kozma, J. (1994) Milyen a jó szociális munkás, vagy ki tud démont űzni? (What is a good social worker like or who is able to fight with demons?) *Esély,* 4, 63–70.

Kozma, J. (1996) Szürke minden teória. (Every theory is dull) *Esély,* 2, 101–116.

Lefever, R. (2007). *Kényszeres segítés. (Compulsive help)* Pécs: Faculty of Humanities, University of Pécs; The Leo Amici 2002 Foundation.

Maschi, T., Youdin, R., Sutfin, S. & Simpson, C. (2012) Social worker as researcher integrating research with advocacy (Chapter 1.) *Social Work Research and Evaluation: Foundations in Human Rights and Social Justice.* Boston: Pearson.

McAdams, D. (2006) The redemptive self. Generativity and the stories Americans live by. *Research in Human Development,* 3 (2–3), 81–100.

McNeill, C., Erskine, A., Ellis, R., & Traynor, M. (2018) Developing nurse match: A selection tool for evoking and scoring an applicant's nursing values and attributes. *Nursing Open* 6 (1). https://doi.org/10.1002/nop2.183

Mihálka, M. (2015) A kiégésről – nemzetközi és hazai kutatási kitekintés. (On burn-out – an international and domestic review) *Acta Sana* 10 (2), 7–20.

Nagy, K. (2003) Pályaorientációs vizsgálatok szociális munkások körében. (Career oreintation among social workers) *Szociális Munka.* 4, 27–47.

Navrátil, P., & Bajer, P. (2018) Social Construction of Social Work Identity in the Processes of its Institutionalisation. *Annals of Social Sciences & Management studies.* 1. 10.19080/ASM.2018.01.555563. https://www.researchgate.net/publication/333399273_Social_Construction_of_Social_Work_Identity_in_The_Processes_of_its_Institutionalisation

Németh, L. (2014) Hova jutott a szociális szakma a rendszerváltástól napjainkig? (What is the development of social work since the transition of the social system?) *Esély,* 3, 95–99.

Pataki, É. (2013) *A szociális identitás szerepe a szociális hivatásban.* (The role of social worker identity in the social professions) MACSGYOE XX. Szakmai konferencia. Siófok, 2011. május 11-13.

Payne, M. (2014) European social works and their identities. *ERIS Web Journal,* 2, 2–14. http://periodika.osu.cz/eris/dok/2014-02/1-payne-european-social-work-and-their-identities.pdf

Pilinszki, A., Béres, O., Sipos B., & Ittzés, G. (2004) Mit értékelnek a szociális munkások? Mesterképzésben részt vevő szociális munkások értékrendjének sajátosságai. (What are the values of social workers? Characteristics of the value system of social workers in postgraduate training) *Esély,* 5. 87–94.

Pusztai, G. (2013). A felsőoktatás munkára felkészítő szerepe a hallgatók értelmezésében. (The role of higher education in preparing for the world of work – as understood by students.) In: Kun AI, Polónyi, I (ed.) *Az Észak-Alföldi régió helyzete: Képzés és munkaerőpiac.* Budapest: Új Mandátum Kiadó, 9–29.

Ruzsa, Á., & Homoki, A. (2015) Szociális munkások szakmai identitásának vizsgálata a Szent István Egyetemen. (Studying social worker identity at the Szent István Unuversity) *A SZIE GAEK TDK műhelyeiben készült tudományos munkák.* https://www.academia.edu/21876054/Szoci%C3%A1lis_munk%C3%A1sok_szakmai_identit%C3%A1s%C3%A1nak_vizsg%C3%A1lata_a_Szent_Istv%C3%A1n_Egyetemen. Last accessed: 24.01.2020.

Saleebey, D. (ed.) (2006) *The Strength Perspective in Social Work Practice.* Boston: Pearson. 1–24

Schön, D. (1983) *The reflective practitioner: how professionals think in action.* New York, Basic Books

Slay, H.S., & Smith, D.A. (2010) Professional identity construction: Using narrative to understand the negotiation of professional and stigmatized cultural identities. *Human Relations* XX(X) 1–23 DOI: 10.1177/0018726710384290 hum.sagepub.com

Straussner, S., Senreich, E., & Steen, J.T. (2018). Wounded healers: A multistate study of licensed social workers' behavioral health problems. *Social Work*, 63(2), 125–133. doi:10.1093/sw/swy012

Szabó, L. (2017) Szociális munkások a terápiák világában. *Párbeszéd* (2) http://parbeszed. lib.unideb.hu/file/2/596367dc68d4d/szerzo/Szabo_Lajos_Szocialis_munkasok.pdf

Szakolczai, Á. (2015) Marginalitás és liminalitás: Státuszon kívüli helyzetek és átértékelésük. (Marginality and liminality. Extra-status positions and their re-evaluation) *Regio.* 2. 6–29.

Szoboszlai, K. (2014) A szociális munka a változások tükrében: kik vagyunk, hol tartunk, és mit kellene tennünk? (Social work in the light of transformations. Who are we, where are we and what should we do?) *Esély* (3) 87–94.

Szöllősi, G. (2012) A *társadalmi problémák (konstrukcionista) elméletének alapjai. (A/constructionist/basis of the theory of social problems.)* Z-Press, Miskolc.

Talyigás, K., & Hegyesi, G. (2014) Honnan indult a szociális munka oktatása és gyakorlata idehaza, és hol tart most? Szubjektív áttekintő és köszöntő. (Where did the domestic education and practice of social work come from and where are they now? A subjective review) *Párbeszéd 1,* 1–2. http://parbeszed.lib.unideb.hu/cikk/cikk/551a4bcae814d

Tinto, V. (1987) *Leaving College: Rethinking the Causes and Cures of Student Attrition.* Chicago, IL: University of Chicago Press.

Turner, V. (1982) *From Ritual to Theatre.* New York, NY: PAJ Publications, 20–60.

van Gennep, A. (1960). *The Rites of Passage.* Chicago, IL: University of Chicago Press

Varga, I. (2008). Lehetséges-e a "minőségbiztosítás" a szociális szférában? (Is quality assurance possible in the social professions?) *Kapocs* (36) http://ncsszi.hu/kiadvanyok/kapocs-letoltheto–lapszamai/kapocs-2008/86/news

Vass, B.Á. (s.d.) *Pályatükör szociális munkások személyes perspektíváiból. Minek látszunk, kollégák?* (Reflections on the profession based on social worker practitioners' perspectives. How are we perceived?) Manuscript, under review.

Webb, S.A. (2017a) Professional identity as a matter of concern. Conference paper: European Social Work. Research Conference, Aalborg University, Denmark, 19th - 21st of April 2017. https://www.scottishinsight.ac.uk/Portals/80/SUIIProgrammes/Integrated%20Health%20and%20social%20care/Stephen%20Webb.pdf? ver=2017-11-15-164150-133

Webb, S.A. (2017b) Matters of professional identity and social work. In: Webb, SA (ed.) *Professional Identity and Social Work.* London: Routledge. 1–18.

Weinreich, P. (2004) Identity structure analysis. In: Weinreich, P., Saunderson, W. (eds.) *Analysing Identity: Cross-Cultural, Societal and Clinical Contexts.* Routledge, London & New York. 7–76.

Weinreich, P. & Saunderson, W. (Eds.) (2004). *Analysing Identity: Cross-Cultural, Societal and Clinical Contexts.* London & New York: Routledge.

Weinreich, P. (2010a). *A Guide to the Generation of a Well-Constructed ISA Instrument. Guidance for Usage of the IPSEUS Software.* Dromore: Identity Exploration Ltd.http://www.identityexploration.com/uploads/files/ISA_identity_instrument_guide.pdf

Weinreich, P. (2010b). A Guide to the Interpretation of ISA results.

Legal sources:

1/2000. (I. 7.) SzCsM rendelet a személyes gondoskodást nyújtó szociális intézmények szakmai feladatairól és működésük feltételeiről (Ministerial decree on tasks and operational requirements of personal care social services)
Learning and outcome requirements. (18/2016 (VIII.05) EMMI, ministerial decree)

Appendix 1

Results of the statistical analysis

Table 13.A1 Differences between social worker degree and other degree professionals – ENTITIES

	t	df	Asymp. Sig. (two tailed)	Effect size (Cohen's d)
Ext_past self	−.661	28	.514 (n.s.)	−
Ext_current self	−1.785	28	.085 (n.s.)	−
Ext_exploratory self 1	−1.792	28	.084 (n.s.)	−
Ext_disliked person	−.133	28	.895 (n.s.)	−
Ext_ exploratory self 2	−1.187	28	.245 (n.s.)	−
Ext_state	−1.217	28	.234 (n.s.)	−
Ext_friend	−1.863	28	.073 (n.s.)	−
Ext_boss	−2.063	28	.049[a]	.08
Ext_admired person	−2.288	28	.030[a]	.08
Ext_people	−.109	28	.914 (n.s.)	−
Ext_future self	−.725	28	.474 (n.s.)	−
Ext_contra ideal self	.238	28	.814 (n.s.)	−
Ext_metaperspective 1	−1.327	28	.195 (n.s.)	−
Ext_ metaperspective 2	−1.703	28	.100 (n.s.)	−
Ext _ideal self	−1.375	28	.180 (n.s.)	−
Inv _past self	.447	28	.658 (n.s.)	−
Inv _current self	−1.189	28	.244 (n.s.)	−
Inv _exploratory self 1	−.997	28	.327 (n.s.)	−
Inv _disliked person	.291	28	.773 (n.s.)	−
Inv _exploratory self 2	−.295	28	.770 (n.s.)	−
Inv _state	−.366	28	.717 (n.s.)	−
Inv _friend	−1.364	28	.183 (n.s.)	−
Inv _boss	−1.293	28	.207 (n.s.)	−
Inv _admired person	−1.837	28	.077 (n.s.)	−
Inv _people	.864	28	.395 (n.s.)	−
Inv _future self	.394	28	.697 (n.s.)	−
Inv _contra-ideal self	1.067	28	.295 (n.s.)	−
Inv _metaperspective 1	−.435	28	.667 (n.s.)	−
Inv _metaperspective 2	−.933	28	.359 (n.s.)	−
Inv _ideal self	−.146	28	.885 (n.s.)	−
Eval_past self	−.616	28	.543 (n.s.)	−
Eval _current self	−1.536	28	.136 (n.s.)	−
Eval _exploratory self 1	−1.916	28	.066 (n.s.)	−

(Continued)

Table 13.A1 Differences between social worker degree and other degree professionals – ENTITIES (*Continued*)

	t	df	Asymp. Sig. (two tailed)	Effect size (Cohen's d)
Eval _disliked person	.512	28	.613 (n.s.)	–
Eval _exploratory self 2	−.848	28	.403 (n.s.)	–
Eval _state	.599	28	.554 (n.s.)	–
Eval _friend	−1.039	28	.308 (n.s.)	–
Eval _boss	−.655	28	.518 (n.s.)	–
Eval _admired person	−1.735	28	.094 (n.s.)	–
Eval _people	−.068	28	.946 (n.s.)	–
Eval _future self	−.154	28	.879 (n.s.)	–
Eval _contra ideal self	−.079	28	.937 (n.s.)	–
Eval _metaperspective 1	−1.383	28	.178 (n.s.)	–
Eval _metaperspective 2	**−2.555**	**28**	**.016**[a]	**.09**
Eval _ideal self	−.631	28	.533 (n.s.)	–
Diff_past self	1.259	28	.219 (n.s.)	–
Diff_current self	.658	28	.516 (n.s.)	–
Diff_ exploratory Self 1	.863	28	.396 (n.s.)	–
Diff_ exploratory self 2	.903	28	.374 (n.s.)	–
Diff_ future self	.654	28	.519 (n.s.)	–
Diff_ contra-ideal self	−.553	28	.585 (n.s.)	–
Diff_ideal self	.863	28	.396 (n.s.)	–

[a] $p < .05$.

Table 13.A2 Differences between social workers and other professionals – EMOTIONAL SIGNIFICANCE and STRUCTURAL PRESSURE – EXTENDED

	t	df	Asymp. Sig. (2-tailed)
ES1	1.482	28	.150
ES2	−.447	28	.658
ES3	.595	28	.557
ES4	.372	28	.713
ES5	−.462	28	.648
ES6	−1.022	28	.316
ES7	.847	28	.404
ES8	.788	28	.437
ES9	−1.278	28	.212
ES10	1.401	28	.172
ES11	−.680	28	.502
ES12	.335	28	.740
ES13	−.376	28	.710
ES14	−.348	28	.730

(*Continued*)

Table 13.A2 Differences between social workers and other professionals – EMOTIONAL SIGNIFICANCE and STRUCTURAL PRESSURE – EXTENDED (*Continued*)

	t	*df*	Asymp. Sig. (*2-tailed*)
ES15	.568	28	.574
ES16	−1.361	28	.184
ES17	.285	28	.778
ES18	.311	28	.758
ES19	−.781	28	.441
ES20	.104	28	.918
ES21	.612	28	.545
SP1	1.951	28	.061
SP2	−.511	28	.614
SP3	−.110	28	.913
SP4	.532	28	.599
SP5	−.878	28	.387
SP6	−.152	28	.880
SP7	−.643	28	.525
SP8	.108	28	.915
SP9	−1.217	28	.234
SP10	.293	28	.772
SP11	−1.398	28	.173
SP12	−.286	28	.777
SP13	−1.568	28	.128
SP14	−1.625	28	.115
SP15	.122	28	.904
SP16	−1.559	28	.130
SP17	.357	28	.724
SP18	−1.321	28	.197
SP19	.983	28	.334
SP20	−.619	28	.541
SP21	1.130	28	.268

	N	#	Polarity	Emotional Significance	Structural Pressure	+ve Component	-ve Component	N	
client as equal	55	01	-1	8,57	67,73	76,71	8,98	4	patronizing and control
continuing education	59	02	-1	9,01	78,32	84,23	5,91	0	finished education
flexible about rules	47	03	-1	6,13	26,07	43,68	17,62	12	rigid about rules
favours self-reflection	59	04	-1	8,82	82,30	85,27	2,96	0	refuses self-reflection
deserving clients only	3	05	1	8,76	76,27	81,92	5,65	56	a chance for everyone
part of clients' lives	1	06	1	8,89	76,66	82,77	6,11	58	client autonomy
interpersonal relations	46	07	-1	6,62	36,47	51,36	14,89	12	societal problems
refuses research	10	08	1	6,76	41,91	54,76	12,85	49	research in pactice
externally formed frameworks	5	09	1	7,61	58,93	67,53	8,60	54	own responsibility for frameworks
respect boundaries	52	10	-1	7,76	50,79	64,19	13,39	7	help at all price
natural skills & practice	20	11	1	7,42	26,39	50,30	23,90	39	a degree in social work
free from own problems	10	12	1	7,37	51,18	62,46	11,27	49	wounded helper
perfect solution	10	13	1	7,80	45,82	61,91	16,09	49	tolerates insecurities
emphathetic	29	14	1	6,14	-2,34	29,55	31,88	30	objective
autonomous decisions	53	15	-1	7,43	56,74	65,51	8,77	6	externally controlled
distance from own ideologies	42	16	-1	5,83	17,05	37,66	20,61	16	teaches own ideologies
critical thinking	47	17	-1	6,76	39,04	53,31	14,27	12	never questions guidelines
societal catch-up	27	18	1	6,47	-3,19	30,74	33,93	31	societal changes
faith in clients' capacity	56	19	-1	7,42	63,86	69,02	5,16	3	people cannot change
spiritual orientation	55	20	-1	7,74	63,96	70,70	6,74	4	welfare and success
team player	52	21	-1	7,17	50,17	60,93	10,76	7	can count only on oneself

Figure 13.A1 Preferences of the 59 respondents.

Table 13.A3 Differences between social workers and other professionals – MAJORITY AND MINORITY GROUP RESPONSES

	t	df	Asymp. Sig. (2-tailed)	Effect size (Cohen's d)
+ve Component 1 'clients are equal'	1.866	28	.073 (n.s.)	–
+ve Component 2 'practitioners should be involved in continuing education'	–.512	28	.613 (n.s.)	–
+ve Component 3 'SW should be flexible about rules and regulations'	.170	28	.866 (n.s.)	–
+ve Component 4 'self-reflection is an important professional resource'	.529	28	.601 (n.s.)	–
+ve Component 5 'people should be worthy of help'	–.735	28	.468 (n.s.)	–
+ve Component 6 '(an SW) should become a central part of their client's lives'	–.520	28	.607 (n.s.)	–

(Continued)

Table 13.A3 Differences between social workers and other professionals – MAJORITY AND MINORITY GROUP RESPONSES (*Continued*)

	t	df	Asymp. Sig. (2-tailed)	Effect size (Cohen's d)
+ve Component 7 'the development of interpersonal relationships is more effective'	.021	28	.983 (n.s.)	–
+ve Component 8 'research is not part of practical work'	.332	28	.742 (n.s.)	–
+ve Component 9 'frameworks of SW should be formed independently of practitioners'	−1.395	28	.174 (n.s.)	–
+ve Component 10 'the helping process has boundaries and limitations'	.713	28	.482 (n.s.)	–
+ve Component 11 'natural skills and practice make a good SW'	−1.276	28	.213 (n.s.)	–
+ve Component 12 'those who have had experienced serious problems themselves cannot become good helpers'	−.083	28	.934 (n.s.)	–
+ve Component 13 'must find the perfect solution to every human problem'	−1.248	28	.222 (n.s.)	–
+ve Component 14 'empathetic'	−1.158	28	.257 (n.s.)	–
+ve Component 15 'autonomous'	.303	28	.764 (n.s.)	–
+ve Component 16 'able to distance themselves from personal ideologies'	−1.800	28	.083 (n.s.)	–
+ve Component 17 'able to think critically'	.388	28	.701 (n.s.)	–
+ve Component 18 'major task is to promote societal catch-up'	−.886	28	.383 (n.s.)	–
+ve Component 19 'must have faith in clients' positive capacity'	.483	28	.633 (n.s.)	–
+ve Component 20 'life has a meaning beyond the individual'	−.447	28	.658 (n.s.)	–
+ve Component 21 'team player'	1.031	28	.311 (n.s.)	–
−ve Component 1 'clients need patronizing and control'	−1.749	28	.091 (n.s.)	–
−ve Component 2 'practitioners do not need continuing education'	.331	28	.743 (n.s.)	–
−ve Component 3 'SW should always conform themselves to rules and regulations'	.651	28	.520 (n.s.)	–

(*Continued*)

Table 13.A3 Differences between social workers and other professionals – MAJORITY AND MINORITY GROUP RESPONSES (*Continued*)

	t	df	Asymp. Sig. (2-tailed)	Effect size (Cohen's d)
−ve Component 4 'those who work hard have no time to think about themselves'	−.454	28	.653 (n.s.)	−
−ve Component 5 'everyone deserves a chance'	.928	28	.361 (n.s.)	−
−ve Component 6 '(an SW) should promote client autonomy'	−.800	28	.431 (n.s.)	−
−ve Component 7 'the treatment of societal problems is more effective'	2.405	28	.023[a]	.52
−ve Component 8 'there is no high-level practice without research'	.209	28	.836 (n.s.)	−
−ve Component 9 'practitioners have a responsibility in forming the frameworks of the profession'	.664	28	.512 (n.s.)	−
−ve Component 10 'an SW must help at all price'	.399	28	.693 (n.s.)	−
−ve Component 11 'a degree in SW is a must'	1.266	28	.216 (n.s.)	−
−ve Component 12 'earlier difficulties in life can become an important professional resource'	.541	28	.593 (n.s.)	−
−ve Component 13 'sometimes must tolerate insecurities and not knowing'	1.780	28	.086 (n.s.)	−
−ve Component 14 'objective'	2.059	28	.049[a]	.76
−ve Component 15 'externally controlled'	.351	28	.728 (n.s.)	−
−ve Component 16 'teaches the clients their own professional ideologies'	.920	28	.366 (n.s.)	−
−ve Component 17 'never questions professional guidelines'	−.236	28	.815 (n.s.)	−
−ve Component 18 'major task is to promote societal changes'	1.493	28	.147 (n.s.)	−
−ve Component 19 '(think/s) people cannot change'	−1.597	28	.121 (n.s.)	−
−ve Component 20 'welfare and success matter'	.774	28	.445 (n.s.)	−
−ve Component 21 'can count only on oneself'	−1.043	28	.306 (n.s.)	−

[a] p < .05.

Table 13.A4 Parameter ranges for the 59 respondents

Parameter	Range	Mean	Std	Min	<Lo	Hi>	Max
Self							
s eval		0.52	0.60	−1.00	−0.09	1.00	1.00
id diff		0.32	0.12	0.00	0.20	0.44	1.00
Entity							
ego-inv.		3.89	0.92	0.00	2.97	4.81	5.00
Eval		0.39	0.59	−1.00	−0.20	0.98	1.00
	High			0.98			1.00
	Moderate			0.20			0.98
	High			−0.20			0.20
	Neg			−1.00			−0.20
splits		0.47	0.32	0.00	0.16	0.79	1.00
construct							
sig		7.45	1.92	0.00	5.53	9.37	10.00
pres		57.97	31.40	−100.00	26.57	89.37	100.00
	Pressured			92.15			100.00
	Core			65.82			92.15
	Secondary			34.42			65.82
	Conflicted			−34.42			34.42
	Contradictory			−100.00			−34.42
imp		0.01	0.61	−1.00	−0.59	0.62	1.00
ident							
ideal		0.58	0.31	0.00	0.27	0.89	1.00
contra		0.30	0.27	0.00	0.03	0.56	1.00
empathy		0.55	0.32	0.00	0.23	0.87	1.00
conflict		0.30	0.17	0.00	0.12	0.47	1.00

14 Reflective practice and professional identity

Stuart Lane and Christopher Roberts

Reflection and reflexivity ensure and enable the optimal development of a person's learning and understanding of their professional identity, and reflective practice is the cornerstone of maintaining this development throughout your career. Good communication, including non-verbal aspects such as tone of voice and facial expressions, along with the giving and receiving of honest feedback, and the ability and desire to immerse in metacognition are vital to establishing the development of effective reflective practice. Reflective practice involves an action-based set of ethical skills and is a skill which can be focussed and polished.

Reflective practice is a concept that is documented and extensively discussed, as well as being a recommendation and requirement of professional organisations of healthcare governance. The GMC (general medical council) has a reflective practice statement, which outlines the principles and importance of the concept.[1] The statement gives a positive summary of the experience of being a doctor and highlights some of the potential difficulties – 'Medicine is a lifelong journey, immensely rich, scientifically complex and constantly developing'. It is characterised by positive, fulfilling experiences and feedback but also involves uncertainty and the emotional intensity of supporting colleagues and patients. This statement outlines that the expectations should be that there will be difficult periods of a clinician's practice, and therefore an ability to synthesis and appraise the context of these periods is vital. The GMC statement is clarified further by stating that 'Reflecting on these experiences is vital to personal wellbeing and development, and to improving the quality of patient care. Experiences, good and bad, have learning for the individuals involved in the wider system'. The key aspects of this statement regarding reflective practice are that it benefits the practitioner, colleagues and patients; hence, the importance in developing this skill.

The GMC guidelines are the most publicised and discussed in the world and were recently updated in response the recent high-profile case involving Dr Bawa-Garba, a junior doctor who was convicted of manslaughter by gross negligence in November 2015 and removed from the medical register in January 2018 following a High Court judgement. This led to concern from doctors who felt that they could no longer reflect honestly, openly and safely.[2] Dr Bawa-Garba's medical defence organisation confirmed that her e-portfolio (or the duty consultant's trainee encounter form) did not form part of the evidence before the court and jury, and the GMC also confirmed that it will never ask a doctor to provide his or her reflective statement when investigating a concern about them, or ask for this to be provided by Royal Colleges or third parties. However, doctors' reflections can form an important part of a doctor's defence in fitness to practise hearings and can be used to demonstrate remediation and current safe practice.[2] This has reignited the debate and reconfirmed the need for reflective practice in a doctor's ongoing professional development.

The pertinent question for healthcare practitioners then becomes 'How do I reflect effectively?', and furthermore who decides whether the reflection is appropriate and adequate? There are many guides available for clinician to use to assist with their reflective practice, some of them are straightforward lists, and the important aspect is to avoid turning it into a 'tick-box' exercise. Koshy et al. describe a list a pertinent questions for any episode of a clinician's practice that they might decide to reflect on: What, where and who – the situation, how did it make you feel – your emotional state, why did it happen – making sense of the situation, could you have done anything differently – critical review and development of insight, what will you do differently in the future – how will this change your practice, re-enforcement – what happens when you put this into practice.[3] Although this list or personal questions can appear to be a 'tick-box' list, there is a difference. First, the question themselves raise the issue of how this impacts future practice, and second and a more pertinent factor is what you do with these reflections in the future. If they are not revisited at a different time, in a different context and potentially with a different person, then there may be no real learning. This whole process can take time and effort to improve.[3] If framed in this way, reflective practice can be seen and encouraged as part of normal clinical practice, which were the recommendations of Adams et al. when studying junior doctors who were working independently for the first time in the setting of an emergency department.[4] The three pertinent findings of their qualitative analysis with regard to the clinical reasoning of the junior doctors were as follows: (1) Inexperience can lead to 'misframing' – this refers to juniors anchoring their diagnosis using a heuristic 'system 1' approach as described by Daniel Kahneman.[5] This led to finding (2) diagnostic time outs should be encouraged – which refers to juniors having time out to consider and explore their diagnosis using a heuristic 'system 2' approach as once again described by Daniel Kahneman.[5] This ultimately led to finding (3) juniors should be given protected time for case follow-up – referring to the ability for junior doctors to critically reflect on their clinical reasoning in the presence of senior colleagues, so they have the ability to consider not just the pathological diagnosis they arrived at, but also how they arrived at it. The journey is more important than the destination, meaning it is more important that they consider how they think. Thinking about how you think is referred to as metacognition.

Metcalfe and Shimamura define metacognition as 'cognition about cognition', or 'knowing about knowing'.[6] It can take many forms, including knowledge about when and how to use strategies for learning or problem solving. Metacognition refers to a person's knowledge concerning their own cognitive processes, or anything related to them, e.g. the learning-relevant properties of information or data. Flavell classified metacognition into three components[7]; metacognitive knowledge is what individuals know about themselves and others as cognitive processors; metacognitive regulation is the regulation of cognition and learning experiences through a set of activities that help people control their learning; metacognitive experiences are those experiences that have something to do with the current, ongoing cognitive endeavour.

Metacognition refers to a level of thinking that involves active control over the process of thinking that is used in learning situations. Looking at how you approach a learning task, monitoring comprehension and evaluating the progress towards the completion of a task are skills that are metacognitive in their nature. The process of metacognition is important when it comes to the discussion of self-regulated learning. Engaging in metacognition is a salient feature of good self-regulated learners, and groups reinforcing collective discussion of metacognition are a salient feature of self-regulating social groups, and ultimately in the context of this chapter, reflective practice.

Metacognition is also one of the forms of reflection described by Hodges. Hodges described that the four different aspects may have different purposes and different uses, especially from an educational perspective.[8] The four aspects of reflection are metacognition; mindfulness; psychoanalysis and confession. Metacognition is concerned what you are thinking *about*, whereas mindfulness is concerned with *how* you think as you go about what you are doing.[9] You can be engaged in your work mindfully without attending to your thought processes themselves. Learners, who are beginning to think about thinking for the first time, will need to pay lots of attention to their thinking, with the intent to understand how they are thinking and to modify this thinking as required. As they master those alternative patterns of thought, the need for metacognitive reflection as a steering mechanism diminishes.[9] As clinicians begin to consider the implications of their learning on future clinical situations and practice, and they become more attuned with metacognition and connecting their new experiences to previous or future life experiences, they begin to move between reflection as metacognition, and reflection as mindfulness.

Schon describes this difference between immediate reflection and delayed reflection in a different narrative, where he calls immediate reflection 'reflection-in-action', and later reflection 'reflection-on-action'.[10] Reflection-in-action occurs immediately by improvising an 'on the spot experimentation', thinking and testing out, refining and retesting various solutions for the problem. Reflection-on-action occurs when individuals reflect after the problem, examining what they did, how they did it and what alternatives existed.[10] Most of us reflect in-action and share it with our colleagues at the time. All of us reflect-on-action but are usually not provided with a system to learn from this reflection. However, Schon states that reflection needs to go further than reflection-on-action and needs to go to the level of critical reflection, where one's own conceptual framework must be questioned: why did I do what I did?[9] Individual observations are laden by prior conceptualisation and interpretation; therefore, learners need strong guidance of one's peers and facilitators to truly reflect on themselves. Schon believes it is highly unlikely that an individual would be able to observe unbiased experiences, reflect openly on these, conceptualise new ideas and principles and apply these new concepts actively, without the pressure of inadequacy and facilitation through others. This reinforces the idea that not only do doctors need to reflect beyond the event, but also that it should be facilitated with other colleagues.

Reflection-in-action takes place while participants were involved in the situation and involved using analysis of observation, listening and/or touch or 'feel' to problem solve. It appears equivalent to metacognitive reflection in Hodges model. Reflection-on-action involves stepping back from the situation, meaning that it happens at some time after the situation has occurred. Therefore, it demands a time commitment, and the skills to do so. Reflection-on-action is how people develop critical reflection, but not all people achieve this.[10] The mindfulness perspective of reflection in Hodge's model appears to be the bridging-link between reflection-in-action and reflection-on-action, since mindfulness begins to link the experience to events, and this leads to ongoing reflection beyond the event: reflection-on-action.

With the theory for reflective practice and organisational guidelines well established, reflective practice is current occurring in all parts of the healthcare environment, and within all healthcare disciplines. In 2016, Fragos undertook an umbrella review of reflective practice in healthcare education, looking at the following aspects: which definitions and models are currently in use; how reflection impacts design, evaluation and assessment and what future challenges must be addressed. In a search of the last 50 years of literature, he uncovered 443 reviews of reflective practice. The results indicated that theoretical models current used still originate from an epistemology of practice as envisaged by Dewey and Schon, including elements of critical reflection, although there is currently a theoretical paradox being observed between the theoretical underpinnings of reflection and its current research or application.[11] These approaches likely indicate a departure from the original theory; however, despite this reflection is having a continuous impact on education, design and assessment. Many reflective techniques used in healthcare education have been associated with deep learning, understanding, attitudes, beliefs and satisfaction, and reflection appears to be positively associated with various learning outcomes.[11]

Assessment of reflective practice has also become a large discussion point among the academic community, and there are numerous assessment rubrics currently being used to assess refection by healthcare students and healthcare professionals. Ryan and Ryan describe the '4Rs of reflective practice': reporting, relating, reasoning, reconstructing, and the rubric scales each category on a descriptive scale of 'above expectation, sufficient, minimal, or unacceptable'. On an educational basis, this allows leaners who are developing reflective practice as to the areas they should aim their reflection, giving them a clear template to guide them, and educators a categorised template to mark them. Some educators feel that giving a clear template to learners who are being assessed on reflection can lead learners to 'say what they think people want to hear', and this is indeed a concern since the essence of reflection lies within the professional themselves, and the role of educators is to set healthcare students and practitioners on the right path, and give them guidance so that they can maintain it, as it is not possible to facilitate every person's reflection at all times. This is an intrinsically internal process that needs to be conceptualised within the person themselves. This process begins by the clinician defining to themselves what reflection and reflexivity mean to them.

Reflexivity is a term which stems from qualitative research, and within this field there are many definitions. One definition is 'Reflexivity is an attitude of attending systematically to the context of knowledge construction, especially to the effect of the researcher, at every step of the research process'.[12] Malterud outlines why reflexivity is important; 'A researcher's background and position will affect what they choose to investigate, the angle of investigation, the methods judged most adequate for this purpose, the findings considered most appropriate, and the framing and communication of conclusions'.[13] There is an assumption among researchers that bias or skewedness in a research study is undesirable. However, preconceptions are different from bias, unless the researcher fails to mention them. Different researchers will approach a study from different positions or perspectives, which can lead to the development of different, although equally valid, understandings of a situation under study. Understanding something about the position, perspective, beliefs and values of the researcher is an issue in all research, but particularly in qualitative research, where the researcher is often constructed as the 'human research instrument'.[14]

The previous examples are the definitions of reflexivity according to researchers, and it means different things to different people. However, the principles discussed should not be unique to research, and as a researcher and a clinician, I believed that I needed to define to myself what I understood by and practiced when I discussed reflexivity. By outlining reflexivity in one's own terms, it demonstrates that you understand the principles deeply, and that I conducted all aspects of your clinical practice with integrity. My interpretation and definition of reflexivity is shown next.[15]

Reflection involves looking back and thinking about an event, whereas reflexivity goes beyond reflection and deeply analyses the situation, subsequently changing future situations accordingly if required. It is this deeper analysis and alteration of future environments that makes reflexivity invaluable. Therefore, rather than being a specific stage in the research process, it should be a constant ongoing dynamic, occurring throughout the research. This makes true reflexivity difficult if not impossible.

Reflexivity is constantly challenging the obvious and making it explicit. In addition, by doing this, it will ensure that the research is honest and true, which I believe is its value and importance. Reflexivity needs to be analytically addressed rather than just simply acknowledged.

Now that we have considered the need to self-define reflection and reflexivity, we will move on to how reflective practice can be influential on, and influenced by professional identity, and we will approach this by considering a concept known as the competency matrix. The competency matrix is a learning development theory that is referred to frequently in healthcare learning, especially in the context of simulated learning environments; however, there are some flaws in the current theory that are preventing the recognition of optimal reflective practice.

The ability or inability to recognise one's limitations, and therefore subsequent learning, is described in a learning framework called 'the competency matrix', which relates to the learning a new skill, behaviour, ability or technique.[16] The framework is outlined in Figure 14.1.

Learners begin at stage 1: 'unconscious incompetence'. As their skills increase, they enter stage 2 of 'conscious incompetence'. With greater skill acquisition, they attain stage 3 of 'conscious competence'. Finally, as they master their skill, they attain stage 4 of 'unconscious competence'. This framework has a vitally important aspect. When students learn, they commonly wish to know how their learning is progressing, and this is often done by the form of assessment.[18] Awarding students marks or grades, such as 7/10 or 56%, does not give the learner any indication of what they actually need to do to improve their score if they were to do the assessment again. This is the basis of the newer paradigms of assessment such as programmatic assessment,[19] which many medical schools are developing and implementing into their new curriculums. This narrative feedback encourages students to not simply settle for a 'pass mark' and develops a desire to reflect on performance and improve. Therefore, the ability for a learner to move through this matrix requires an ability to recognise which part of the matrix they are currently situated at. Levels 2 and 3 are usually very obvious to learners, however levels 1 and 4 are not, and having two distinct ends to learning suggests that there is a very obvious beginning and end, which in course is far too simple.

Consider this model with a person learning to drive a car. Before learning to drive, many people have been in a car and sense that driving might be relatively

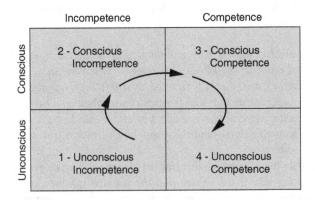

Figure 14.1 The conscious competency learning matrix – the four stages of learning.[17]

easy to do. This is stage 1, where they are not aware of how difficult it can be for the person who has never done it before. When they actually have their first lessons, they realise how difficult it is and they become aware of how unskilled they are, and they realise that they have a lot to learn. This is stage 2. As they continue to learn to drive, every step is very deliberate; however, they begin to learn, and they recognise that they are driving the car well. This is stage 3. Finally, they get to a point where driving is no longer deliberate thought, they change gear and brake automatically without thinking. They are at stage 4 and no longer aware of their own competence. However, if the person ages and loses reflexes and abilities, this level of skill will change, or even if they simply change the car and become unfamiliar with their environment.

The learning can also be displayed in a time cycle, with time learning on the *x* axis, and level of learning on the *y* axis, as seen in Figure 14.2. This model displays the 'dip' that people describe as they attempt to acquire a new skill. The 'dip' actually reflects a person's appreciation of what they know and therefore relates to their confidence rather than their knowledge, as they do not lose skills as they start to develop a new skill, although they may relearn what they previously thought they knew.

This lack of reflection for ongoing learning from this early model of the competency matrix is one of the significant flaws. Level 4 of 'unconscious competence' has also been described as 'mastery'.[20] This phrase suggests that the learner can learn no more, they have mastered their skill. This has obvious risks in the field of medicine, where disease concepts and knowledge, investigations and management are continually changing. If a practitioner does not maintain their level of skill, they will no longer have 'mastery' of their subject, and this can easily occur if apathy or complacency start to creep into a doctor's practice.[21] Therefore, this suggests that reflective practice is a requirement if a practitioner has to maintain

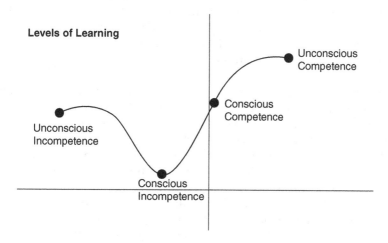

Figure 14.2 Level of learning and the competency matrix.

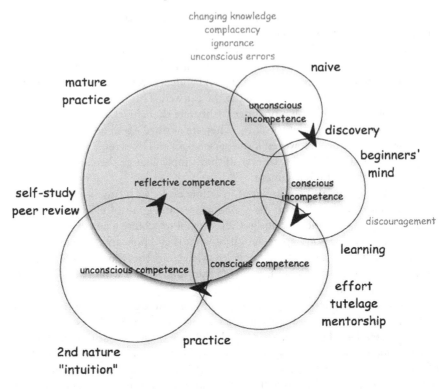

changing knowledge
complacency
ignorance
unconscious errors

naive

mature
practice

unconscious
incompetence

discovery

beginners'
mind

self-study
peer review

reflective competence

conscious
incompetence

discouragement

learning

unconscious competence

conscious competence

effort
tutelage
mentorship

practice

2nd nature
"intuition"

Figure 14.3 Reflective competence as a fifth level of the competency matrix.

their mastery; however, as stated in the previous paragraph, the practitioner needs to have reflection at both ends of the matrix (stages 1 and 4), as well as throughout the middle stages of 2 and 3. Therefore, reflective practice needs to be an ongoing process throughout a practitioner's career, always present in the background or even the forefront of their thinking. This led to the development of a more recent version of the matrix, displayed in Figure 14.3.

Regarding teaching and learning, this fifth stage of competence has been described as 'conscious competence of unconscious competence', which is a person's ability to recognise and develop unconscious incompetence in others and themselves.[21] More simply, it is described as reflective competence, as seen in the diagram. The ability to recognise one's ongoing learning needs and the accumulation of one's knowledge and application is a major aspect of emotional intelligence, and furthermore to recognise it in others is an even greater level of emotional intelligence. The link here can be seen to the two previous articles, of how emotional intelligence for your learning and that of others is intertwined with situational awareness (within the learning environment) and intellectual humility (in your rate of acquisition of knowledge versus what there is still to learn). Having learned a skill, many learners will forget what they went through to learn it, and how they mastered it – they have forgotten the theory and application and they just become functional. This has a major impact if they are trying to teach it to somebody, as they will struggle to impart knowledge if they cannot recall how they amassed it. Therefore, they can make worse teachers than someone who has good ability at the conscious competence stage.[22]

There are also another three aspects of learning that are neither demonstrated nor explained by this framework. First, while the diagram demonstrates an overlap between each of the stages of competency model, as stated earlier reflective competence should occur at all stages, in some circumstances learners are not always 'unconsciously incompetent' from the beginning and accept that they do not know about what they are attempting to learn, so they are 'consciously incompetent' from the beginning. However, in other clinical circumstances they are 'unconsciously incompetent', suggesting that their place on the competency matrix has to be related to the context of what they are learning. Therefore, the diagram relates to a specific person learning a specific task. This problem has commonly been related to younger learners, which can be derogatory as they may well be more willing to accept that they have a lot to learn, compared with a more experienced learner who might believe they cannot be taught anything new.

Second, in some cases where the leaner is at a level of being 'consciously competent', they become 'unconsciously incompetent' as further learning is attempted. This is related to the previously mentioned intellectual humility and aligns with overconfidence as somebody acquires a new skill. Reflective competence should not be considered a fifth stage that occurs once a leaner has attained 'unconscious competence', but rather a background quality that is always present.

Third, while the initial diagram talks about learners going back from stage 4 to stage 3 and then stage 2, this only occurs if the person possesses reflective competence. If they do not possess this quality, they can regress from stage 4 of 'unconscious competence' directly to stage 1 of 'unconscious incompetence' without even realising. The current diagram does not show a link between unconscious competence and unconscious incompetence for when reflective competence is lost, and this process may occur. The point at which the transition from unconscious incompetence to conscious competence occurs has often been called the 'light-bulb moment',[23] but the light-bulb might not flash in the opposite direction, going from unconscious competence to unconscious incompetence, if the learner does not possess reflective competence.

What this learning model demonstrates is that whether or not a learner is actually ready to learn may not be so straightforward. The ability to possess the correct mindset to learn links with the previous discussion regarding intellectual humility and situational awareness, whereas a growth mindset is about how you apply oneself to the learning environment once you are immersed in it, the competency matrix, and especially the beginning of the matrix, influences your ability to learn before you have even entered the learning environment. Since mentors and educators are not always present in a learner's development, it is therefore imperative that they impart the ability and the desire for the learner to develop and continue to possess reflective competence throughout their learning.

If learners have the intellectual ability and a desire to learn, and also possess reflective competence, then they should eventually develop unconscious competence – mastery. If learners start to learn, but become overconfident in their learning and their abilities, that means they have lost the ability of reflective competence and will once again be unconsciously incompetent. If learners develop 'mastery' of the process and they maintain reflective competence, they will recognise when they are beginning to lose or have lost their 'mastery', meaning they can choose to reharness their skills or not to.

Therefore, the important aspect for learners and facilitators is not just ensuring how learners negotiate the competency framework, but how they are cognitively situated before they commence the learning process, and how they will remain cognitively situated throughout their ongoing learning. To re-conceptualise the competency framework, I have developed what I believe to be a more accurate representation of the competency framework of learning. This model was developed from exploring the experiences of medical interns who had been involved in open disclosure communication, apologising for errors that happened to patients while receiving healthcare. This model addresses the limitations to the previous framework of our understanding of the competency matrix, which I highlighted as:

1   Context specific to the task being performed by the learner.
2   Learners falling back directly from unconscious competence to conscious incompetence due to lack of appropriate reflection.
3   Learners who are aware that they are consciously incompetent from the beginning and are ready to learn.
4   The place of rationalisation and cognitive dissonance.
5   Learners making mistakes as they progress from conscious incompetence to unconscious competence.
6   The concept of the learners' state of mind before they enter the competency matrix, i.e. in this study 'readiness' to apologise.
7   Contextualised reflective practice can be expressed as a model shown in Figure 14.4.

As previously stated, the mindset of learners before they undergo a learning experience is vital, and the context of this research project, this mindset was labelled 'readiness to apologise'.

I have listed a ten-point description of what this model demonstrated for this study:

1   Everybody starts off as a learner, but it must be contextualised for the task. This accommodates point 2 of the six-point list. In the case of our study, it was the ability to communicate open disclosure about a medication error with a patient or their family member, among medical interns.
2   If the intern possesses the correct mindset, which in our study we have labelled 'readiness to apologise', then they will move towards the upper part

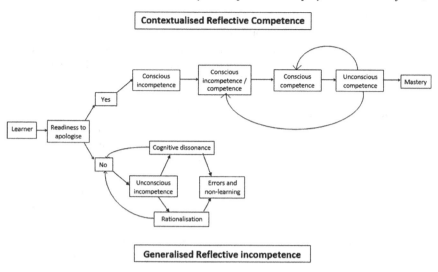

Figure 14.4 Learning model for 'contextualised reflective practice.'

of the diagram. If they do not possess the mindset of 'readiness to apologise', they will move towards the lower part of the diagram. This accommodates point 6 of the six-point list.

3 If the intern does not possess 'readiness to apologise', they will progress to the bottom part of the diagram, leading to unconscious incompetence, and they will and commit errors. The outcome of these errors will be 'non-learning', as they are unconsciously incompetent.

4 When these learners demonstrate unconscious incompetence and commit errors, they may experience cognitive dissonance, demonstrate rationalisation or neither. This accommodates point 5 of the six-point list. The result of all three is that as they go back to the NO of 'readiness to apologise'. This keeps them on the bottom part of the diagram.

5 The bottom part of the diagram is described as having a mindset of 'generalised reflective incompetence' – which can be practically explained as reflecting with the wrong people, at the wrong time, in the wrong manner or a mixture of all three.

6 If the intern does possess the mindset of 'readiness to apologise', they will progress to the upper part of the diagram, leading conscious incompetence, a willingness to learn and an acceptance that they make mistakes and learn from them. This accommodates point 1 of the six-point list.

7 As the intern progresses through the various stages of competency, they go through learning stage where they are aware, they are getting it right sometimes and wrong at other times. This is a new middle-stage in diagram, reflecting a hybrid learning stage. The previous model of having the learner at either conscious incompetence or conscious competence is too binary and

does not reflect most learners' experience of developing a skill. This accommodates point 3 of the six-point list.

8　As they develop their skills further, they progress through conscious competence, to unconscious competence, and ultimately they achieve 'mastery'. Variations of daily performance are seen, when learners who have previously attained a certain level of competency are having a bad day. This is not because the person has not developed the ability to consistently perform the task, they are simply not performing at their usual level. This is demonstrated by the arrows going backwards from unconscious incompetence and conscious competence to conscious incompetence.

9　The upper part of the diagram is described as having a mindset of 'context reflective competence' (CRC), which can be practically explained as reflecting with the right people, at the right time, in the right manner or a mixture of all three.

10　Because they have CRC for that specific task, they remain on the upper part of the diagram, whatever their level of attained competency or actual daily performance. If they lose the mindset of 'readiness to apologise', they transfer to the bottom part of the diagram and head towards unconscious incompetence.

If learners have the intellectual ability and a desire to learn, possess CRC and demonstrate a 'readiness to apologise', then they should eventually develop unconscious competence – mastery. If learners start to learn but become overconfident in their learning and their abilities, that means they have lost the ability of CRC and will then therefore lose their 'readiness to apologise' and move to the bottom level of the learning model. If learners develop 'mastery' of the process, if they still possess CRC they will recognise that they are beginning to lose or have lost their 'mastery', they will still possess the 'readiness to apologise' and will be hopefully able to regain their mastery.

In this study, what this learning model demonstrated beyond the ten-point description was that 'readiness to apologise' is a construct that is complex and difficult to define; however, it is related to certain cognitive frameworks which have been identified in elsewhere in this chapter. Examples of cognitive frameworks that might influence the 'readiness to apologise' are intellectual humility; situational awareness; the development of a 'growth mindset'; belongingness and the development of professional identity. What the data from the study suggested was that appropriate personal critical reflection, mentorship and guidance are required to ensure that learners stay on the correct level of the framework (the upper level). Since mentors and educators are not always present in a learner's development, it is therefore imperative that they impart the ability and the desire for the learner to develop and continue to possess CRC.

Therefore, the important aspect for learners and facilitators is not just the ensuring how learners negotiate the competency framework, but also how they are cognitively situated before they commence the learning process, and how they will remain cognitively situated during their ongoing learning. This shows that reflective practice and professional identity are inextricably linked and influence each other. The way in which you reflect forges your professional identity, and your professional identity and the way you view your learning experiences influences the way you reflect. What I hope I have demonstrated is that a huge amount of responsibility for ongoing learning and development rests with the learner themselves, and not with assessment organisations and accreditation bodies. It is useful to know about theory and concepts such as the competency matrix, intellectual humility, growth mindset and situational awareness; however, the most important aspect is how you personally utilise them and develop them within your own learning and professional practice. The vital personal recognition is that your learning is there to help others, your patients. Your patients are the ultimate beneficiary of your learning and development, which is why it is paramount that you start to ensure it develops optimally as early as you can in your career. This requires reflecting with the right people at the right time in the right manner, including yourself.

References

1. https://www.gmc-uk.org/education/standards-guidance-and-curricula/guidance/reflective-practice/the-reflective-practitioner—guidance-for-doctors-and-medical-students

2. https://www.bma.org.uk/collective-voice/influence/key-negotiations/training-and-workforce/the-case-of-dr-bawa-garba/reflective-practice

3. Koshy K, Limb C, Gundogan B, Whitehurst K et al. Reflective practice in health care and how to reflect effectively. Int J Surg Oncol. Jul 2017; 2(6): e20.

4. Adams E, Goyder C, Heneghan C, Brand L et al. (2015) Clinical reasoning of junior doctors in emergency medicine: a grounded theory study. Emerg Med J emermed-2015-205650.

5. Kahneman D, & Tversky A. Choices, values, and frames. Am Psychol. Apr 1984; 39(4): 341–350.

6. Metcalfe J, & Shimamura A. Metacognition: knowing about knowing. Cambridge, MA: MIT Press. 1994.

7. Flavell J. Metacognition and cognitive monitoring. A new area of cognitive-development inquiry. Am Psychol. 1979; 34: 906–911.

8. Hodges B. Scylla and Charybdis. (2010) Canadian Conference on Medical Education. Available at: http://www.mededconference.ca/assets/de%20Discourses%20of%20Self%20Reflection%20v5%20ENG%20April%202010%20FINAL_Brian%20Hodges.pdf

9. Van Gelder T. Mindfulness versus metacognition, and critical thinking. May 27 2009. Available at: http://timvangelder.com/2009/05/27/mindfulness-versus-metacognition-and-critical-thinking/

10. Schon D. Educating the reflective practitioner. San Francisco, CA: Jossey-Bass Publishers. 1987.

11. Fragos K. Reflective practice in healthcare education: an umbrella review. Educ Sci. 2016; 6(3): 27. https://doi.org/10.3390/educsci6030027

12. Ryan, M., & Ryan, M. ALTC project: developing a systematic, cross-faculty approach to teaching and assessing reflection in higher education: final report. 2012. Retrieved from http://www.olt.gov.au/resource-developingsystematic-cross-disciplinary-approach-teaching-and-assessing-reflective-writing

13. De Witt L, & Ploeg J. Critical appraisal of rigor in interpretive phenomenological nursing research. Journal of Advanced Nursing. 2006; 55(2): 215–229.
14. Koch T, & Harrington A. Reconceptualizing rigour: the case for reflexivity. J Adv Nurs. 1998; 28(4): 882–890.
15. Gadamer H. Philosophical Hermeneutics. 1976.
16. Lane AS, & Roberts C. The use of the learning pathways grid to ensure reflexivity and optimise data collection in face-to-face interviews and focus groups. Int J Qual Methods. 2018; 17: 1–8.
17. Conscious competence learning model. four stages of learning theory – unconscious incompetence to unconscious competence matrix – and other theories and models for learning and change. Available at: http://www.psychology-solution.com/confidence/competence
18. The four stages of learning – http://aucklandmagicianblog.com/the-four-stages-of-learning/
19. Wormald BW, Schoeman S, Somasunderam A, & Penn M. Assessment drives learning: an unavoidable truth? Anat Sci Educ. Sep-Oct 2009: 199–204.
20. Van der Vleuten C, Schuwirth L, Driessen E, Dijkstra, J et al. A model for programmatic assessment fit for purpose. Med Teach. 2012; 34(3): 205–214.
21. Barrett L. The structure of current affect: controversies and emerging consensus. Curr Dir Psychol Sci. 1999; 8(1): 10–14.
22. https://www.businessballs.com/self-awareness/conscious-competence-learning-model/
23. Baume D. A dynamic theory of organizational knowledge creation. Organ Sci. 2004; 5: 14–37.

15 Crisis in teacher identity

ISA guided mentorship and teacher turnover

Graham Passmore and Julie Prescott

Introduction

This chapter aims to provide three sections of text that, in turn, consider the meaning of professional identity, its measurement, and mastery of it. The opening section of the chapter considers how professional identity is paramount for student teachers and the teaching profession. In doing so it provides the reader with an overview of professional identity in teaching, considering its relationship to issues of stress, burnout and retention in the profession.

The body of the chapter describes the application of Weinreich's (2003) Identity Structure Analysis (ISA) to the examination of an idiographic ISA report of one teacher and a nomothetic ISA report of five teachers. The idiographic ISA analysis is provided to inform the reader how measurement of an individual's identity can inform a mentoring structure by revealing conflicts and stresses such that professional identity development might be impacted. Each section of the idiographic analysis considers just one or two ISA parameters. The sections terminate with consideration of ways and means whereby schools might use information in the ISA analysis for mentorship sessions that hold potential for guiding the professional development of the teacher. A summary of the ideographic report is offered that can be delivered in a mentorship session. Analysis of the nomothetic report is presented in similar fashion, but here the sections terminate with advisements for guiding the development of the group of teachers. The latter advisements say something about the nature of the teacher's professional identity crisis. The idiographic and nomothetic analyses speak to the measurement of professional identity. Further, the analyses exemplify the application of a template that simplifies and expedites the presentation of ISA findings. The analytical template can be thought of as a manual for the interpretation of ISA.

The conclusion to the chapter further explores how ISA-derived knowledge of professional identity can be applied within mentorship sessions to mediate the negative effects of high stress in the workplace. The combined approach of ISA and mentorship is also discussed in terms of professional development programmes and mentoring schemes that aim to increase the retention of qualified teachers. That is, the combination of ISA and mentorship is offered as an approach that holds potential for offsetting the perennial problem of teacher turnover. Within the chapter we examine this potential by comparing findings in the idiographic and nomothetic reports pointing to similarities across conflicted ISA constructs, patterns of identification and shifts in empathetic identification patterns. The comparison is offered as very preliminary commentary on the nature of teacher identity crises as they manifest in ISA analyses. The teacher in crisis is assumed to be a teacher in danger of succumbing to turnover.

Finally, the concluding sections of the chapter consider how the revelations of ISA analyses can be applied in mentorship and professional development sessions. They further discuss how professional identity can be enhanced and maintained through mentoring. That is, the authors argue that the professional identity of teachers can be enhanced through a mentoring process that is structured and guided through an ISA approach. This ISA combined with mentoring approach can be either through an individual mentoring or a group approach. The intent of the combined approach is to provide means whereby the mentor and mentee teacher are moved some way towards mastery of the development of professional identity. Prior to extensive testing in the field, the combined approach can only be said to hold potential for movement towards such mastery. However, pointing the reader towards this potential may be enough to move the field towards greater application of the combined approach and thus greater exploration of its potential.

Overview of professional identity in teaching

Identity is a fluid and dynamic process where an individual will choose behaviour relevant to a salient identity in a given context (Stryker & Burke, 2000). Identity theorists argue that individuals invest more time and energy in their more salient identities (Greenhaus & Powell, 2003). According to social identity theorists, identity is developed and formed via the social roles and categories an individual belongs to (Ashforth & Mael, 1989). The numerous roles that individuals hold form a person's sense of self and within these roles are expectations and behaviours individuals adhere to (Ashforth & Mael, 2001; Tajfel & Turner, 1979; Turner et al., 1987). Self-categorization theory posits that people categorize themselves on a personal level (individual) as well as a group level (group membership) and dependent on which category is salient, and it is the category that is salient that determines whether a person behaves on an individual or group level (Turner et al., 1987). Research has found improved teacher identity to be important for student teachers and retention in the profession (Friesen & Besley, 2013). Indeed, Fresen and Besley suggest that student teachers need to learn how to be a teacher as well as how to teach and that the identity of being a teacher is equally as important to a teacher as the knowledge and skills of how to teach.

It is argued that teacher identity develops and is shaped through the interactions with others within the professional context (Beijaard, Meijer, & Verloop, 2004; Beauchamp & Thomas, 2009). As highlighted, this development of an identity as a teacher is a central process in becoming a teacher (Alsup, 2005; Friesen & Besley, 2013). Having a strong sense of professional identity has been found to contribute to teacher retention, enabling student teachers to feel a sense of control and resilience (Bieler, 2013) as well as promoting well-being and effectiveness in student teachers (Sammons et al., 2007). Conversely, a lack of identity can cause stress. Any self-discrepancy in how an individual believes they are (actual self) with how they would like to be (ideal self) can cause an individual negative effects such as stress (Haywood, Slade, & King, 2006), low self-esteem (Higgins, Klein, & Strauman, 1985), as well as mental health issues such as depression and anxiety (Higgins et al., 1985; Kinderman & Bentall, 1996; Pierce, Strauman & Lowe-Vandell, 1999), as well as negatively impacting general well-being (Heidrich, 1999). Stress particularly has been found to negatively impact teacher retention (i.e. Lachman & Diamant, 1987); it is highlighted as an issue of concern for the profession (Beijaard et al., 2004).

An organization or profession is a social category with which individuals can identify, with job role being one of the most important social categories (Hogg & Terry, 2000). The more an individual identifies with the organization or profession, the more they will act in accordance to the group's norms and values resulting in stronger support for the organization or profession (Hogg & Terry, 2000), resulting in low employee turnover and increased job satisfaction (Van Dick et al., 2004). This has been found to be the case with student teachers (Hong, 2010).

Identity development within the teaching profession takes time and may involve a number of periods of exploration, uncertainty and conflict (Meijer et al., 2011). This period of exploration and perhaps conflict as purported by Meijer et al. (2011) could benefit student teachers through mentor support as expressed in the authors recent publication (Passmore, Prescott, & Turner, 2019). The authors have recently purported that teacher identity development and the mentoring process could be embedded within the student teachers' education via what we can call here as the ISA process. The ISA process involves the integration of ISA analysis into a mentorship framework. The ISA process allows for deep exploration and an understanding of, perhaps, covert conflicts that can be addressed through mentoring. Mentoring is recognized as a powerful tool in developing teacher identity, allowing for professional learning and professional identity development to occur (Liu & Fisher, 2006; Ticknor, 2014; Timoostsuk & Ugaste, 2010). Due to the potential importance of mentoring in identity development and maintenance, there is a need to maximize it in promoting the identity development of student teachers (Yuan, 2016) and ultimately reducing dropout from the profession (Hong, 2010).

In essence, an individual's degree of identification with an organization yields important organizational outcomes such as commitment, loyalty and motivation (Ashforth & Mael, 1989; Elsbach, 1999). In terms of the teaching profession, professional development should encourage the awareness of identity development and how this is shaped (Rodgers & Scott, 2008; Pleasance, 2016). Awareness of professional identity may enable teachers to deal with change within education (Beijaard et al., 2000) through reflective practice and as an on-going activity (Antonek et al., 1997). This chapter advocates further the ISA process as an appropriate support for identity development through its support and mentoring from both an idiographic and nomothetic approach, in order to help recognize and address teacher stress, points of conflict and crisis in terms of identity with the profession and ultimately help retention issues within the profession. It should be noted at this point, that there is a differentiation between mentoring for the individual and professional development for a school or group. The text beyond the analyses focuses on the use of idiographic reports for the individual. Nomothetic reports we view as being implemented in school-wide professional development sessions wherein teachers are made aware of their stresses and given the task of formulating plans to tackle them. This chapter includes a nomothetic analysis alongside an idiographic analysis simply to see if similarities exist and if they point to the nature of teacher crises. This chapter has two main functions. First, it points to the nature of a teacher crisis in general and then moves on to suggest a path for mentorship guided by ISA for individuals.

Instrument design

The constructs and entities of the teacher instrument represent a simplified version of a more complex earlier version. Simplification was required to accommodate issues of language across the participants of the Hong Kong study. The entities of the simplified version fully represent the domains of self and work, but home entities are restricted to the person to whom the participants feel closest and thus to the person most likely to influence identity formation in that domain. The constructs of the simplified instrument represent themes that research (Armor et al., 1976) suggest as being of import.

Design of the study

Eighteen Hong Kong teachers in three school (six teachers per school) were rated by their principals as 'good or average/weak'. They completed the instrument, and an initial ISA analysis was used to compare the groups of teachers according to their rating. In this work, the Hong King data is revisited with a focus on five of the original 18 who were identified as being in a state of crisis. ISA analyses of these teachers' identities are presented later. In an earlier work (Passmore, Prescott, & Turner, 2019) we made use of a template (Weinreich, 2013 personal communication) that streamlines the ISA report interpretation process. It considers core ISA parameters in the following order:

- Core and conflicted dimensions of identity
- Idealistic identification (II) and contra-identification (CI) with influential others
- Empathetic identifications for two current entities of self and one past entity of self
- Identity conflicts for 2 current entities of self and one past entity of self
- Evaluations of, and ego involvement with, influential others
- Evaluations of entities of self and identity diffusion

Idiographic analysis of one teacher

Structural pressure (SP) and emotional significance

Emotional significance: minimum value = 0.00, maximum value = 100.00

The emotional significance of a construct used in appraisal of the teacher's social world is defined as the strength of affect associated with the expression of the construct. The index of standardized emotional significance can range from 0.00 (no significance) to 10.00 (maximal significance).

Structural pressure: minimum value = −100, maximum value = +100

SP reflects the consistency with which a construct is used to evaluate entities. High SP constructs are used in consistent manner to evaluate others. They represent the core, stable evaluative dimensions of the identity under consideration. Low SP constructs are used to evaluate others in different ways depending on circumstance and context. Low SP suggests an area of stress and indecision; a conflicted dimension liable to poor decision-making. Core and conflicted constructs for the teacher are presented in Table 15.1.

Table 15.1 Core and conflicted values and beliefs

Pole 1	Pole 2	Structural pressure	Emotional significance
Core constructs			
Is straightforward with people	Plays games with people	93.62	10.00
Feels there is a lot I can do to get students to value learning	Feels there is little I can do to get students to value learning	72.89	7.29
Sides with society's disadvantaged	Sides with the advantaged in society	70.81	7.08
Becomes closely involved with students	Maintains a formal relationship	66.99	6.70
Believes there is no finer job than teaching	Believes there are better jobs than teaching	54.70	5.47
Depends on others in making decisions	Prefers to work things out alone	38.44	5.79
Conflicted constructs			
Communicates well with parents	Is remote from parents	−24.72	6.81
Takes issue with the way things are	Supports the way things are	−31.58	7.27
Deals with awkward people by appealing to everyday rules	Confronts awkward people	−38.12	7.35
Puts the needs of students first	Puts personal needs first	−84.69	9.43

Core constructs

The primary core constructs of this teacher concern: playing games with people, feeling there is little he can do to get students to value learning, siding with the disadvantaged in society, maintaining a formal relationship with students, believing there are better jobs than teaching and preferring to work things out alone. Interestingly one of the constructs (plays games with people) is subject to very high structural pressure suggesting that it is a black and white and pivotal issue of the teacher's identity. The remaining core constructs are subject to lesser but still significant structural pressure. Significant SP suggests the teacher will adhere to the behaviours of the favoured poles of these constructs most of the time. Two themes dominate the teacher's core constructs. Team player is represented by, believes there are better jobs than teaching and plays games with people. Relationship with students is represented by, sides with the disadvantaged in society and maintains a formal relationship with students. Of the remaining core constructs, the teacher feels there is little they can do to get students to value learning is part of the theme, approach to classroom management and teaching and prefer to work things out alone is a construct of the approach to problem-solving theme. The pivotal construct of the teacher's identity (pays games with people) is subject to maximal emotional significance. Each of the remaining core constructs is subject to moderate emotional significance. Two of the findings discussed before are worthy of additional note. That the teacher believes that there are better jobs than teaching suggests a lack of commitment to the job. That he feels there is little he can do to get students to value learning points to a deficiency in his sense of efficacy as a teacher. These findings speak to the teacher's potential to leave the teaching profession.

Conflicted constructs

Two of the conflicted constructs fall in the theme approach to classroom management and teaching (communicates well with parents, confronts awkward people). The construct, supports the way things are, is in the team player theme and, puts the needs of students first, is a construct of approach to problem solving. Putting the needs of students first is by far the most conflicted construct and is the only one that has high emotional significance. Moderate emotional significance is associated with each of the remaining conflicted constructs suggesting that the teacher may or may not be aware that they represent areas of difficulty.

In ISA, developing paths for professional development begins by considering ways and means to help the teacher cope with the issues that surround conflicted constructs. This is the case as conflicted constructs represent components of teaching where teachers are unsure and where, as a result, they will likely be amenable to suggestions for improvement (this is especially the case if the constructs are associated with significant emotional significance as the teacher will likely be aware that the issues represent a problematic area). Conversely, in the case of emotionally significant, core constructs, teachers are sure of their thinking and as such suggestions for change are likely to be unappreciated and resisted. To counter this resistance, ISA recommends linking a conflicted construct to one that is core. This act of connection provides teachers with more to think about than the issues that surround core constructs and thus more to think about than the issues that dominate their thinking.

Turning to how the above information could be used in mentoring sessions to help this teacher feel sure in stance towards conflicted constructs focus on the most conflicted construct, puts the needs of student first. The high emotional significance of this construct suggests that he will be aware that it represents a troublesome issue and as such he will likely welcome attempts to firm up his understanding. Begin by asking him to describe situations that have caused stress when it comes to putting his own or the needs of his student first. With this information in hand, work to develop plans for improvement and then implement the plans in later mentoring sessions such that he is guided to firmer ground. The planning process might require that the mentor work with the teacher to develop a set of rules or examples that the teacher can implement. Conversely a mentor could ask the teacher to list his issues around how to prioritize needs, and in the mentoring sessions, discussion of these matters could be used to devise solutions for implementation by the teacher. Linking a conflicted to a core construct might be accomplished by asking the teacher a question that associates, puts personal needs first, with the pivotal core construct, plays games with people. For example, can you describe situations where putting your students' needs before your own impacts your ability to play games with them? Here again the information that turns up could be used to generate plans for future mentoring.

Idealistic and contra-identifications

II: minimum value = 0.00, maximum value = 1.00
    CI: minimum value = 0.00, maximum value = 1.00
    IIs reveal a person's role models and indicate the characteristics a person will seek to emulate over the long term. CIs indicate negative role models (Table 15.2). Negative

Table 15.2 Idealistic and contra-identifications

Entity	II	CI
School principal	0.42	
Closest family member	0.42	
A disruptive student	0.42	
A person I do not like	0.33	
A person I admire	0.33	
A good student	0.33	
A person I do not like		0.67
A disruptive student		0.58
A good student		0.58
Closest family member		0.50

characteristics these people possess are characteristics the teacher will wish to shun over the long term.

The teacher exhibits significant II with school principal, closest family member and a disruptive student. Relative to me at work, the school principal is seen to exhibit superior behaviours regarding the following: plays games with people, feels there is little the teacher can do to get students to value learning, sides with the disadvantaged in society and prefers to work things out alone. These findings are targets for mentorship as they represent long-term behavioural aspirations for the teacher. However, some of the noted behaviours are not socially admirable traits (playing games with people is a questionable trait as is feeling there is little a teacher can do to get students to value learning). Further, a person I do not like, and a disruptive student are not typically admired entities. For the teacher under consideration, a mentor would work to determine the cause of deviations from the expected and then as per the other conflicted constructs work to develop a set of plans that can set the teacher along a better path.

Identity crises can be short-term affairs involving a teacher in the work of locating and coming to grips with a new set of values and beliefs. Alternately, crises can come to represent long-term issues where the teacher cannot on their own resolve the issues to hand. In the case of short and long-term crises, ISA-guided mentorship may prove valuable in locating a path forward.

Significant CI (negative identification) is registered for a person I do not like, a disruptive student and a good student. Note that the good student and the disruptive student are subject to both idealistic and contra-identification. We will compare the scores of me at work to the disruptive student. In this comparison, the latter entity is seen to do the following: prioritize, student welfare, become closely involved with students and depend on others in making decisions. Becoming closely involved with students and depending on others in making decisions are positions that run counter to the position the teacher holds for these core constructs. Mentoring here would focus on helping the teacher see why disruptive students might behave as perceived. Success in this regard could increase the teacher's ability to empathize with these students and as a result better reach and teach them.

Empathetic identifications

Empathetic identification: minimum value = 0.00, maximum value = 1.00

Although IIs represent long-term aspirations, empathetic identifications are of the here and now. Change in empathetic identifications across context and mood states reflects potential for change in behaviour.

Current empathetic identifications based in 'me at work', are closest family member (0.80), a disruptive student (0.80), and a person I do not like (0.70)

Current empathetic identifications based in 'me at home' are school principal (0.75), a person I admire (0.50), and typical artists today (0.50)

Past empathetic identification based in 'me as a student teacher' are a disruptive student (0.93), closest family member (0.83), a person I do not like (0.83), and a good student (0.75)

At work, both now and in the past, there are similar levels of empathic identification with the same entities (a good student does not appear in the empathetic identification pattern in the workplace at present) of the instrument. Note, however, the shift in empathetic identification in the home where the school principal is the main target of empathetic identification. At home, the teacher also identifies with entities that are typically admired; a person I admire and typical artists today. The shifts in empathetic identification reflect potential to change behaviour when moving between home and work. Empathetic identification with entities that are not typically admired in the workplace may indicate that something in this domain is preventing him from behaving as he would wish. Here again, mentoring would adopt the tack of using this information to develop pointed questions that uncover causes of the potential for behavioural change. The information so uncovered would then be used to direct the formation of plans for future mentoring.

Conflicted identifications

Conflicted identification: minimum value = 0.00, maximum value = 1.00

Conflicted identification references the combination of contra- and empathetic identification; being 'as' another while at the same time wishing to disassociate from those characteristics that are seen to be held in common.

Current identification conflicts based in 'me at work' are a person I do not like (0.68), a disruptive student (0.68), a good student (0.64), closest family member (0.63), and typical scientists today (0.55).

Current identification conflicts based in 'me at home' are none.

Past identification conflicts based in 'me as a student teacher' are a person I do not like (0.75), a disruptive student (0.73) good student (0.66), closest family member (0.65), and typical scientists today (0.54).

The current pattern of conflicted identification in the workplace matches the pattern that existed in the past. The suggestion is that these conflicted identifications are long-standing, that they are unresolved and, therefore, that they require mentorship.

Conflicted identifications like conflicted constructs represent arenas around which a framework for mentorship can be focussed. Negative behaviours this teacher sees in himself and in a person I do not like include dealing with people straightforwardly, feeling there is a lot he can do to get students to value learning, becoming closely involved with students, prioritizing student welfare, siding with the advantaged in society and believing that there is no finer job than teaching. Mentorship would work to explore the teacher's issues around these constructs to uncover useful places to start a mentorship conversation for future growth.

Evaluation of and ego involvement with others

Evaluation of the following: minimum value = −1.00 maximum value = +1.00

Ego involvement with the following: minimum value = 0.00 maximum value = 5.00

Evaluation of others refers to a summation of the positive and negative scores associated with each entity. Entities as a result can have a positive or negative value.

Ego involvement refers to the overall responsiveness to an entity in terms of the extensiveness in quantity (number of characteristics possessed) and strength (where the rating of each characteristic lies along the zero-centre scale) of the attributes they are rated as possessing.

A person I do not like (evaluation of −0.32) (ego involvement: 5.00)

A good student (evaluation of −0.35) (ego involvement: 4.66)

A disruptive student (evaluation of 0.00) (ego involvement: 3.79)

School principal (evaluation of 0.12) (ego involvement: 3.79)

A person I admire (evaluation of −0.30) (ego involvement: 3.28)

Typical scientists today (evaluation of −0.36) (ego involvement: 2.76)

This teacher holds all entities of interest to a moderate degree of evaluation. Ego involvement with all entities of interest is also moderate except in the cases of a good student and a person I do not like where it is high. That ego involvement is highest for a person I do not like suggests that the teacher will be more motivated to avoid the behaviours associated with this negatively evaluated entity than he will be to behave as per a more admired entity such as school principal.

Evaluation of self, extent of identity diffusion and identity variant

Self-evaluation: minimum value = −1.00, maximum value = 1.00

Identity diffusion: minimum value = 0.00, maximum value = 1.00

Self-evaluation refers to measurements wherein characteristics associated with the various entities of self (me as I was, me as I am) are compared to characteristics associated with the ideal aspirational self (me as I would like to be). They can be positive or negative in value.

Identity diffusion in ISA is a measure of the extent of a person's conflicts of identification.

Identity variants in ISA are reported in a table that places the various entities of self within an identity variant category according to their combination of self-evaluation and diffusion. The central identity variant (indeterminate) is considered optimal. Interpreting the table requires consideration of why and how the placement of the entities of self-differs from the optimal (Figure 15.1).

Me at home

Self-evaluation:	0.55
Identity diffusion:	0.25
Identity variant:	Defensive/indeterminate

Defensive High Self-Regard	Confident	Diffuse High Self-Regard
Defensive	Indeterminate	Diffusion
Defensive Negative	Negative	Crisis

Figure 15.1 Classification of identity variants.

Me at work
Self-evaluation: −0.16
Identity diffusion: 0.52
Identity variant: Crisis
Me, as a student teacher
Self-evaluation: −0.23
Identity diffusion: 0.53
Identity variant: Crisis
Me, as I would hate to be
Self-evaluation: −0.50
Identity diffusion: 0.52
Identity variant: Crisis
Me, as I would like to be
Self-evaluation: 1.00
Identity diffusion: 0.40
Identity variant: Confident

Most of the teacher's identity variants fall within the crisis cell of Figure 15.2. Self-evaluation of me at work is essentially the same as me as a student teacher suggesting he does not feel he is not moving towards his goals in the workplace. He feels better about self in the home than he does at work and there are fewer conflicted identifications in this domain. In the home, self-evaluation is normal, whereas it is low for all other entities of self other than me as I would like to be where it is too high (in the confident cell of Figure 15.2). The implication behind the confident rating is that the teacher has failed to fully think through expectations for his future performance. Mentoring to temper those expectations is recommended. Mentoring to help the teacher overcome his conflicted identification patterns (along the lines described in the text previously) is also recommended to increase his self-evaluation and thereby move his identity variants towards the desired indeterminant cell of Figure 15.2.

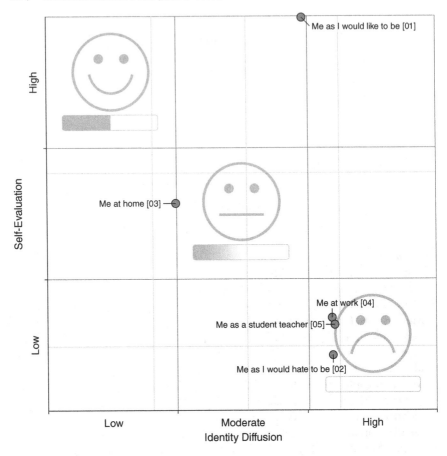

Figure 15.2 Identity variant summary of the five teachers in crisis.

Nomothetic analysis of five teachers

Structural pressure (SP) and emotional significance

Refer to Table 15.3.

Table 15.3 Core and conflicted values and beliefs of the nomothetic analysis

Pole 1	Pole 2	Structural pressure	Emotional significance
Core constructs			
Believes there is no finer job than teaching	Believes there are better jobs than teaching	35.29	7.29
Is straightforward with people	Plays games with people	28.08	7.71

(*Continued*)

Table 15.3 Core and conflicted values and beliefs of the nomothetic analysis (*Continued*)

Pole 1	Pole 2	Structural pressure	Emotional significance
Feels there is a lot I can do to get students to value learning	Feels there is little I can do to get students to value learning	25.09	7.27
Follows a firm agenda when dealing with difficulties	Deals with difficulties creatively	19.79	7.95
Becomes closely involved with students	Maintains a formal relationship	14.82	7.38
Conflicted constructs			
Depends on others in making decisions	Prefers to work things out alone	3.25	5.03
Sides with society's disadvantaged	Sides with the advantaged in society	2.81	6.81
Puts the needs of students first	Puts personal needs first	−26.39	8.44

Core constructs

The primary core constructs of the five teachers in crisis concern: believing there are better jobs than teaching, playing games with people, feeling there is little they can do to get students to value learning, dealing with difficulties creatively, and maintaining a formal relationship with students. Interestingly, all the listed constructs are subject to moderate structural pressure and are in fact secondary constructs for the teachers. The lower SP suggests that the teachers will not adhere strictly to the behaviours of the favoured poles. Two themes dominate the teachers 'core' constructs. Team player is represented by believes there are better jobs than teaching and plays games with people. Relationship with students is represented by deals with difficulties creatively and maintains a formal relationship with students. The remaining 'core' construct, feels there is little they can do to get students to value learning, is part of the theme, approach to classroom management and teaching. Each 'core' construct is subject to moderate emotional significance. Two of the previous findings are worthy of additional note. That the teachers believe there are better jobs than teaching suggests a lack of commitment to the job. That they feel there is little they can do to get students to value learning points to a deficiency in their sense of efficacy as teachers. The latter two findings speak to the teachers' potential to leave the teaching profession. The latter two findings were also present in the ISA analysis of the individual teacher in crisis.

Conflicted constructs

Most of the conflicted constructs fall in the theme relationship with students (sides with the advantaged in society and puts the needs of students first). The construct prefers to work things out alone is in the approach to problem-solving theme. Moderate emotional significance is associated with all the conflicted constructs (puts student or personal needs first is borderline high). Interestingly, the teachers' relationship with students is both a core and a troublesome theme. That the construct puts the needs of students first is subject to a destabilizing level of structural pressure, and that it experiences the most emotional significance suggests it is the most stressful arena for the teachers.

Begin the mentoring process by helping the teachers feel sure in their stance towards the conflicted constructs. Focus on personal needs first. It is likely that they are aware that this construct represents a problem area. They may or may not be aware of their potential to vacillate over the remaining conflicted constructs given the attendant moderate emotional significance. Ask the teachers to describe situations that have caused stress when it comes to putting their own or the needs of their student first. Develop a set of rules or examples for the teachers to follow and introduce them in mentorship sessions. If preferred, ask the teachers to list their issues around how and when to prioritize their own or their students' needs. Thereafter work with the teachers discussing these matters and devising solutions that the teachers feel comfortable implementing. To link a conflicted construct to one that is core construct asks the teachers a question that associates 'puts personal needs first' with the core construct 'believes there are better jobs than teaching'. For example, can you think of situations where putting your own needs over the needs of your students reduces your impression of the value of teaching as a career? Here again, use the information that turns up to generate plans for future mentoring.

Idealistic and contra-identifications

The teachers exhibit moderate (not significant) II with the entities listed in Table 15.4. Strongest positive affiliations are with the school principal and typical scientists today. Relative to me at work, the school principal is perceived to exhibit one superior behaviour: takes issue with the way things are. Typically, raw scores associated with II reveal long-term aspirant behaviours and as such they are considered suitable targets for mentorship.

The negative identifications listed in Table 15.4 are also moderate (CI with a person I do not like and a good student are borderline significant). Relative to

Table 15.4 Idealistic and contra-identifications

Entity	II	CI
School principal	0.38	
Typical scientists today	0.38	
A disruptive student	0.37	
A person I do not like	0.37	
A person I do not like		0.55
A good student		0.53
A disruptive student		0.45
A person I admire		0.43
Closest family member		0.42

me at work, the good student prioritizes student welfare, feels there is a lot the teachers can do to get students to value learning, depends on others in making decisions and feels there is no better job than teaching. Feeling there is a lot the teachers can do to get students to value learning and that there is no better job than teaching are positions around core constructs that run counter to the teachers' preferred thinking. It may be that mentoring for these constructs holds the key to the teachers' CI pattern with the good student. Depending on others in making decisions is a conflicted construct for the teachers, and so it may also serve as a useful target in mentorship sessions. The approach to mentorship is the same as per other ISA findings. Question the teachers about the stresses they feel (or get the teachers to generate a list of stresses). Work to develop plans that may work to offset those stresses.

Empathetic identifications

Current empathetic identifications based in 'me at work', are a person I do not like (0.78), a disruptive student (0.75), typical scientists today (0.69), a good student (0.66) and closest family member (0.65).

Current empathetic identifications based in 'me at home' are school principal (0.55) and a person I admire (0.54).

Past empathetic identification based in 'me as a student teacher' are a person I do not like (0.79), closest family member (0.73), a disruptive student (0.72), a good student (0.68) and typical scientists today (0.65).

In present and past times at work, we see similar levels of empathic identification with the same entities. It should be noted that significant empathetic identification for the teachers begins at 0.73 and that some of the entities listed previously are subject to moderate empathetic identification. Note the shift in the empathetic identification pattern in the home. Note also that the teachers feel more 'as' entities that teachers would be expected to model when they are in the home (school principal, a person I admire). The shift in empathetic identification suggests potential for the teachers to change behaviour when moving between their home and work environments. The shift in empathy towards typically admired entities in the home suggests that something in the work place is preventing the teachers from behaving as per expectations. Finally note that a shift in empathetic identification from work to home was exhibited by the teacher of the ideographic identification. Just as was the case of the ideographic identification, mentorship should focus on why the change in empathetic identification occurs. Ask the teachers why they feel as certain entities in the workplace and different entities in the home. Use the information the teachers provide to guide future mentorship sessions.

Conflicted identifications

Current identification-conflicts based in 'me at work' are a person I do not like (0.64), a good student (0.58), a disruptive student (0.57) and typical scientists today (0.56).

Current identification-conflicts based in 'me at home' are a person I admire (0.48) and school principal (0.45).

Past identification-conflicts based in 'me as a student teacher' are a person I do not like (0.65), good student (0.59) a disruptive student (0.57) and typical scientists today (0.55).

For these teachers significant conflicted identification begins at the 0.61 level. The above data, therefore, suggests that the teachers' only truly significant conflicted identification is with a person I do not like in the work environment; both now and in the past. This entity is subject to more contra than II suggesting that the conflicted identification pattern is negative in its nature. Behaviours the teachers do not like that are seen in me at work and in a person I do not like include dealing with people straightforwardly and feeling there is a lot they can do to get students to value learning becoming closely involved with students. Uncovering the teachers' issues around these constructs would be a good place to start a mentorship conversation for future growth.

Evaluation of and ego involvement with others

A person I do not like (evaluation of −0.19) (ego involvement: 4.41)
  A good student (evaluation of −0.25) (ego: 3.93)
  A disruptive student (evaluation of −0.05) (ego: 3.77)
  School principal (evaluation of 0.00) (ego: 3.57)
  Typical scientists today (evaluation of −0.14) (ego involvement: 3.94)

The teachers' hold all entities of interest to a moderate degree of evaluation. That said, a person I do not like, and a disruptive student are the most negatively evaluated. Ego involvement with all entities of interest is moderate. Ego involvement is highest for a person I do not like. It is the case then that the teachers' will be more motivated (highest ego involvement) to avoid the behaviours they associate with the entity a person I do not like than they will be motivated to behave as per an admired entity. Mentorship to address the conflicted identification pattern with a person I do not like will work to concomitantly offset the evaluation findings.

Evaluation of self, extent of identity diffusion and identity variant

Me at home

Self-evaluation: 0.16
Identity diffusion: 0.37
Identity variant: Negative/Indeterminate

Me at work

Self-evaluation: −0.15
Identity diffusion: 0.53
Identity Variant: Crisis

Me, as a student teacher

Self-evaluation: -0.07
Identity diffusion: 0.53
Identity variant: Crisis
Me, as I would hate to be
Self-evaluation: −0.37
Identity diffusion: 0.51
Identity variant: Crisis
Me, as I would like to be
Self-evaluation: 0.91
Identity diffusion: 0.36
Identity variant: Confident

The crisis cell of Figure 15.3 dominates the location of the teachers' identity variants. The teachers' do not feel they are moving towards life goals in the work place as the self-evaluation of me at work is slightly lower for me as a

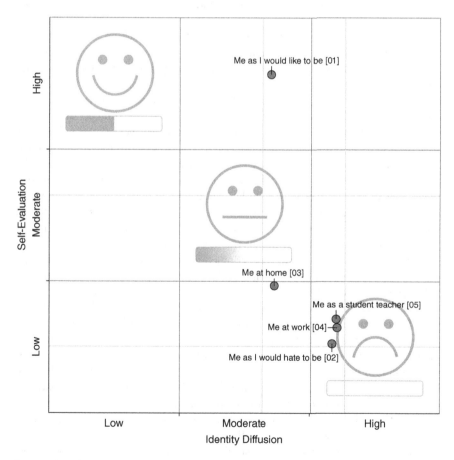

Figure 15.3 Identity variant summary of the five teachers in crisis.

student teacher. They do feel better about self in the home than they do at work and there are fewer conflicted identifications in this domain. However, even in the home, self-evaluations are on the low side. Me as I would like to be is in the confident cell of Figure 15.3 (self-evaluation that is too high). Focus mentoring on tempering expectations for future performance in the classroom. In addition, focussed mentoring by the teachers helps to overcome their conflicted identification patterns. Doing so ought to work to increase their self-evaluation and lift identity variants towards the indeterminant rating.

The nature of teacher identity crises

This section of the work compares the nomothetic and ideographic analyses to generate preliminary comments about the nature of teacher identity crises as they manifest in ISA. Both analyses turned up high levels of conflicted identification with others and attendant's low self-evaluation. Further, both conflicted identification patterns stemmed from identifications with others that were primarily contra in their nature.

Following are the fully four core constructs of the five teachers, and the individual teacher was found to overlap: playing games with people, feeling there is little they can do to get students to value learning, maintaining a formal relationship with students and feeling that there are better jobs than teaching. Given that only six constructs were core to the individual teacher's identity, 66.67% of his core constructs matched those of the teachers. That said, the structural pressure associated with the core constructs of the five teachers was significantly lower than the structural pressure associated with the core constructs of the individual teacher. This finding is perhaps to be expected given that structural pressure represents the extent to which a construct is applied consistently across the entities of the instrument (there is similarity but not complete agreement across the five teachers which manifests as reduced structural pressure). There is less overlap across the conflicted constructs of the two analyses. That said, it is interesting that putting personal needs, or the needs of students first, is the most conflicted construct in both cases.

Across the idealistic, contra- and conflicted identification patterns of the one teacher and the group we again see similarities. Both analyses present with II towards a disruptive student and a person I do not like. Regarding contra-identification, the teacher and the group exhibit agreement in being negative towards a person I do not like, a disruptive student, a good student and closest family member.

Regarding empathetic identification: closest family member, a disruptive student and a person I do not like are in play for the one teacher and the group in the workplace both now and in the past. More interesting is the fact that the one teacher and the group both exhibit drastically different empathetic patterns of identification across the work and home domains. It is suggested that for the one teacher and the group, something in the workplace is preventing the performance of preferred behaviours. Finally, regarding conflicted identifications, the one teacher and the group exhibit similar patterns in the workplace both now and in the past (a person I do not like, a disruptive student, a good student and typical scientists today). In the home the conflicted identification analyses do show differences across the one teacher and the group. There is a lack of conflict in the home for the group whilst the one teacher has issues with a person I admire and the school principal. Future work with greater number of teachers in crisis is recommended to determine whether these patterns of persist.

Rationale for the complementary nature of ISA guidance and mentorship

This section of the chapter considers the complementary nature of ISA summaries and mentorship. Mentoring has a number of personal and professional developmental prospects (Barker, 2006). Generally defined as a relationship with an individual, usually with advanced knowledge or experience and more often than not in a more senior position, mentorship actively provides assistance and support to enhance the career development of an individual, the mentee or protégé with less knowledge and experience (Kram, 1985; Hayden, 2006). It is viewed as an experience that enables individuals to bridge the gap between education and real-world experience (Barker, 2006). According to Kram (1985), mentoring provides two functions. The career development function enables individuals to learn about professions from the profession, whereas the psychosocial function to mentoring enhances confidence and competence of the mentee. In relation to student teachers, mentoring has been viewed as a key factor to their success (He, 2009), with the mentoring relationship having the potential to influence the retention of student teachers (Ingersoll & Smith, 2003), and the mentoring relationship has been found paramount to the development of identity as a teacher (Izadinia, 2013). The mentoring role for student or pre-service teachers is an important role, and the enhancement of the mentoring role and mentoring process to improve and sustain student teachers is an important consideration for research in the field. ISA can be utilized in a way that guides and supports the mentoring process, providing support for both the mentor and the mentee.

A proposed complementary application of ISA analysis and mentorship

As highlighted in the brief overview of professional identity and the teaching profession at the start of this chapter, professional identity is important for student teachers and this can be facilitated through a successful mentoring process. A well-structured and well-planned mentoring programme has been viewed that has the potential to develop confidence (Hudson & Peard, 2005, cited in Perkins, 2015) and also influence the quality of teacher education (Hudson & Hudson, 2010) as well as improve classroom practices (Hudson & McRobbie, 2004). Interestingly, mentors tend not to receive any professional development in order to facilitate the mentoring process to support student teachers or more junior members of the teaching profession (Hudson & Hudson, 2010). Therefore, there is no standard or adequate guidance offered which could result in a compromise in quality. Indeed, research has highlighted various challenges with mentorship including the power imbalance negatively impacting the relationship and process (Boz & Boz, 2006; Ongondo & Borg, 2011). Recent research has found negative mentoring experiences impinge upon the professional learning, growth and overall teacher identity of pre-service language teachers (Yuan, 2016), suggesting a need to get it right. A positive relationship whereby the mentee viewed their expectations as having been met increases student teachers' confidence. Conversely, a negative relationship decreases student teachers' confidence (Izadinia, 2015).

Recent UK research by the National Foundation for Education (Worth et al., 2017) suggests there has been a more rapid rise (since 2010) in the number of teachers leaving their school in contrast to a slight rise in those leaving the profession during this period. Teachers leaving the profession is problematic, but teachers moving schools also negatively impacts the schools financially in terms of recruitment costs, as well as staffing uncertainty (Worth et al, 2017). Mentoring can help increase career self-efficacy (Day & Allen, 2004), which, in turn, can enable professional identity development (He, 2009).

Student and early career teachers are more likely to experience higher levels of stress in terms of any discrepancy between beliefs and realities of being a teacher (Pillen et al, 2013). In turn, conflicts between beliefs and expectations can lead to identity development and or confirmation (Zembylas, 2005). The high levels of emotional labour involved in teaching has been associated with burnout and retention issues (Schutz & Zembylas, 2009), this is particularly so for student teachers (Nichols et al., 2017). In a recent study, Vahasantanen and Hamalainen (2019) explored teachers' professional identities with teachers working in vocational education in Finland. Findings suggested the nuances in the development of professional identity needs consideration at an individual level and that the development of professional identity is imbued with emotion. The authors argue for social support such as mentoring in order to support professional identity development. The ISA process would facilitate a mentoring process tailored for individual needs. The recognition of emotional labour involved in teaching roles is becoming more at the forefront of research. From a counselling psychology prospective, Hanley (2017) has recently put forward a framework for supervising teaching staff whose role involves supporting the emotional well-being of young people and young adults. Recognizing the lack of support teachers receive for emotional labour, his framework suggests that teachers should engage in reflexive activities, and he also suggests group supervision to support as well. Again, this point of view suggests there is an increasing need for teachers to be supported which we advocate can be achieved, at least partially, through a form of ISA guided mentorship on either an individual or group level.

Conclusion

The aim of this chapter was to provide the reader with an overview of professional identity in teaching, considering a number of issues such as stress, burnout and retention in the profession. The chapter hoped to demonstrate how important professional identity development is to retain student teachers in the profession. Through Weinreich's (2003) ISA, we hoped to demonstrate how professional identity can be measured and how this approach can support teachers in developing their professional identity. In particular, the chapter wanted to consider how the professional identity of teachers can be supported through mentoring, and in writing this chapter, the authors wanted to put forward a case for using ISA to guide the mentoring process. Through this guided mentoring approach, support and structure is provided for both mentor and mentee, providing both parties with a direction guided by ISA analysis. The chapter has discussed the idiographic ISA report of one teacher and the nomothetic ISA report of five teachers. This first ISA analysis provides the reader with an understanding of how measurement can be obtained on an individual's identity in order to inform a mentoring structure to aid conflicts and stresses which may impact professional identity development. The second ISA analysis enabled an initial consideration of the nature of the teacher identity crises.

References

Alsup, J. (2005). *Teacher identity discourses: Negotiating personal and professional spaces.* Lawrence Erlbaum Associates, Mahwah, NJ.

Antonek, J. L., McCormick, D. E., & Donato, R. (1997). The student teacher portfolio as autobiography: developing a professional identity. *Modern Language Journal*, 81(1), 15–27.

Armor, D., Conroy-Oseguera, P., Cox M., King, N., McDonnell, L., Pascal, A. Pauly, E., & Zellman, G. (1976). Analysis of the school preferred reading programs in selected Los Angeles minority schools (Report No. R-2007-LAUSD). Santa Monica, CA: Rand Corporation.

Ashforth, B. E., & Mael, F. (1989). Social identity theory and the organization. *Academy of Management Review*, 14(1), 20–39.

Ashforth, B. E., & Mael, F. (2001). *Role transitions in organizational life: an identity-based perspective.* London, Lawrence Erlbaum Associates.

Barker, E. R. (2006). Mentoring – a complex relationship. *Journal of the American Academy of Nurse Practitioners* 18: 56–61.

Beauchamp, C., & Thomas, L. (2009). Understanding teacher identity: an overview of issues in the literature and implications for teacher education. *Cambridge Journal of Education*, 39 (2); 175–189.

Beijaard, D., Verloop, N., & Verloop, N. (2000). Teachers' perceptions of professional identity: an exploratory study from personal knowledge perspective. *Teaching and Teacher Education*, 16(7), 749–764.

Beijaard, D., Meijer, P. C., & Verloop., N. (2004). Reconsidering research on teachers' professional identity." *Teaching and Teacher Education* 20(2): 107–128.

Bieler, D. (2013). Strengthening new teacher agency through holistic mentoring. *English Journal*, 102(3), 23–32

Boz, N., & Boz, Y. (2006). Do prospective teachers get enough experience in school placements? *Journal of Education for Teaching*; 32(4) 353–368.

Day, R. & Allen, T.D. (2004). The relationship between career motivation and self-efficacy with protégé career success. *Journal of Vocational Behavior* 64: 72–91.

Elsbach, K.D. (1999). An expanded model of organizational identification. *Research in Organizational Behavior*, 21, 163–200.

Friesen, M.D., & Besley. S.C. (2013).Teacher identity development in the first year of teacher education: a developmental and social psychological perspective *Teaching and Teacher Education*, 36, 23–32. doi:10.1016/j.tate.2013.06.005

Greenhaus, J. H., & Powell, G.N. (2003). When work and family collide: deciding between competing role demands. *Organizational Behavior and Human Decision Processes*, 90: 291–303.

Hanley, T. (2017). Supporting the emotional labour associated with teaching: considering a pluralistic approach to group supervision. *Pastoral Care in Education*, 35(4), 253–266. doi: 10.1080/02643944.2017.1358295

Hayden, J. (2006). Mentoring: help with climbing the career *ladder. Health Promotion Practice* 7(3): 289–292.

Haywood, A., Slade, P. & King, H. (2006). The development of a self-discrepancy scale for use with women. *Health Psychology Update*, 15 (2), 34–45.

He, Y. (2009). Strength-based mentoring in pre-service teacher education: a literature review Mentoring & Tutoring: *Partnership in Learning*, 17(3); 263–275.

Heidrich, S.M. (1999) Self-discrepancy across the life span, *Journal of Adult Development*, 6 (2), 119–130.

Higgins, E.T., Klein, R. & Strauman, T. (1985). Self-concept discrepancy theory: a psychological model for distinguishing among different aspects of depression and anxiety. *Social Cognition*, 3, 51–76.

Hogg, M.A., & Terry, D. J. (2000), Social identity and self-categorization processes in organizational context, *Academy of Management Review*, 25, 121–140.

Hong, J.Y. (2010). Ore-service and beginning teachers' professional identity and its relation to dropping out of the profession. *Teaching and Teacher Education*. 26, 1530–1543. doi:10.1016/j.tate.2010.06.03

Hudson, P., & Hudson, S. (2010). Mentor educators' understandings of mentoring preservice primary teachers. *The International Journal of Learning*, 17(2), 157–170.

Hudson, P., & McRobbie, C. (2004). Evaluating a specific mentoring intervention for preservice teachers of primary science. *Action in Teacher Education*, 17 (2), 7–35.

Ingersoll, R., & Smith, T. M. (2003). The wrong solution to the teacher shortage. *Educational Leadership*, 60(8), 30–33.

Izadinia, M. (2013). A review of research on student teachers' professional identity. *British Educational Research Journal*, 39(4); 694–713.

Izadinia, M. (2015). A closer look at the role of mentor teachers in shaping preservice teachers' professional identity. *Teaching and Teacher Education*, 52; 1–10.

Kinderman, P., & Bentall, R.P. (1996) *Self-discrepancies and persecutory delusions: Evidence for a model of paranoid ideation. Journal of Abnormal Psychology*, 105, 106–113.

Kram, K.E. (1985). *Mentoring at work: developmental relationships in organizational life.* Glenview, IL: Scott Foresman. 7(3): 289–292.

Lachman, R., & Diamant, E. (1987). Withdrawal and restraining factors in teachers' turnover intentions. *Journal of Organizational Behavior*, 8(3), 219–232.

Liu, Y., & Fisher L. (2006). The development patterns of modern foreign language student teachers' conceptions of self and their explanations about change: three cases. *Teacher Development*, 10(3); 343–360.

Meijer, P.C., de Graaf, G., & Meirink, J. (2011). Key experiences in student teachers' development. *Teachers and Teaching: Theory and Practice*, 17(1), 115–129.

Nichols, S.L., Schutz, P.A., Rodgers, K., & Bilica, K. (2017). Early career teachers' emotion and emerging teacher identities. *Teachers and Teaching*, 23(4), 406–421.doi: 10.1080/13540602.2016.1210

Ongondo, C.O., & Borg, S. (2011).'We teach plastic lessons to please them': the influence of supervision on the practice of English language student teachers in Kenya. *Language Teaching Research* 15(4); 509–528.

Passmore, G.J., Prescott, J., & Turner. A. (2019). *Identity Structure Analysis and Teacher Mentorship Across the Context of Schools and the Individual.* London: Palgrave Macmillan

Perkins, T. (2015). Mentoring to alleviate anxiety in pre-service primary mathematics teachers: an orientation towards improvement rather than evaluation. In M. Marshman, V. Geiger, & A. Bennisin (Eds). *Mathematics education in the margins* (proceedings of the 38th annual conference on the Mathematics Education Research Group of Australia), PP. 501–507. Sunshine Coast: MERGA.

Pierce, K.M., Strauman, T.J., & Lowe-Vandell, D. (1999) Self-discrepancy, negative life events and social support in relation to dejection in mother of infants. *Journal of Social and Clinical Psychology*, 18, 490–501.

Pillen, M., Beijaard, D., & Den Brok, P. (2013). Tensions in beginning teachers' professional identity development, accompanying feelings and coping strategies. *European Journal of Teacher Education*, 36(2), 240–260.

Pleasance, S. (2016). *Wider professional practice in education and training.* London: Sage

Rodgers, C. R; & Scott, K. H. (2008). *The development of the personal self and professional identity in learning to teach.* In Cochran-Smith, M; Feiman-Nernser, S; Mcintyre, J; & Demers, K. (eds) *Handbook of Research on Teacher Education.* 3rd ed. New York and London: Routledge

Sammons, P., Day, C., Kington, A., Gu, Q., Stobart, G., & Smees, R. (2007). Exploring variations in teachers' work, lives and their effects on pupils: key findings and implications form a longitudinal mixed-method study. *British Educational Research Journal*, 33(5), 681–701.

Schutz, P.A., & Zembylas, M. (2009). *Advances in teacher emotion research: the impact on teachers' lives.* New York, NY: Springer.

Stryker, S., & Burke, P.J. (2000). The past, present and future of an identity theory. *Social Psychology Quarterly* 63(4): 284–297.

Tajfel, H. & Turner, J.C. (1979). An integrative theory of social conflict. In Austen, W. & Worchel, S. (eds), *The Social Psychology of Inter-Group Relations*, 2nd ed. Chicago: Nelson Hall.

Ticknor, A.S. (2014). Negotiating professional identities in teacher education: a closer look at the language of one preservice teacher. *The New Educator*, 10(4), 289–305

Timoostsuk, I., & Ugaste, A. (2010). Student teacher's professional identity. *Teaching and Teacher Education*, 26(8); 1563–1570.

Turner, J. C., Hogg, M.A., Oakes, P.J., Reicher, P.J., & Wetherall, M.S. (1987). *Rediscovering the social group: a self-categorization.* Oxford, UK, Blackwell.

Vahasantanen, K., & Hamalainen, R. (2019). Professional identity in relation to vocational teachers' work: an identity-centred approach to professional development. *Learning: Research and Practice*, 5 (1), 48–66, doi: 10.1080/23735082.2018.1487573.

Van Dick, R., Wagner, U., Stellmacher, J. & Christ, O. (2004). The utility of a broader conceptualization of organizational identification: which aspects really matter? *Journal of Occupational and Organizational Psychology* 77: 171–191.

Worth, J., De Lazzari, G. & Hilary, J. (2017). *Teacher retention ad turnover research: interim report.* Slough: NFER.

Yuan, E.R. (2016). The dark side of mentoring on pre-service language teachers' identity formation. *Teaching and Teacher Education*, 55; 188–197.

Zembylas, M. (2005). *Teaching with emotion: a postmodern enactment.* Greenwich CT:IAP.

Appendix 1

Table 15.A1 Entities in the teacher instrument

Domain	Label	Classification
Mandatory entities of self		
	Me, as I would like to be	Ideal self
	Me, as I would hate to be	Contra Ideal self
	Me at work	Current self
	Me, as I am at home	Current self
	Me as a student teacher	Past self
Home entities		
	My closest family member	
Work entities		
	A good teacher	
	A good student	
	A disruptive student	
	School principal	
Entities relating to subject taught		
	Typical politicians today	
	Typical scientists today	
	Typical artists today	
Entities of broader society		
	A person I admire	
	A person I do not like	

Table 15.A2 Constructs in the teacher instrument

Theme	Left label	Right label
Team player		
	Is straightforward with people	Plays games with people
	Takes issue with the way things are	Supports the way things are
	Believes there is no finer job than teaching	Believes there are better jobs than teaching
Approach to class management and teaching		
	Prioritizes achievement	Prioritizes welfare
	Feel there is a lot I can do to get students to value learning	Feel there is little I can do to get students to value learning
	Deals with awkward people by appealing to every day rules	Confronts awkward people
	Communicates well with parents	Is remote from parents
Relationship with students		
	Sides with society's disadvantaged	Sides with the advantaged in society
	Puts the needs of students first	Puts personal needs first
	Becomes closely involved with students	Maintains a formal relationship
Approach to problem solving		
	Depends on others in making decisions	Prefers to work things out alone
	Follows a firm agenda when dealing with difficulties	Deals with difficulties creatively

16 Interprofessional education and interprofessional identity

Jacqueline Bloomfield, Carl Schneider, Astrid Frotjold and Stuart Lane

Introduction

Professional identity is developed throughout a person's life and career, and this identity has three distinct elements: in being members of groups (social identity), having certain roles (role identities), or being the unique biological entities that they are (personal identities). With increasing exposure and utilisation of interprofessional education (IPE) amongst healthcare students, all three aspects of their identity formation are altered. With specific reference to a recent empirical study conducted by the authors, the evidence suggests that their professional identity of students can be well formed and even rigidly set, long before they graduate from their respective degrees and begin working within the healthcare environment. This can affect their sense of belonging and the ability to simultaneously identify themselves with both their own profession, and with that of the interprofessional community. Therefore, the need to develop a suitable professional identity and professionalism, in relation to one's colleagues as well as themselves, is essential for ensuring optimal patient care is provided by practitioners working as part of a healthcare team. However, a recent scoping review of literature addressing interprofessional identity raised some surprising and concerning findings. First, despite increasing interest in the subject, no universal definition of interprofessional identity exists. Second, there is no shared understanding of interprofessional identity and its relationship with professional identity. Third, there is currently poor alignment between definitions, conceptualisations, theories, and measures of interprofessional identity.[1] This reinforces the notion that there is still a large amount of work to be embarked upon in the area, and our design and delivery of IPE needs to continue to evolve.

Background

Collaborative practice among healthcare professionals from diverse disciplines is essential for the provision of safe, high-quality patient care, and improved patient outcomes.[2] IPE underpins the development of future collaborative practice among healthcare students and promotes the development of a dual professional and interprofessional identity, which is necessary for effective and cohesive teamwork.[3] Universities, therefore, have a responsibility to provide a pedagogically sound education that adequately prepares students to work in a collaborative context. Historically, IPE has been opportunistic and challenging, with little consideration given to the pedagogical principles required for effective learning. Skill acquisition and the development of interprofessional socialisation (IPS) and competency require reinforcement through educationally sound strategies such as scaffolded learning,[4] yet typically IPE is delivered on an ad hoc basis. IPE is widely mandated in healthcare curricula and professional accreditation standards and is now prioritised in many tertiary institutions across the world.[5] Subsequently, educators are currently faced with the challenge of how to implement this effectively across multiple health disciplines.

IPE, which occurs 'when students from two or more professions learn about, from and with each other', is the foundation for future collaborative practice in the workplace among healthcare professionals.[6] Interprofessional collaboration is vital for the provision of safer, person-centred care and is now a global strategy aimed at improving patient outcomes.[2] IPE is widely recognised as an essential element of pre-qualification curricula across a diversity of healthcare disciplines,[7] and in many countries, its inclusion in healthcare curricula has now been mandated.[8] As such, there is an expectation that educators involved in curriculum development and teaching, in both the classroom and clinical setting, facilitate meaningful opportunities for interprofessional learning for all healthcare students across all disciplines.

A crucial component of education for students in any healthcare discipline is professional socialisation, a process whereby students become acculturated into the work-based values, norms, beliefs knowledge, skills, and roles of the specific profession in which they will qualify.[9] Traditionally, the majority of university-based healthcare education is delivered using a discipline-specific approach,[10] which although necessary for the attainment of discipline-specific knowledge, skills, and professional socialisation, may be detrimental in terms of developing the capabilities for interprofessional collaboration.[3] The development of a strong professional identity, reinforced through profession-specific education may, for example, contribute to professional isolation, feelings of mistrust towards those external to the group, and ineffective communication. Uni-professional education may also, albeit unintentionally, reinforce existing stereotypes and misconceptions about different health professions leading to poor communication and risk to patient safety,[9] whereas group collaboration in IPE enabled students to identify with their profession as well as creating a safe place to gain insight into other professions' competencies. Moreover, students could obtain knowledge about being a professional participant and could enrich their professional identity, as they were involved with students from other professions. IPE groups strengthened professional identity rather than threatened it.[11]

The recent emphasis on the importance of collaborative teamwork for safe patient care has highlighted the need for healthcare students to develop dual professional and interprofessional identities.[12] Khalili et al., who developed a framework to conceptualise IPS, proposed that this process comprises three stages. These include Stage 1: breaking down barriers, Stage 2: interprofessional role learning and collaboration, and Stage 3: dual identity development. It is assumed that, as they progress through each of these stages, students will develop the levels of trust, respect, and equal status required for effective interprofessional collaboration and teamwork in the clinical setting.[13] More recent literature from Joynes has suggested a move beyond dual identity and states that healthcare students need to develop not just a dual identity, but also an interprofessional responsibility. Joynes found that previous conceptualisations of professional identity aligned to a whole profession do not relate to the way in which professionals perceive their identities, with professionals claimed to be more comfortable with their own professional identity, and with working across professional boundaries, than junior colleagues.[14]

Cartwright et al. suggest that exposing healthcare students to IPE at an early stage in their university education will enable then to learn about the importance of teamwork for patient care and subsequently apply this to their practice in the real-life setting.[15] There is, however, limited evidence about how, when, or how best to prepare healthcare students to work together;[6] however, what has been shown is that there is a significant and consistent growth rate in dual identity found among the participants when they are exposed to IPS-based IPE programmes,[16] and early IPS of students supported their learning about the complementary roles of doctors and nurses and enabled them to gain early experiences of interprofessional teamwork.[17]

Historically, IPE within health curricula has been opportunistic with little consideration given to formation of professional identity, with healthcare students educated in discipline-specific silos with minimal interprofessional exposure and socialisation. IPE is fundamental for the development of IPS and is now widely recognised as an important component of healthcare education, although when and how best to implement IPE remains unclear. Current IPE curricula commonly develop by joining multiple activities rather than developing the activities around an established framework.

We considered how institutions should attempt to develop an IPE curriculum, based on established team-working and team-dynamic principles, and devise principles utilising the recognised and established frameworks of Lencioni and Tuckman.

Lencioni's pyramid of team dysfunction

In 2002, American management consultant Patrick Lencioni in his own book 'The Five Dysfunctions of a Team', identified what he believed were the five most important pitfalls of a team.[18] He mapped these out in a pyramid model, to allow people and organisations to work towards a successful and effective team. Lencioni begins by describing the CEO of a Silicon Valley firm, who took control of a dysfunctional executive committee and helped its members succeed as a team, and then offers explicit instructions for overcoming the five human behavioural tendencies that he says corrupt teams (absence of trust, fear of conflict, lack of commitment, avoidance of accountability, and inattention to results).[18] In order to develop the team with the aid of the Lencioni trust pyramid model, it is necessary that all team members are able to and want to work on the team. The realisation that something needs to be changed is important to get more potential from the team.[13] The Lencioni trust pyramid is divided into five layers, starting at the bottom of the model. Like any pyramid, the underlying layers must be sufficiently supported before they can be built on further. The bottom layer of any pyramid is by definition the largest and therefore needs to be able to support all the subsequent structures and building, making it pivotal to the whole structure.[18] Furthermore, each subsequent level has to also be able to support the ones above, making it vital in the subsequent steps. When this is translated to a team environment, this means that the bottom level of team function is fundamental to all subsequent levels, and in order for a team to function effectively, it is all subsequent levels and requirements that need to be established. Lencioni suggests that the pyramid model can be interpreted either negatively and positively, that is to say it can be used in a positive frame to explain how teams function well, and also in a negative frame to explain why team become dysfunctional.[18]

Figure 16.1 is the original diagram from Lencioni, with the aspect of team dysfunction within the pyramid, and the subsequent resulting team behaviour and characteristics to the right of the pyramid.

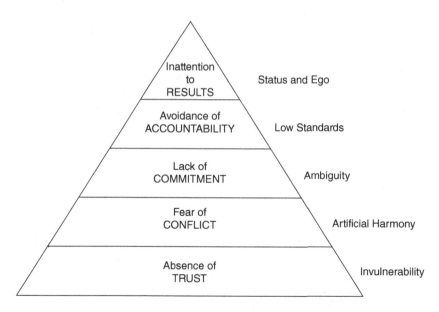

Figure 16.1 The five dysfunctions of a team. The leadership fables of Patrick Lencioni. 2010.

Source: Permission for use granted by Wiley and Sons publishing.

Level 1: trust versus invulnerability

Lencioni proposes that the foundation to all functioning teams, and therefore bottom part of the pyramid, is the ability to establish trust amongst the team. If trust is neither established nor maintained, then the team will never evolve into a functioning team and will fall apart if it had been established. He further states that the way to establish trust is to come from a place of vulnerability. He explains that showing vulnerability, admitting your mistakes or weaknesses, is the way to build trust. This is because he believes trust is a psychological state where you can show and accept vulnerability based on the positive expectation of the behaviour of another. Team members need to know more about each other, their lives, and values, making it easier to describe a team member's strong or weak points, because it is the giving and receiving of constructive feedback about these qualities that builds trust. Vulnerability also means openly admitting to any mistakes or assumptions that have been made, since openly discussing frustrations generates the need for the team to find a solution towards the issue.

Level 2: constructive conflicts versus artificial harmony

Humans are unique; therefore, conflict is inevitable, and will occur regularly even in the most functional of teams. Conflict is often portrayed inaccurately, with many programmes and courses giving suggestions for how to resolve conflict. The perception has unfortunately moved from 'conflict resolution' to 'conflict avoidance'. This leads to the deterioration of relationships and team-functioning, as the strongest teams share their disagreements openly, work through them, and emerge stronger for these having been discussed and resolved. Teams that have healthy conflicts lend themselves to dynamic and creative meetings and look for solutions to the real problem. The trust from the foundation is vital, since without trust, people do not voice their opinion for fear of creating conflict. Conflict is a good thing amongst teams, and it is dealing with conflict well that builds strength within the team. When nobody expresses themselves in the team, there is only artificial harmony and problems are never addressed. It is precisely these constructive conflicts that lead to progress.

Level 3: involvement versus vagueness

This level of dysfunction occurs when people agree on the surface but do not really commit to a decision. They do not feel safe to have their say and want to preserve harmony, with the lack of psychological safety being present because they do not feel trust within the team. Although there may be perceived solidarity within a team, this does not mean that everyone agrees on every aspect. A team in which solidarity is present takes choices without doubting, as arguments from both sides are already heard. Team members are much more likely to buy into a decision when they have had their say, but if there is no debate, their opinions are not included in the decision-making process. When group members are not involved with each other and the work of the team, vagueness prevails, leading to lack of clarity as to which course the team is on. A common misconception is that choosing the 'middle way' is the best option; however, it is more valuable to find out which aspects have priority and what the right direction for the whole of the team.

Level 4: accountability versus low standard

The most effective and highly performing teams are those in which individuals hold one another to account. When people feel uncomfortable having difficult conversations or holding somebody to account, the team won't function well. Accountability is often seen as an individual characteristic; however, the team has collective responsibility. The individual is, of course, responsible for their own behaviour, attitude, and performance; however, this can only be truly reinforced and embedded within the team if the whole team holds each member accountable for those things that the team considers important.

Level 5: results versus status and ego

The final and ultimate level of the pyramid is results. When team members are too busy pursuing their own objectives, the team does not achieve what it needs to succeed. The whole team needs to be clear about collective goals and the importance of results, which can only occur by openly talking, measuring, acknowledging, and rewarding team members for working towards them. A focused team enjoys success and minimises individualistic behaviour. In a group where outcomes are not prioritised, it will be difficult to achieve the objectives, and inevitably personal interest often takes precedence over the collective. An individual team member may seek credit for outcomes achieved by the whole group, further consolidating frustrations within the team. Lencioni states that the term 'team' is used far too often, and there are few groups of people who meet the definition of a team. He draws on comparisons with marriage: 'However much we want to work together, becoming and remaining a team requires dedication and discipline. It is just like a good marriage. A marriage is not just positive by itself. You have to constantly work for it'.

In summary working from the bottom of the pyramid up:

1 Building trust requires vulnerability
2 Healthy conflict implies candid debate
3 Commitment follows healthy conflict
4 To take accountability requires commitment
5 Accountability will lead to a focus on delivering measurable results

Tuckman's model of team development

In 1965, American psychologist Bruce Tuckman published a paper in the journal 'Psychological Bullet-in', titled 'Developmental sequence in small groups'. Previous research had shown that groups go through specific stages when they first form.

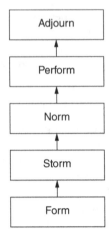

Figure 16.2 Linear representation of the five stages of team development.

Rickards, T., & Moger, S. (2000) Creative leadership processes in project team development: An alternative to Tuckman's stage model. *British Journal of Management*, 11, 273–283.

Tuckman identified these five stages as forming, storming, norming, performing, and adjourning. Figure 16.2 shows a linear representation of these stages. We will now consider each of the stages in greater depth.

Stage 1: forming

Forming occurs when the team meet for the first time and discover their team objectives. This leads to the recognition of the challenges that they will face, and the opportunities that are being presented to them. However, in this stage, team members still behave independently, even though they are introducing themselves to each other and becoming acquainted. Energy and motivation are generally high, and members usually model appropriate behaviour, however still have a large focus on themselves; therefore, the environment plays an important role to model the behaviour of each individual. The major focus of the group is focused on the task they have been set to achieve. To move towards their goal, the members of the group need to progress to the storming phase, which will mean partaking in discussion that may lead to conflict.[19]

Stage 2: storming

The storming stage is the most difficult and the most crucial stage. This stage requires the development of trust in the other members of the group. The team starts to give their opinions and ideas towards the task at hand, which can lead to conflict and disagreement. As conflict and disagreement arise, team members may start to display perceptions or expectations of power differentials and hierarchy within the group. The different team members also start to recognise the different working and communication styles within the group, and they start to draw preferences towards certain people who they feel they can work with to a greater extent within the group. The atmosphere currently is civil and positive, even though they are forming impressions and making assumptions about the other members of the team. Personality clashes and major disagreements need to be addressed and resolved at this stage before the team can progress, and there is a risk that the team may never progress beyond this stage. Team performance may decrease at this stage as energy is invested in activities that are unproductive, and the teams that do progress past this stage may re-enter it if new challenges or disputes arise. To move through this phase, team members must work to overcome obstacles and accept individual differences. Tolerance and patience are key to ensuring this occurs. Team members need to feel that they are in a place of psychological safety and respect within the team, and this allows the development of trust that facilitates healthy robust discussion.[19]

Stage 3: norming

When the team emerges from the storming stage, some degree of cohesion and unity has been established. Agreement has been reached regarding allocation of specific roles within the team, and there is a mutual commitment to achieving the team objective. The interpersonal disagreements have been resolved, and the negotiated conflict results in stronger intimacy and cooperation between team members. During this stage, the team is productive as all team members take responsibility and are motivated to achieve the team's goals. Tolerance and patience are plentiful, as team members' idiosyncrasies have been accepted and moved beyond. However, risk still exist within this stage, as members can become focused on avoiding further conflict that may have occurred in the storming phase, and any conflict that does arise can push the team back into the storming phase.[19]

Stage 4: performing

In the performing stage, consensus and cooperation have been well established, and the team is mature, organised, and well-functioning. Team members focus on achieving common goals and are motivated and knowledgeable about how to achieve them. The focus shifts away from individuals acting individually for themselves, to team members acting individually in the interests of the team without direction and supervision. Problems and conflict may still occur; however, these are dealt with efficiently and effectively. Even the most effective teams may regress to the previous stages in specific circumstances, however if the basic structure and culture has been established, they will be able to negotiate their way back through the stages to the performing stage.[19]

Stage 5: adjourning

Tuckman and Mary-Ann Jensen added a fifth stage to the original four stages, that of adjourning. At this stage, most of the team's work has been completed, and as this occurs, team members may leave or be assigned to other tasks. There is a need for recognition and celebration at this stage to remind the team of the productive nature of their efforts. If the team is fully disbanded, people can move on with positive memories of the nature of the team; however, if the team is continuing with different members and it re-enters the storming phase, then desire for the previous team dynamic can occur. For this reason, some aspects of this stage have also been labelled 'the mourning phase'.[19]

Figure 16.3 shows a summary of the five stages, with the two of the pivotal points where team development can falter, highlighted: the continuation of the 'storm stage', and the inability to exceed normal performance levels.

Combining Lencioni and Tuckman's frameworks to design an IPE curriculum

As stated earlier, IPE curricula have traditionally been developed in academic silos, and with no structure or framework of thought as to how they are placed within the respective curricula. When we consider the two frameworks of Lencioni and Tuckman, we can see the similarities that exist between the principles that ensure the frameworks are navigated and negotiated. We see and hear the repetition of aspects such as trust and healthy conflict, and the need for group not just individual commitment, leading to a combined individual and group accountability, which ultimately produces the desired results. Designing an IPE curriculum to

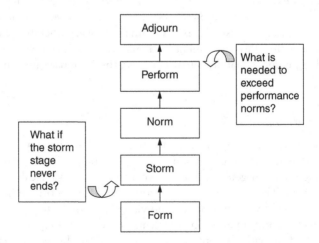

Figure 16.3 Five stages of team development, with two pivotal points.

Rickards, T, & Moger, S. (2000) Creative leadership processes in project team development: An alternative to Tuckman's stage model. *British Journal of Management*, 11, 273–283.

mirror both the development of a functioning and a highly performing team is not without logistical, political, pedagogical, and resource challenges, however with a combined recognised framework to refer to, and team desire to make it happen is feasible. The need for a highly dedicated, functioning, and performing interprofessional team, to create educational activities to develop future highly dedicated, functioning, and performing team, is not without its irony. We will consider this development using Tuckman's team development as the baseline and considering how the Lencioni pyramid of establishing functionality aligns.

The first part should be the easiest, getting the students together in one place at the same time to allow forming to occur. This obviously depends on the will and motivation of the team members and the wider team members around them to ensure the success of the IPE initiative. Meeting and greeting are typically easy with enthusiastic healthcare students, who usually have an established educational goal, which is to learn how to improve patient care and outcomes. In alignment with to Tuckman's model, progressing the students through the subsequent storming phase is the most challenging. As previously described, this needs the establishment of trust and the ability to engage in healthy conflict and negotiations. From a curricula perspective, this will require the development of pedagogical activities that both achieve this and establish this for future sessions. As the storming aspect is the most crucial, and can take the longest amount of time, healthcare curricula that try to align with this should also align with the appropriate timelines. Take, for example, a Faculty of Health within a large university that comprises numerous disciplines each of which runs a 4-year master's degree course for students. It is important that the time spent on storming activities should be appropriate to the length of the course. So, whilst the first 6 months of the degree would focus on the forming aspects of future healthcare teams, the subsequent 18 months of associated activities would focus on the storming aspects of the future healthcare teams. For teams to enter the norming phase, they commit to the team outcomes and become accountable; however, this needs to be aligned with increasing clinical knowledge and immersion, which would be in the later stages of the degree. Finally, for the team to be performing, as they are all focused on results and patient outcomes, this needs to be close to graduation, as they are preparing to enter the workforce. However, Stage 5 will occur here, as the students will more than likely complete their degrees, and then commence work with new colleagues from the variable healthcare disciplines. Therefore, it is vital that by the time they have entered the workforce, they have developed their dual identity, as both a healthcare practitioner and as an interprofessional team member.

Our own empirical research into IPE socialisation and development of a dual identity

The need to develop a dual identity in healthcare has been discussed previously; however, the way in which that is achieved has not yet been adequately addressed. Based on our framework of combining Lencioni and Tuckman, we believe that the key element in ensuring an IPE curriculum is successful for all healthcare disciplines is the establishment of trust between the team members. For this to occur, there needs to be early exposure to one's future fellow future healthcare professionals. We devised an IPL workshop involving the disciplines of nursing, pharmacy, and medicine which occurred in the first 6 weeks of their respective pre-qualification postgraduate master's degrees. The workshop was specifically designed to establish an early introduction to students from other healthcare disciplines, with the aim of increasing an awareness of each other, and promoting trust for the future activities, which would allow the storming phase to begin.

Outline of study

Between March 2018 and May 2019, we conducted a study, using a mixed method exploratory design. This comprised the administration of pre and post-questionnaires and discipline-specific focus groups. The study was undertaken in conjunction with the implementation of large-scale IPE workshops. During the first semester of 2018 and again in 2019, IPE workshops were delivered to all students enrolled in the first year of three pre-qualification graduate entry degree programmes within the Faculty of Medicine and Health at a large university in Sydney. This workshop included students enrolled in the Master of Nursing (n = 461, 45.7%), Master of Pharmacy (n = 103, 10.2%), and Doctor of Medicine (n = 444, 44%) with a total number of 1008 of students across 2 years participating. The IPE workshop, which comprised three separate stations, was developed and facilitated by academics from schools of nursing, pharmacy, and medicine and was focused on promoting IPS. Students, who were randomly allocated into mixed discipline groups of between six and eight members, were instructed to work together to complete the activities at each station. These activities focused on teamwork, communication skills, and developing an awareness of professional roles. They also aimed to enhance the development of interprofessional collaboration and socialisation by emphasising the importance of trust and mutual respect for each profession. The duration of the workshop was 3 hours in total which include pre-briefing (30 minutes), three activities (25 minutes each), and debriefing (30 minutes).

Data collection

Prior to the commencement of the workshop, students completed an anonymous paper-based pretest questionnaire. This included items about gender and discipline. Students were also asked to create a unique code that could be used to match their post-test questionnaires. Following the workshop, students were invited to complete a post-test questionnaire. Questionnaires were collected at the end of the session and matched according to the unique identification codes. The pre and post-questionnaire comprised the Interprofessional Socialisation and Valuing Scale (ISVS-9). This validated self-reporting scale developed by King, Orchard, and Khalli, which consisted of nine items with each item rated on a seven-point

Likert scale (1 = not at all; 7 = to a very great extent).[12] The reliable and validated instrument, which was refined from the original 21-item self-report measure as two short-form questionnaires for use in pre-post-test studies, is designed to measure IPS among healthcare students and their readiness to function in interprofessional teams.[12] Items sought to capture respondent beliefs, attitudes, and behaviours at baseline and at post-intervention periods. The scores of the nine items were tallied to generate an overall score with higher scores indicating a stronger belief, attitude and/or behaviour indicative of IPS and behaviour.[20] The questionnaire-administered pre-workshop included demographic items about gender and discipline. The post-intervention questionnaire included an additional two close-ended and five short response questions. These questions sought to obtain further information from the students' regarding their perceived benefits and challenges of the workshop and its impact on future work in the professional healthcare setting. Data were analysed using SPSS v. 24 (SPSS Inc., Chicago, IL, USA). Descriptive statistics (frequency and percentages) were used to describe participant characteristics including gender and specific discipline. Paired t-tests were used to compare the pre and post-questionnaire data generated from each discipline, and t-tests were used to compare groups. A p value of 0.05 indicated statistical significance. Responses to the open-ended questions were analysed using content analysis as described by Elo and Kyngäs. Responses for all open-ended questions were pooled for analysis, iteratively coded, and analysed for categories. Illustrative quotes were identified and reported for each major category.

Results

When the pre-workshop questionnaires were analysed, no statistically significant differences (p > 0.05) were detected when the mean scores of the nursing (5.25, SD 0.83), medical (5.44, SD 0.78), and pharmacy (5.47, SD 0.71) were compared. When pre and post-workshop questionnaire data were compared within disciplines, both nursing (p < 0.05) and pharmacy (p = 0.05) had significantly higher post-questionnaire mean scores. The post-questionnaire score for medical students was lower than the prequestionnaire score, although this difference was not significant (p = 0.11). When the post-questionnaire scores were compared between the three disciplines, significant differences were found between the scores of nursing and medicine students (p < 0.001) and between those of the pharmacy and medicine students (p < 0.001). No difference, however, was found when the post-test scores of nursing and pharmacy students were compared (p = 0.11).

In total, 545 post-questionnaires were completed. Reported responses from participants' regarding their overall experience of the workshop showed that the majority (80.8%, n = 440) rated their experience as either very good or good, 16% (n = 87) rated their experience as average, and less than 3% (n = 15) reported that their experience was poor or very poor. Furthermore, 64.5% (n = 352) of participants who responded indicated that the workshop had changed how they considered other health professionals, while 34% (n = 186) reported that it had not. Content analysis of the two open-ended questions included in the post-questionnaire pertaining to why considerations had changed were varied, but included responses related to the development of a greater understanding of the importance of teamwork and communication. Examples of responses included:

> *If all healthcare professionals worked together in teams, then the outcome is better care for patients.*
>
> *Female nursing student*

> *Need to rely on all medical professionals to effectively communicate.*
>
> *Male medical student*

Participants also remarked on how the IPE workshop had led to their increased awareness of the breadth of roles of their colleagues, examples being:

> *It gave me a better understanding of differences in roles and showed me how holistically nursing students think compared to some others.*
>
> *Female pharmacy student*

> *It changed my perception of pharmacists as pill-retailers and pencil-pushers. They are actually a very important part of patient contact with crucial responsibilities.*
>
> *Female medical student*

Some students reported that the IPE workshop had a positive effect on dispelling professional healthcare stereotypes that are often portrayed and reinforced within general society. These included traditional hierarchies and gender-based roles. For example:

> *It gave me a better understanding of differences in roles and showed me how holistically nursing students think compared to some others.*
>
> *Female pharmacy student*

> *It changed my perception of pharmacists as pill-retailers and pencil-pushers. They are actually a very important part of patient contact with crucial responsibilities.*
>
> *Female nursing student*

> *I thought that medical students would try to be 'know-it-alls' and assert their hierarchy, but I was wrong.*
>
> *Female nursing student*

However, contrary to this, other responses from students highlighted the perceived sense of dominance of the medical students that reinforced these long-held hierarchal stereotypes. For example:

> *Assertion of professional dominance was much more prominent than expected.*
>
> *Female nursing student*

I felt that medical students still held themselves as the leaders of the group which is not always ideal in the workplace as they do not hold all the expertise.

Female nursing student

I didn't expect the nursing students to respect me by default- was a bit odd.

Female medical student

Responses pertaining to what they had learned align with the important elements of collaborative practice including the importance of teamwork, shared understanding and mutual respect and effective communication. For example:

To work as a team and build on each other's strengths and weaknesses.

Male nursing student

The value of all healthcare professionals in the healthcare system and their role in patient-centred care.

Male medical student

Understanding that most professionals are aware of their abilities and that interdisciplinary communication is welcome.

Female nursing student

Discussion of study

Teamwork and collaborative practice are the cornerstone of high-quality patient care, and it is imperative that healthcare students from all disciplines receive adequate preparation for these roles through educational opportunities that facilitate IPS. The aim of this study was to examine the effect of a large-scale interprofessional workshop on IPS in first year nursing, pharmacy, and medicine students. Findings revealed that the majority of students rated the workshop positively and reported that it had changed their views of other health professionals. This finding provides evidence of the perceived educational value of the workshop by students and supports the notion that healthcare students should be exposed to IPE early stage in their university education.[12] Providing opportunities for students from different health disciplines to mix and socialise from the beginning of their studies may facilitate the development of role understanding clear communication, and mutual respect, all of which are fundamental requisites for effective collaborative practice.

The ISVS-9 was used to measure changes pre and post-workshop in the beliefs, behaviours, and attitudes that underpin IPS and findings were mixed. Interestingly, nursing students started with lower pretest scores than both the medicine and pharmacy students, yet their scores increased significantly following the IPE workshop. This is a positive finding in that nurses represent the largest sector of the professional healthcare workforce, and subsequently play a considerable role in the provision of patient care (reference). Findings showed an improvement in attitudes of the nursing students towards students in other disciplines. This may demonstrate the value of IPE for nursing students for the development of confidence, assertiveness, and a positive attitude towards teamwork. Participation in IPE may assist nursing students to prepare for more effective communication and teamwork with students from other health professions, thereby enhancing their future contribution to collaborative patient care.[21] This is especially pertinent in light of historical stereotypes and hierarchies that have been associated with the medical profession and traditional unequitable team membership.[22]

An unexpected study finding were the lower scores achieved by the medical students on the ISVS-9 scale following the interprofessional workshop. Although this difference was not significant and may be related to the comparatively small number of medical students, compared with others, it is noteworthy. A possible explanation for this was that the medical students had an important assessment due at the time the IPE workshop was run, which may have influenced its perceived value. This emphasises the importance of timing of IPE activities to ensure that all students are able to attend and engage without distraction of other commitments.

Patient safety is a major priority within healthcare systems globally, and IPE is now widely recognised as the cornerstone for the IPS and development of team working skills required for future collaborative practice among healthcare professionals. As IPE is now a mandatory component of many healthcare curricula, it must be delivered and implemented based on sound pedagogical principles. Attitudes are resistant to change and skill development requires reinforcement. Utilising a spiral approach to curriculum development may be a way to, therefore deemed an appropriate way, to incorporate IPE into healthcare courses. Developed originally by Bruner, a spiral curriculum provides the opportunity for students to learn through 'reiterative revisiting of topics, subjects or themes throughout the course'.[23] Through this approach to learning, students progressively build upon previously acquired knowledge, deepening their knowledge with each subsequent encounter.[24] Introducing IPE activities at an early stage of their healthcare education, as was done in this study, provides opportunities for the initial development of IPS among healthcare students. Importantly, it would also provide the foundation from which deeper concepts related to teamwork and collaborative practice, utilising known teamworking frameworks such a Lencioni's pyramid of team dysfunction and Tuckman's framework of team formation, allowing more complex IPE opportunities to be scaffolded over time.[25]

Summary of chapter

To overcome the difficulty of IPE curricula being developed in academic silos, we constructed a pedagogical and philosophical framework that combined Lencioni's five-level model of team function with Tuckman's model of five stages of team formation, to better understand how IPE teams could be more effectively formed and developed. By recognising the five stages at which a team develops, we recognised that we could design new activities that ensured student interaction allowing the five stages of team development: forming, storming, norming, performing and adjourning. Furthermore, by recognising the five levels at which teams can become dysfunctional, we aligned the current and new activities with developing student awareness and learning of these levels, ensuring learning outcomes were avoidance of these problems. We developed this framework based on findings from our own empirical research that demonstrated the development of a dual professional and interprofessional identity, as well as reinforcing the notion of interprofessional responsibility, as essential parts of learning to become a healthcare professional with the ability to engage in collaborative practice. Collaborative practice among healthcare professionals requires effective teamwork, which is predicated on students in different disciplines learning together to develop trust, respect, and an understanding of each other's roles. Innovative ways to implement and deliver IPE are therefore essential.

References

1. Tong, R., Brewer, M., Flavell, H., & Roberts, L. D. (2020) Professional and interprofessional identities: A scoping review. *Journal of Interprofessional Care*. DOI: 10.1080/13561820.2020.1713063.
2. World Health Organization (2010). *Global Status Report on Noncommunicable Diseases 2010*. Geneva: World Health Organization. http://www.who.int/nmh/publications/ncd_report_full_en.pdf.
3. Lockeman, K. S., Appelbaum, N. P., Dow, A. W., Orr, S., Huff, T. A., Hogan, C. J., & Queen, B. A. (2017) The effect of an interprofessional simulation-based education program on perceptions and stereotypes of nursing and medical students: A quasi-experimental study. *Nurse Education Today*, 58, 32–37.
4. Thislethwaite, J. E. (2015) Interprofessional education and the basic sciences: Rational and outcomes. *Anatomical Science Education*, 8(4), 299–304.
5. Zook, S. S., Hulton, L. J., Dudding, C. C, Stewart, A. L., & Graham, A. C. (2018) Scaffolding interprofessional education: Unfolding case studies, virtual world simulations and patient-centred care. *Nurse Educator*, 43(2), 87–91.
6. Stehlik, P., Frotjold, A., & Schneider, C. R. (2018) Effect of hospital simulation tutorials on nursing and pharmacy student perception of interprofessional collaboration: Findings from a pilot study. *Journal of Interprofessional Care*, 32(1), 115–117.
7. Reid, A. M., Fielden, S. A., Holt, J., Maclean, J., & Quinton, N. D. (2018) Learning from interprofessional education: A cautionary tale. *Nurse Education Today*, 69, 63–71.
8. Dematteo, D. J., & Reeves, S. (2013) Introducing first year students to interprofessionalism: Exploring professional identity in the "enterprise culture": A Foucauldian analysis. *Journal of Interprofessional Care*, 27(1), 27–33.
9. Khalili, H., Orchard, C., Spence Laschinger, H. S., & Farah, R. (2013) An interprofessional socialization framework for developing an interprofessional identity among health professions students. *Journal of Interprofessional Care*, 27(6), 448–453.
10. Lapkin, S., Levvett-Jones, T., & Gilligan, C. (2013) A systematic review of the effectiveness of interprofessional education in health professional programs. *Nurse Education Today*, 33, 90–102.

11. Haugland, M., Brenna, S. J., & Aanes, M. M. (2019) Interprofessional education as a contributor to professional and interprofessional identities. *Journal of Interprofessional Care*. DOI: 10.1080/13561820.2019.1693354.

12. King, G., Orchard, C., Khalili, H., & Avery, L. (2016) Refinement of the interprofessional socialization and valuing scale (ISVS-21) and development of 9-item equivalent versions. *Journal of Continuing Education in the Health Professions*, 36(3), 171–177.

13. Stanley, K., & Stanley, D. (2019) The HEIPS framework: Scaffolding interprofessional education starts with health professional educators. *Nurse Education in Practice*, 34, 63–71.

14. Joynes, V. C. T. (2018) Defining and understanding the relationship between professional identity and interprofessional responsibility: Implications for educating health and social care students. *Advances in Health Sciences Education: Theory and Practice*, 23(1), 133–149.

15. Cartwright, J., Franklin, D., Forman, D., & Freegard, H. (2015) Promoting collaborative dementia care via online interprofessional education. *Australasian Journal of Ageing*, 34(2), 88–94.

16. Khalili, H., & Orchard, C. (2020) The effects of an IPS-based IPE program on interprofessional socialization and dual identity development. *Journal of Interprofessional Care*. DOI: 10.1080/13561820.2019.1709427.

17. Arnold, C., Berger, S., Gronewold, N., Schwabe, D. et al. (2020) Exploring early interprofessional socialization: A pilot study of student's experiences in medical history taking. *Journal of Interprofessional Care*. DOI: 10.1080/13561820.2019.1708872.

18. Lencioni, P. (2002) *The Five Dysfunctions of a Team*. New York: Wiley Publishing.

19. Tuckman, B. W. (1965) Developmental sequence in small groups. *Psychological Bulletin*, 63(6), 384–399.

20. King, G., Shaw, L., Orchard, C. A., & Miller S. (2010) The Interprofessional Socialisation and Valuing Scale: A tool for evaluating the shift towards collaborative care approaches in health care settings. *Work*, 35, 77–85.

21. Wong, A. K. C., Wong, F. K. Y., Chan, L. K., Chan, N., Ganotice, A., & Ho, J. (2017) The effect of interprofessional team-based learning among nursing students: A quasi-experimental stud. *Nurse Education Today*, 53, 13–18.

22. Meleis, A. I. (2016) Interprofessional education: A summary of reports and barriers to recommendations. *Journal of Nursing Scholarship*, 48(1), 106–112.

23. Harden, R. M., & Stamper, N. (1999) What is a spiral curriculum? *Medical Teacher*, 21(2), 141–143.

24. Masters, K., & Gibbs, T. (2007) The spiral curriculum: Implications for online learning. *BMC Medical Education*, 7, 52. DOI: 10.1186-1472-6920-7-52.

25. Shrader, S., Hodgkins, R., Laverentz, D., Zaudke, J., et al. (2016). Interprofessional Education and Practice Guide No. 7: Development, implementation, and evaluation of a large-scale required interprofessional foundational programme. *Journal of Interprofessional Care*, 30(5), 615–619.

17 Psychometric measurement of professional identity through values in nursing and medicine

Roger Ellis and Elaine Hogard

Introduction

Measuring Professional Identity is a central theme of this book, and its importance is discussed in the first chapter. First, it is important that a potentially nebulous concept such as Professional Identity should be grounded in some way in observable actions and events. The more precisely these events can be described the better, and ultimately this points to some form of measurement. Second, if the professional training curriculum claims to develop professional identity, then it will be necessary to operationalise and assess this, and this again points to some valid and reliable from of measurement.

In this book, we have covered three approaches to measuring professional identity: observational methods, consultative methods and psychometric methods. This chapter is concerned with the psychometric measurement of professional identity and values or rather a specific method using Identity Structure Analysis (ISA), and its associated measurement approach Ipseus. So first we outline the theoretical and psychometric basis of ISA/Ipseus. Then we give an example of its use in Nursing to develop an instrument called Nurse Match (NM). NM is described in detail and its evaluation summarised. Finally, we describe a potential use in Medicine to develop Medi Match (MM). This project is underway, and we describe progress to date.

Our interest in the measurement of professional identity led us to review the methods available for the measurement of identity in general to see how these might be applied to professional identity. Having surveyed over 50 reports of identity measurement (Passmore, Ellis, & Hogard, 2014), we chose Weinreich's ISA/Ipseus approach (Weinreich and Saunderson, 2012) for several reasons. First, his theory is, in part, a synthesis of three major theoretical perspectives, namely Erikson (1968), Kelly (1955) and Festinger (1957). Second, the linked software, Ipseus, is a framework software; rather than being a dedicated instrument in itself, it provides a basis for developing customised instruments appropriate for particular applications. Third, ISA/Ipseus is theory-based and its reports relate to key identity parameters from ISA, which in its turn draws on major theoretical perspectives regarding identity. Fourth, it is highly functional in that it not only facilitates the development of customised instruments but also presents the instrument to respondents in an attractive onscreen fashion, records and analyses their responses and produces a report regarding key identity parameters. Fifth, its reports can be used to test hypotheses or offer quantified comparisons of candidates with an ideal.

An Ipseus instrument is a form of questionnaire and requires respondents to apply a number of bipolar constructs representing ways of thinking and values to a number of entities that are significant persons in the relevant social environment and also aspects of self. These judgements are recorded in the test software and then processed to yield scores on relevant variables including the favoured poles on the constructs/values and the significance of the constructs in the respondent's world view. The instrument thus gives a quantified profile of the respondents' value orientation. Each profile can be compared – matched – with a predetermined ideal profile.

Given these advantages, ISA/Ipseus has been used by us and our colleagues to develop a number of Professional Identity measures including ones for nursing, social work and school teaching. These are described in other chapters in this book. In this chapter, we are going to concentrate on two measures called NM and MM. NM has been developed over a period and formally evaluated as an aid to selection. The Match label refers to the fact that results from respondents can be compared with ideal results. Thus, applicants for Nursing programmed are matched and compared with ideal Nurses. MM is our latest project and is in its first stages, but its purpose will be to aid the selection of medical students by profiling the values they hold and how these match with the ideal.

In the introductory chapter, we suggested that professional identity has three main components: knowledge, competence and values. Thus, a professional's identity is made up of what they know, what they can do and what values they subscribe to. NM and MM are concerned primarily with measuring values. Values are fundamental beliefs that determine behaviour in a range of situations. Values have an ethical dimension and are sometimes referred to as professional ethics. They are assumed to have a degree of permanence. Values themselves are hypothetical constructs and are not directly observable but have to be inferred from consistencies in observable behaviour. When a value points clearly to a set of behaviours or at least a behavioural disposition, they may be called attributes. While they are considered important in courses of professional training, they pose problems for teaching, learning and assessment. They also pose a problem in selection where it will be important to choose applicants whose values are considered appropriate for the profession for which they will train. The idea of our match instruments is that they can contribute useful information to inform both the selection process and the subsequent development of professional identity pre and post registration...

We have developed NM over a 5-year period, and the project arose from two concerns. The first problem was that the behaviour of a small number of practising nurses suggested that they did not hold the right values and that this should have been detected when they first applied for a programme (Report of Mid Staffordshire Trust, 2013). As a result in the United Kingdom, all nursing programmes had to consider how they took values into account in their selection. The second related problem was that the present methods used to assess values including typically interviews and the assessment of a personal statement (PS) were of dubious validity and reliability. From this arose the need for a valid, reliable and feasible psychometric test that could be a part of the selection procedures.

Before describing and evaluating NM in detail, we will describe Weinreich's ISA and its associated measure, Ipseus, more fully.

Theorising and measuring identity

There is a substantial literature regarding identity and its measurement. In the next section, we briefly review this literature focusing on three foundation theorists and conclude this review with a description of a particular comprehensive theoretical framework regarding identity known as ISA together with its associated measuring tool – Ipseus.

We were looking for a tool that would validly, reliably and feasibly measure identity and identity change. Such a tool could be used to assess applicants to Nursing programmes. If used in a before and after design, it could chart changes in identity associated with an intervention program. It could also feedback insights to participants to aid their development and allow a categorisation or typology of participants to be adduced and related to process and outcomes. It would have to provide better data than other means of investigation including conventional questionnaires. ISA/Ipseus seemed worth exploring for a number of reasons that are considered next. A number of theorists have addressed the notion of identity and the associated concept of self. Some brief consideration of three-key approaches will serve as a prelude to the exposition of the ISA framework that we found to be unusually comprehensive in its synthesis of a number of perspectives on identity and self.

Within the number of psychological orientations that address identity and the related idea of self, Burns (1979) found three broadly defined perspectives emerging:

- the psychodynamic approach to identity (Erikson, 1963,1968)
- the personal construct theory (PCT) view of identity and self (Kelly, 1955; Fransella, 1981)
- the cognitive–affective consistency approach to the relationship between self's cognitions of people and self (Festinger, 1957)

Erikson (1963, 1968) focuses on the lifespan development of identity from a predominantly psychodynamic viewpoint but conceptualised within a cultural context. Erikson's definition of identity spans one's past sense of self, current self as determined by self and significant others and one's expectations for the future. Erikson's sophisticated and influential conceptualisation of identity emphasises that identity formation is a process that begins with partial identifications in childhood and proceeds through more complex identifications in adulthood that may be integrated into a coherent identity or may involve crises with identity conflicts.

The PCT of Kelly (1955), Fransella (1981), has as its fundamental postulate that individuals interpret or construe the world, rather than observing it directly. This construal constitutes their identity. Thus, rather than an objective world that people have to comprehend; comprehension is an actively constructed process that determines the world as we know it.

PCT has three major characteristics. First, there are its philosophical roots in 'constructive alternativism'; that is, the view that we construct a world of meanings and an identity from a number of possible alternatives. Second, there is PCT itself, which Kelly expresses formally as a series of postulates and correlates that express the nature of constructs, the elements to which they are applied and their interrelations. Elements may be persons, things or ideas and constructs are the bipolar dimensions used to construe and make sense of the elements. Central to PCT is the powerful conception of the discrete 'bi-polar personal constructs' – the individual's unique framework/template for anticipating and interpreting people and events. Thus, for example, the people I know might be considered as elements, and the constructs I use to make sense of the people might include such bipolar dimensions as good/bad, friendly/unfriendly, clever/stupid etc.

Third, there is Kelly's method that allows the eliciting and analysing of an individual's constructs. Called the repertory grid test, it is based on the identification of differences and similarities between triads of elements. In this test, the individual is presented with elements in threes – the triads – and asked to indicate how two are similar and one is different from the other two. This elicits constructs that can then be applied to all relevant entities. Using this approach iteratively reveals the key constructs used by an individual to make sense of, and to construct, their world.

Festinger's (1957) theory of cognitive dissonance concentrates on circumstances when the cognitions and feelings that constitute identity are incompatible with each other or one's behaviour. There is, he would argue, a pressure or tendency to realign one's attitudes and cognitions so as to decrease dissonance. For example, the inclination to believe good things about an admired person is strong, and one may reject or distort contrary evidence about that person to avoid dissonance. There is a process of adjustment whereby incompatible elements are made compatible by adjustment to one or both. Thus, if there are bad facts known about an admired person, there are at least three possible adjustments: the person is seen as less good, the bad facts are seen as less bad or a more complex conceptualisation of the person is developed admitting a combination of good and bad facets.

Some understanding of what these theorists had to say about identity will help in understanding ISA, and particularly the results of an ISA/Ipseus instrument since Weinreich's ISA is largely based on these foundation theorists. Concepts from these theorists are expressed through the parameters of an Ipseus report and thus what the instrument can tell us about the respondent or group of respondents. Key parameters include identification with key individuals and evaluation of those individuals and self. Of particular relevance to this project is the information given on the use of constructs, the significance of constructs to the respondents' world view, the emotional significance of constructs, the preferred poles of constructs and conflicts or tensions in identifications and construct use.

Having surveyed over 50 reports of identity measurement to identify what seemed the best approach to explore professional identity and values (Passmore et al, 2014), we chose Weinreich's method for a number of reasons. First, his theory is, in part, a synthesis of three major theoretical perspectives, namely Erikson, Kelly and Festinger. Second, the linked software, Ipseus, is a framework software in that rather than being a dedicated instrument in itself, provides a basis for developing customised instruments appropriate for particular applications. Third, it is theory-based, and its reports relate to key identity parameters from ISA that in its turn draws on major theoretical perspectives regarding identity and the use of constructs/values. Fourth, it is highly functional in that it not only facilitates the development of customised instruments but also presents the instrument to respondents in an attractive on-screen fashion, records and analyses their responses and produces a report regarding key identity parameters. Fifth, the approach and the Ipseus reports represent a unique integration of qualitative (emic) and quantitative (etic) measures. Sixth, the Ipseus reports allow for both idiographic individual identity analysis and nomothetic group analysis. Seventh, the approach has been proven in more than 50 studies of identity in a number of fields and applications including ethnic and national identity, education, counselling, social work and professional identity, but only recently in Nursing (Parry, 2011). This project is built on Parry's work that developed an identity instrument to explore the identities of nursing students and led to a categorisation of learning types.

Identity Structure Analysis (ISA)

Three things need to be addressed in understanding ISA/Ipseus. First is the theory of identity itself called ISA. Second is the associated measuring tool, Ipseus, that facilitates the exploration of identity and is based on ISA. Third is the report that comes from a completed Ipseus instrument and which can be used both ideographically and nomothetically to identify key features of identity, including values, in individuals and groups. This can be used for exploratory purposes or to test hypotheses. It can also be used to compare a respondents profile with an ideal profile. Ultimately it will be this report that forms the basis of the results that will be available from the use of the instrument with individuals and groups.

ISA is a comprehensive theoretical framework for the understanding of identity and represents a unique synthesis of key theorists in the area. It draws particularly on the psychodynamic approach to identification and identity development of Erikson, Kelly's Personal Construct Theory and Festinger's ideas of cognitive/affective dissonance and consonance. Other contributory theories include Marcia's development of Erikson, the symbolic interactionism of Cooley and Mead, Goffman's dramaturgical approach and Harré's agentic theories. Three main features of ISA and subsequently Ipseus and its reports can be traced to these three foundation theories.

One idea from Erikson is that our identity is based on a complex pattern of 'identifications' 'with significant others throughout our lives. We form an identity based on positive identifications with those we wish to be like and negative identifications with those we don't wish to be like. This brings in a second key idea that of evaluation which is judging aspects of ourselves and significant others as relatively good or bad. People appraise the circumstances in which they are involved in order to bring meaning to the circumstance against the greater background of how they appraise self in relation to their social world. A third idea from Erikson is that our identity is constantly open to change and development as we form new identifications and is subject to periodic crises when there is a mismatch or contradiction between these identifications.

Kelly's Personal Construct Theory has influenced ISA/Ipseus in two ways. First, it emphasises that our identity is constructed through the ways in which dimensions of meaning called constructs are applied to the physical and social world represented by entities. Second, the repertory grid approach determined the structure of the Ipseus instrument that requires respondents to apply a number of constructs chosen for their relevance to the area under investigation to entities consisting of significant others in the area and aspects of self.

Festinger's idea of cognitive and affective dissonance or consonance underpins the dynamics in identity that move to achieve some harmony between identifications and constructions to resolve tensions and conflict.

Integrating these three theories, the concept of 'identity' in ISA is defined as

> ... the totality of one's self-construal, in which how one construes oneself in the present expresses the continuity between how one construes oneself as one was in the past and how one construes oneself as one aspires to be in the future.

The Ipseus identity measuring instrument

An Ipseus instrument is in the form of a fairly lengthy questionnaire requiring judgements to be made by respondents regarding entities and constructs, a notion derived from Kelly's Personal Construct Theory.

It is constructed using Ipseus software available from identityexploration.com.

Typically, an Ipseus instrument will consist of about 20 entities and 20 constructs. Completing the instrument requires each construct to be applied to each entity. Thus, in a 20 × 20 instrument, 400 judgements would be required. Each item in an Ipseus instrument requires a judgement to be made of how a particular construct applies to a particular entity. This judgement is described by Weinreich as a mini discourse. An example from the NM instrument is given as follows in Box 17.1.

In constructing each judgement (or discourse as Weinreich calls them) in the instrument, the Ipseus software allows the syntax to be adjusted from the basic constructs and entities to ensure normal usage. Each judgement of an entity using a construct are located on a nine-point scale, each end of which represents the

---

BOX 17.1

A Nursing Ipseus Discourse

In this judgement, the construct –
Believes that the safety of patients must come before everything else ....
*Accepts that realistically patient safety will sometimes suffer as a result of pressures
on the health service*
Is applied to the entity – *A Great Nurse*

---

opposing poles of the construct and are represented numerically as +4 and −4. The remaining seven points represent degrees of relative applicability of the construct with ranges from +3 to +1 through 0 to −1 to −3. These judgements constitute the raw data from an Ipseus instrument.

While an Ipseus instrument has certain predetermined structural characteristics and mandatory requirements, it is primarily tailored to the particular topic being explored. Thus, constructs and, to a degree, entities are selected to reflect the topic area and, particularly, the themes that the investigator wishes to explore. In this project, the topic area is the professional identity and values of nurses. The themes reflect those features of this professional identity that the researchers deem important.

In considering the professional identity of nurses, a number of themes emerged from a literature review, from interviews and from the judgements of an expert group. A number of qualitative judgements were involved in prioritising these themes and selecting those that were translated into constructs for the instrument.

The area and focus of the project determined the relevant social domains and objects of thought. Thus, the Nurse Identity project included domains of other nurses, associated clinicians and patients. Each domain generates one or more entities hence 'other clinicians' included 'a clinician I admire' or 'a clinician I would not wish to be like'. All Ipseus instruments have to include mandatory anchor entities including a past self, a present self and a future self. These might be represented as entities: 'me as I was', 'me as I am at present' and 'me as I would like to be'. Entities, then, describe other people and/or a setting. Constructs are represented as a pair of opposing statements on a notional dimension. Together, the entities and constructs create a series of situations or discourses to which each participant is asked to respond. The instrument is presented through an interactive program where all the judgements are recorded. The software then processes the data regarding the judgements and yields a report where a number of variables are expressed in verbal, numerical and graphical form. The results may be used in an exploratory way or may be assessed against predictions to test out hypotheses. The constructs and entities chosen for the NM instrument are set out in subsequent tables.

Ipseus report

Each judgement made by the respondents is recorded in the software that then carries out the calculations dictated by its algorithms. The software will then generate a report that shows results for the various ISA/Ipseus parameters including:

- Favoured poles of constructs
- Significance of constructs in world view (structural pressure)
- Consistency of use of constructs
- Emotional investment in constructs
- Ego identification with entities, that is the importance attached to an entity and the understanding of it
- Evaluation of entities as relatively good or bad
- Idealistic identification with entities, that is the extent to which one wants to be like an entity
- Contra-identification with entities, that is the extent to which one does not want to be like an entity
- Empathetic identification with entities that is the extent to which one believes oneself to be like an entity
- Conflicted identification with entities that is ambivalence in identification
- Identity Diffusion that is the total of conflicted identities
- Self-evaluation

The most important parameters relating to values are those concerned with constructs including favoured pole, structural pressure and emotional significance. The favoured pole indicates whether the candidate subscribes to the value or rejects it. The structural pressure indicates how important the construct/value is in the respondent's world view, that is cognitively. The emotional significance indicates how important the construct is affectively, that is, to the respondents' feelings.

The Nurse Match instrument

Introduction

Having given an outline of the ISA/Ipseus approach, we will now describe the project to develop the NM instrument to measure and explore the identities of nurses, nursing students and, in particular applicants to Nursing programmes. The instrument focuses on the values held by respondents regarding Nursing. The conceptualisation and construction of the instrument have raised a number of issues, and these are identified and explored theoretically and empirically. The instrument and its development are located in the theoretical and empirical literature regarding identity and its measurement. The particular theoretical and empirical framework chosen for the instrument ISA/Ipseus is that of Saunderson and Weinreich

(2012), and the steps in the development of an Ipseus instrument are described in detail. An evaluation of the instrument and its use for selection is reported.

The project is concerned with the development of an instrument to measure and explore professional identity in Nursing (PIN). Encompassed by the notion of professional identity are the values, beliefs and attitudes that underpin the professional behaviour of nurses. The instrument is intended to meet the need for a method to measure candidates' values as a component of values-based recruitment (VBR). Since the instrument will allow comparison of respondents with ideal models, it is called NM.

Value-based recruitment

Following the UK Francis Report of a public inquiry into the failings at Mid Staffordshire NHS Foundation Trust (2013) and widespread concerns that standards of nursing care may be falling, there has been increased emphasis in the United Kingdom on the need for reliable and valid instruments to measure professional identity and values for selection and developmental purposes. An appropriate instrument would profile the values and attitudes of applicants to Nursing programmes to determine their suitability. It could also be used during the programme to determine progress towards an appropriate standard and in professional development programme to assess the maintenance and development of professional identity and values.

While there is broad agreement that the values that underpin nursing practice are important, there is no agreement regarding their conceptualisation or expression. The same problems exist with the broader notion of professional identity. There is limited evidence or empirical research into the concept of professional nursing identity or nursing values. Given the dearth of research, it is hardly surprised that there is a limited number of instruments available to measure professional Identity and values in Nursing and none that meet the necessary standards of psychometrics (Warren, 2014).

Notwithstanding the lack of suitable instruments, there is now a requirement in the United Kingdom that schools of nursing should build some form of VBR (Erskine, 2014) into their admission procedures. VBR can include conventional semi-structured interviews, multiple mini interviews (MMIs), scenarios and simulations. These practices can in principle be supported by or replaced by reliable and valid psychometric tools (Erskine, 2014).

The NM project has developed such a psychometric tool/instrument using the well-established theoretical perspectives of ISA and its associated psychometric technology, Ipseus (Weinreich, 2012). ISA is a wide-ranging theory of identity that integrates the perspectives of a number of key theorists including Erikson, Kelly, Festinger and Goffman. Ipseus is comprehensive software that facilitates both the development and the administration of the instrument. In addition, it records and analyses responses to produce a quantified report regarding key variables. This ISA/Ipseus approach has been used widely in a variety of settings but not previously in Nursing (Parry, 2011).

An Ipseus instrument consists of a number of constructs that are bipolar dimensions of thought and entities that are objects of thought drawn from relevant social domains and aspects of self. Completion of an instrument requires the application of the constructs to each of the entities using a nine-point scale to indicate how the construct applies. The responses to these judgements are then analysed by the specially developed programme to yield identity parameters indicating how respondents use constructs and relate to entities. Scores and qualitative descriptors regarding these parameters give a uniquely detailed identity profile and a description of how the respondent is positioned in relation to key values. The constructs used in the NM instrument are based largely on values that are considered important for Nursing.

Match software (Erskine, 2014) allows systematic comparison of identity profiles with a model identity profile or profiles. In this case, the comparison and match would be between the profiles of applicants to Nursing and students enrolled on Nursing programmes on the one hand with experienced and successful Nurses on the other. The title NM is intended to capture the capacity of the instrument to make these comparisons of respondents with ideal model identities.

The project has followed a number of stages including instrument development based on a comprehensive literature review and ethnographic work to determine the most appropriate constructs/values and entities, piloting of the instrument and field-testing and initial standardisation of the instrument. Reporting procedures from the standardised instrument have been developed to ensure its functionality and fitness for purpose. The procedures involved in these stages are described as follows.

Constructing the Nurse Match instrument

As explained above, an Ipseus instrument consists of entities and constructs selected for their relevance to the area being investigated. Completing the instrument requires a respondent to apply each of the constructs to each of the entities. On the basis of these judgements, the Ipseus software then produces a report in terms of the ISA variables. This transformation from responses to parameters is carried out with the application of algorithms set out in Chapter Three of Weinreich (2012).

Constructs are dimensions of thought and entities are the objects of thought. The task for those constructing an instrument is to determine the most appropriate sets of constructs and entities. The process is to identify the relevant social domains and represent these as entities and to identity relevant themes and represent these as bipolar constructs. This process is primarily qualitative in nature and requires a number of informed decisions from those devising the instrument. We wanted the constructs in the NM instrument to reflect the values that are considered important in Nursing. The process of constructing the NM instrument required the following steps that are standard for any Ipseus instrument. They are set out by Weinreich (2014).

- Decide on the subject matter of the project, in this case the Professional Identity of Nurses
- Gather background information, using different sources to avoid crude stereotyping, from the local context for the project's participants the media, as in commentaries about like individuals and groups fieldwork, such as discussion groups and interviews, with similar people a review of 'the literature' on the subject matter, such as research reports
- List the main themes emerging from this information
- List the social domains of relevance to one or other theme
- Edit themes into phrases or discourse texts and seek out a contrast for each, so as to form two 'poles' of a 'bipolar construct'
- Use the Ipseus editing facilities to create the customised identity instrument containing the above-identified themes and domains, so that, in the matrix of themes and domains, the project participant has the opportunity to appraise the relevant social world aspect by aspect
- Present the identity instrument on screen using Ipseus, one judgement at a time made up of a bipolar construct expressed as contrasting phrases and an entity. The construct has to be applied to the entity.

Determining social domains and hence entities was a relatively straightforward process. An Ipseus instrument requires a number of mandatory entities related to self, which are fundamental to the framework and methodology. In addition to these mandatory elements, entities were required which reflected the key social domains in the area of study, in this case, Nursing.

The identification of themes and subsequently constructs is the most demanding part of the test construction and required a number of qualitative judgements regarding the salience of theories and constructs to the Nursing identity being studied. It is not straightforward to translate a value into a plausible construct where both poles are credible and acceptable.

For the NM instrument deciding on themes and subsequently constructs for this project involved four main processes.

1 A review of the literature on professional identity and values in Nursing covering the last 15 years (Warren, 2014).
2 Focus groups with practising nurses (n = 30) and service users (n = 10), postgraduate diploma nurses in mental health (PG DIP n = 25) and third-year adult mental health branch students (n = 20), adult and child preregistration nurses years 2 and 3 (n = 20).
3 Elicitation from focus groups of Key Quality Indicators concerning professional identity and nursing values using 'sticky note' technique.
4 Scrutiny of themes and constructs by two expert groups.

From these four sources, 109 potential themes were identified. An expert panel then sorted the themes into four categories to indicate their relative salience for PIN. A second expert group then had the task of reducing the themes to a number nearer 20, which represented the most salient that could be used to generate around 20 bipolar constructs.

The first approach to this qualitative reduction task was to identify obvious duplications. The next stage was to validate the priority categorisations from the first group. This validation was done first by ensuring that the themes related clearly to a behavioural disposition which would be likely to impact on practice. A number did not meet this criterion. The remaining themes were then assessed for their perceived salience to the practice of nursing. There were five members in the group and the selected themes reflected a consensus between these experts. The chosen themes were then expressed as bipolar constructs.

At the end of this process, a first proto-instrument existed which was then checked out with the first expert group.

It should be clear that the current drive to measure nursing values and hence identity requires an in-depth approach both conceptually and methodologically. ISA and its associated Ipseus Instrument represent such an approach providing a unique integration of qualitative and quantitative parameters. Initial results from the use of the instrument suggest it has a useful discriminatory power. Further work will explore the correlational and predictive validity of the instrument and develop its use in recruitment and in charting development in preregistration and post registration education. The instrument has been constructed on the basis of a partnership between Identity Exploration Ltd and a number of Nursing Departments in Higher Education. Any readers interested in participating in such a partnership to further develop and trial the instrument would be welcome to contact either of the authors.

Evaluation of Nurse Match

Having developed the NM instrument, the next stage was to test and evaluate it in practice. We were fortunate to receive a grant to evaluate the use of the instrument in the selection of students for nursing programmes in Northern Ireland. The following is a summary of the report produced at the conclusion of this evaluation.

The NM instrument is a specially constructed test based on the well-established ISA theory and its associated Ipseus software for test construction and scoring. Ipseus instruments measure aspects of identity including the values that make up identity. The values measured by NM are based on the five attributes proposed in 2013 by Gateway, the committee responsible overall for nurse recruitment in Northern Ireland in Northern Ireland. These attributes plus an additional one concerned with communication provided a framework for the ideal profile against which the respondents profile could be matched. The test yields a score on individual values and an overall score on the set of values. This score can then be used to select applicants to proceed to the next stage of selection.

The PS used prior to NM is submitted by applicants as part of their Universities and Colleges Admission System (UCAS) application. Applicants for Nursing are encouraged to focus their statement on this profession. The statements are then marked by Nursing faculty using a scoring grid related to four attributes: personal desire for a career in nursing, motivation for nursing, expectations of the course and nursing as a profession and decision-making affecting self and others

The marked PS yields a score that can be used to screen applicants. The PS has been used as a basis for initial screening at Queen's University Belfast (QUB) and Ulster University (UU) since 2012.

The evaluation is structured using the well-established Trident Method that focuses evaluation questions on Outcomes; Process and Stakeholder Perspectives.

The major outcome evaluated is the fitness for purpose of the test for initial applicant screening. The test is also evaluated with regard to its compliance with psychometric standards and hence its psychological probity and defensibility as a basis for decisions. The processes required for the tests are evaluated with regard to feasibility and cost effectiveness. With regard to stakeholder perspectives, the acceptability of NM to applicants is evaluated. Additionally, the data are analysed to explore gender differences and the provisional identification of leadership potential.

The evidence for the evaluation comes from two pilot uses of NM first in 2015 with a group of first-year students at QUB and second in 2018 with applicants to nursing programmes at QUB and the UU; from an analysis of NM and PS against APA psychometric standards and from surveys of the views of those who completed the instrument in the two pilots.

Outcomes

The primary evaluation question regarding outcomes was the extent to which the instrument was fit for the purpose of ranking a set of applicants using valid and reliable criteria including he values they held relevant to Nursing. On the basis of this ranking, applicants could be selected to proceed to the next stage of selection. The selection instrument should be fair, transparent and defensible through meeting internationally recognised standards for a psychometric instrument. That is, the instrument should have psychometric probity.

In the 2015 study the NM instrument was found to have:

- discriminated effectively and efficiently between year 1 nurses in terms of the professional quality of their inherent nursing values and attributes;
- created suitability scores (S^{TOT} scores) for candidate screening purposes;
- produced suitability scores that closely approximated normal distributions;
- proved valid and reliable: robust in quantitative and qualitative terms;
- been administered, scored and interpreted in a standard manner;
- been easy to understand and complete and well received by participants.

In the 2018 study, funded by the Burdett Trust, the NM psychometric test was found to have:

- screened applicants effectively and efficiently in terms of the professional quality of their inherent nursing values and attributes;
- measured the overall professional quality of applicant's values in terms of a single suitability score (S^{TOT});
- the S^{TOT} score for overall suitability had a normal distribution: symmetry and shape were within limits for skewness and kurtosis;
- was shown to be robust in quantitative and qualitative terms; valid and reliable (internally consistent);
- was administered, scored and interpreted in a standard manner;
- was easy to understand and complete and well received by most applicants;
- was a more effective, robust and valid screening tool than the PS;
- provided data that on analysis can inform staff appraisal and the management process.

On the basis of these two studies, it was established that the NM instrument offered a standardised, effective, user friendly, screening test for values and attributes.

We were told by the universities concerned that in 2014 an evaluation was undertaken of 2 years' use of the PS and the conclusion was that the data suggested this was an effective approach to streamline the number of individuals offered an interview. We were unable to locate an evaluation report with these conclusions.

It is clear that both NM and the PS are fit for purpose in the sense that they provide a score that can be used in the initial screening of applicants to Nursing programmes. However, the measures are quite different in the extent to which they meet psychometric standards of validity and reliability and hence are fair, transparent and defensible in use. NM demonstrates psychometric probity whereas PS does not.

There is no requirement to use a Value Recruitment instrument at this stage of selection. However, it is an advantage that NM has been specially devised to be such an instrument and is based on the Gateway attributes. PS is not a VBR instrument but rather an assessment of knowledge and commitment to Nursing in a PS included in the UCAS application.

So, two measures were assessed in detail, the PS and NM, with regard to the extent they meet APA standards for psychometric tests. While NM has been designed as a test following well-established principles and practices, PS is more an opportunistic use of a statement required as part of a UCAS application for a university place and the marking of that statement while functional was not designed as a psychometric measure. Nevertheless, it could be argued that the fairness and defensibility of PS would require it to meet psychometric standards.

The study showed in evidenced detail that while NM measures up well to APA standards of validity and reliability, there are serious weaknesses in PS with regard to both validity and reliability. Practically this means that it would be difficult to justify PS as a measure used to exclude applicants whereas the use of NM would be justified by its psychometric probity.

Process

This is a brief description of the process involved in using PS or NM as part of the selection procedure for entry to undergraduate Nursing programmes. Along with the descriptions, some comparisons are made of the resource implications of the two approaches.

PS has been used as part of the selection procedures of QUB and UU since 2012. Applicants for undergraduate programmes through the UCAS are required to complete a PS to support their application. This is described by UCAS as 'a chance for you to articulate why you'd like to study a particular course or subject, and what skills and experience you possess that show your passion for your chosen field'.

Support for the production of the PS is provided by UCAS and often by the careers teachers of secondary schools and colleges. The production of the PS is cost neutral for universities. There is no guarantee that a statement was actually produced by the applicant.

Following a decision by Gateway in 2012 PSs of applicants to UU and QUB are marked and used for the initial screening. Marking is undertaken by faculty in Nursing and is on a four-point scale against each of four criteria. These are personal desire for a career in nursing, motivation for nursing expectations of the course and nursing as a profession, decision-making affecting self and others.

These criteria, whilst relevant in themselves, are not conceived as VBR and do not relate to the five attributes proposed by Gateway in 2014. There is clearly a cost involved in this marking in terms of the time of nursing faculty. This has not been quantified at this point but clearly it could be in terms of number of PSs marked, average time per marking and cost of the total time as a proportion of lecturer cost. For faculty who have to meet the demands of teaching, research and professional updating, this marking probably has an opportunity cost.

NM requires applicants to complete an internet-based instrument. This takes about 40 minutes in a computer-equipped classroom. In principle, the instrument could be completed on any device with internet access and in whatever circumstances suited the applicant. The instrument has been completed by 291 respondents in two pilots described in published reports.

The responses of each applicant are stored on a server, and initial scoring and reporting is carried out through the Ipseus software that produces an overall score and scores for six values. The cost of this for each candidate will be between £30 and £50 depending on the depth of reporting required. This cost could be met by the receiving university or by each applicant and compared with the cost of marking PS.

Stakeholder perspectives

A formal survey was undertaken of those who completed NM in the two pilots. Details are given in the following reports but in summary participants reported the instrument as being

1   easy to understand (97%) and could be responded to intuitively (93%)
2   quite easy to complete (94%); quite difficult to complete (19%)
3   identified most important nursing values (83%) and contain no irrelevant issues (88%)
4   was interesting, to complete (65%)
5   required extra time to complete (6%)

Further analyses

Additionally, the data from the second pilot were further analysed to identify gender differences and to explore an approach to identifying leadership potential. These two studies were suggestive of further studies that might be undertaken to identify indicative results. McNeill in Chapter 11 describes such a study regarding leadership potential.

Conclusions and recommendations

NM is a psychometric instrument that measures the value orientation of respondents. It has been devised to measure orientation towards the five Gateway attributes plus an additional attribute teamwork. It has proved valid, reliable and practical. Scores from the instrument can be used for an initial screening of applicants which is value based. Its use is defensible since it has demonstrated psychological probity.

The PS has been used for 6 years to screen applicants and the scores from its marking allow this. It is not a measure of values but rather of knowledge of and motivation towards Nursing and the training programme. Against psychometric standards, the PS has problems of validity and reliability. The poor inter-marker reliability found is a particular cause for concern. Its defence would pose problems.

Marking the PS places considerable demands on faculty staff time. While this has not been costed for the evaluation, it is likely to be significantly more expensive than NM the costs of which could be met by applicants.

On this basis of this assessment, it was recommended that NM should be used for the initial screening of applicants for initial training in Nursing at QUB and UU.

Developing the Medi Match instrument

The impetus to develop MM at the Northern Ontario School of Medicine came from similar concerns to those which led to NM. That is that while prospective medical students were selected on academic achievement and to a lesser extent interpersonal competence, there was little data on the values to which they subscribe and their conjunction with the distinctive mission of the school. The school had attempted to assess values and in particular commitment to rural medicine and working with first nation communities throughout Ontario through the scrutiny of PSs and through interviews but had doubts about the validity and reliability of these approaches for this purpose. The school thought a more cost-effective approach might be to require applicants to complete an appropriate psychometric test assuming a suitable one was available. We were asked to consider how our NM approach might apply to Medicine.

The decision was informed by an earlier project in the school that had produced a proto Ipseus instrument. This had been constructed by a postgraduate student to assess the values held by students in the programme and how these related to the values of exemplary clinicians. Conceived originally as a PhD project, this had to be set aside for resource reasons. Nevertheless this had been a useful start and we include some material from this project and its proto-instrument later in the chapter to exemplify the approach.

Funding was found to commence a new project at NOSM. With the full support of a representative Steering Group, we are developing a new test that we have called MM. Our aim is to build into the selection procedures evidence of the medically related values held by applicants and the extent to which these match those which an ideal clinician should hold. We wanted the test to be tailored in part to the particular values that would be consistent with the distinctive regional mission of the school.

While recognising existing methods for value-based selection including interviews, PSs and MMIs, we wanted to develop a psychometric test that would be fit for purpose in that it would provide a valid, reliable and feasible indication of the values held by applicants. We wanted the test to provide a fair and defensible input to the selection process.

We could not find a test that met our requirements (Passmore et al., 2014) but were of course familiar with the earlier attempt to develop an instrument in the School. This and our experience in developing NM confirmed that we should use the identity theory called ISA and its associated measurement approach Ipseus (Weinreich, 2012). We knew of course how this approach had been used to develop a VBR instrument for Nursing programmes and that this had been piloted successfully. We decided to use a similar approach to develop a MM instrument with values relevant to our programme and its regional role.

The first phase of developing any Match instrument is determining the values that the tool will measure.

Examples of values deemed important in Medicine range from attempts to describe a small number of fundamental values to longer lists that aim to be comprehensive at a more detailed level.

Four basic principles to guide the professional approach to patients and their care are autonomy, justice, beneficence and avoidance of maleficence. Each of these principles can of course be broken down into more specific values. As the analysis becomes more detailed and fine-grained, values get closer to specific behaviours and shade into competencies. For example, autonomy for the patient requires informed consent and decision-making, and freedom from coercion. Informed consent requires knowledge of procedures and risks and effective communication. Freedom from coercion requires respect for persons and sensitivity to feelings.

As an example of a longer list of values, the UK Medical Schools Council Assessment Alliance has produced a list of core values and attributes needed to study medicine. The distinction between value and attributes is an interesting one in that values are beliefs that may not lead to action whereas attributes are behavioural dispositions reflecting values. Attributes should be manifest in assessable behaviour.

The list includes:

- Motivation to study medicine and genuine interest in the medical profession
- Insight into your own strengths and weaknesses
- The ability to reflect on your own work
- Personal organisation
- Academic ability
- Problem solving
- Dealing with uncertainty
- Manage risk and deal effectively with problems Statement on the core values and attributes needed to study medicine
- Ability to take responsibility for your own actions
- Conscientiousness
- Insight into your own health
- Effective communication, including reading, writing, listening and speaking
- Teamwork
- Ability to treat people with respect
- Resilience and the ability to deal with difficult situations
- Empathy and the ability to care for others
- Honesty

Producing a convincing list of values and attributes is one thing; determining the evidence that will give valid and reliable evidence of their existence is another. The above list was produced to inform the application process for Medicine that raises the question of how data might be gathered for selection.

Selection in NOSM is the culmination of the Application Process when decisions are made as to who should be admitted to the programme. Selection should be based on valid and reliable evidence about a candidate. This evidence is evaluated against standards and in comparison, with other candidates in the context of the number of places available. This process has been transparent, fair and legally defensible.

Selection should be predictive of success on the programme and ultimately as a medical practitioner. Medical programmes consist of academic and practical learning components together with the development of a professional identity and its values.

Selection for the academic component is the most straightforward since it can be based on national examination results and also on dedicated tests for prospective medical students. Using these results for selection meets the requirement for transparency, fairness and defensibility.

Gauging potential for practical learning and professional development is more problematic. The applicant may be required to produce evidence of relevant practical activities.

Evidence may be drawn from a wide range of experiences including:

- Work experience placements
- Experience of paid employment
- Volunteer work
- Participation in social activities
- Educational experience

But the availability, acceptability and evaluation of this evidence are relatively unreliable and dubiously valid and certainly cannot count as a measure of values held by applicants.

Practical assessments may be built into selection through simulations or even preliminary Objective Structured Clinical Examinations. Use can also be made of MMIs where each interview requires a practical response. Face-to-face interviews may include an assessment of communication skills.

Assessing the values held by applicants and their potential for developing the values central to a professional identity is particularly difficult. This approach to selection is called VBR (Health Education England, 2014). VBR is an approach that attracts and selects students, trainees or employees on the basis that their individual values and behaviours align with the values of the selecting organisation.

Medical values are of course not directly observable but have to be inferred from behaviour in the professional role. Clearly this is not feasible for applicants. Methods that are used to assess values prior to selection include

- Structured interviews;
- MMIs;
- Selection centres; and
- Situational Judgement Tests (for screening).

Scoring these activities depends on valid and reliable inference from behaviour by trained observers. The candidate's response to questions or in a PS depends on their ability to reflect on their own values. This self-report evidence is of doubtful validity since it assumes that applicants are able to reflect on their values and that they will report them honestly rather than saying what they believe is required. A more cost-effective approach may be to require applicants to complete an appropriate psychometric test assuming a suitable one is available.

So, at the Northern Ontario School of Medicine, we are developing such a test that we have called MM. Our aim is to build into our selection procedures evidence of the medically related values held by applicants and the extent to which these match those which an ideal clinician should hold. We wanted the test to be tailored in part to the particular values that would be consistent with the distinctive regional mission of the school.

As described earlier in this chapter, an Ipseus instrument is not a conventional questionnaire. The instrument is made up of bipolar constructs derived from the chosen values that have to be applied to entities. The bipolar constructs represent dimensions of thought representing particular values; the entities represent people and aspects of self. Completing an instrument requires each construct to be applied to each entity. Through these mini dialogues applying constructs to entities the respondent's value position can be calculated with scores on individual values and an overall score.

MM is being custom designed and built using the Ipseus software framework. The form the instrument will take can be exemplified through the earlier discontinued project at NOSM. This project had produced an instrument that required the application of 20 bipolar constructs representing medical attributes and values to 12 entities from personal, home and work domains. The value constructs used in this early MM instrument were derived from a literature search, consultation and trials with experienced and well-respected clinicians; moderated by the insights of the expert research team. The following are some examples of possible constructs in relation to values.

Value: Commitment to research-based medical knowledge as a basis for practice
Construct:
Believes that practical skills must be based on theory............Believes practical skills are based on common sense and experience

Value: Independence and self determination
Construct:
Believes a senior person should never be challenged.......... Believes a senior person should be challenged if they are incorrect

Value: Realistic approach to work
Construct:
Would take shortcuts to achieve a target............... Would always make sure everything is done thoroughly

The entities included at present are:

> Ideal self
> Self at work
> Self at home
> Me 2 years ago
> Me in 5 years' time
> The person I most dislike

A model medical practitioner
A clinical manager
A typical patient
A bad medical practitioner
My best friend
My parents

In the instrument, each construct is presented as a connecting two contrasting points of view. In applying a construct to an entity respondents use a nine-point, semantic differential scale with a centre zero and four points on either side indicating the positive or negative appropriateness of the pole for the entity being appraised. Centre zero is used by the respondent if they cannot decide between polar values.

The entities in the instrument are aspects of self and people from the work-place and home context. Respondents are asked to appraise aspects of self and other people in terms of the attributes or values they perceive them to have or hold. For example, 'At work I … am prepared to challenge someone more senior if I feel it is in the interests of the patient/… would not challenge someone more senior in any circumstances'.

A conventional questionnaire would ask direct questions regarding the values held by a respondent. The MM instrument approached the values less directly by requiring the respondent to apply each value in a number of dialogues appraising a range of people. From the algorithms in the Ipseus software, indications can be given of the respondents preferred value poles and the significance of the value to the individual.

This proto-instrument identified as MM One provided useful background for the new project. The present stage of the current project, as we write, is concerned with gathering the views of key stakeholders including community stakeholders on the values that will inform the instrument. This is being done through interviews and focus groups culminating in a Delphi survey.

MM Two is then still at an early stage of development, but it is anticipated that like NM it will be a useful measure of values that could play a part not only in selection but in charting progress towards a professional identity and subsequent professional development. Any medical educators interested in the project should contact Professor Hogard at NOSM.

References

Burns, R. B. (1979). The Self-Concept in Theory: Measurement, Development and Behaviour. Harlow: Longman.

Erikson, E. H. (1963). Childhood and Society. New York, NY: Norton.

Erikson, E. H. (1968). Identity, Youth and Crisis. New York, NY: Norton.

Erskine A (2014) Match Factsheet Identity Exploration Ltd. identityexploration.com

Festinger, L. (1957). A Theory of Cognitive Dissonance. Evanston Row, IL: Peterson.

Fransella, F. (1981). Personal construct psychology and repertory grid technique. Methuen, London

Health Education England (2014) Values Based Recruitment Framework. London: HMSO.

Kelly, G. A. (1955). The psychology of personal constructs. New York, NY: W. W. Norton

Parry, C, (2011) Unpublished PhD: Internal Representation in Nurse Education: Imagery and Identity University of Chester UK.

Passmore G, Ellis R, Hogard E, (2014) Measuring Identity: A Review of Published papers SHEU Occasional paper 12 Buckinghamshire New University.

The Mid Staffordshire NHS Foundation Trust (2013) Report of the Mid Staffordshire NHS Foundation Trust Public Enquiry Chaired by Robert Frances NHS London

Warren J (2014) A Review of the Concepts of Professional Identity Held by Nurses and their Measurement: Occasional Paper, Strategic Planning Office, University of Chester

Weinreich P and Saunderson W (2012) Analysing Identity: Cross- Cultural, Societal and Clinical Contexts. RKP, London

Weinreich P (2014) Guidance for Constructing and Ipseus Instrument IEL Belfast.

18 Explicating professional identity through consultative methods

Elaine Hogard and Roger Ellis

Introduction

One obvious way to explore professional identity is to ask the professionals themselves. The broad range of social science methods available to do this includes interviews, focus groups and questionnaire surveys. This chapter describes four more specialized consultative approaches which can be used to make professional expertise more explicit. The methods are what I have called reconstitutive ethnography, together with critical incident technique (CIT), an expert system approach and the Delphi technique.

We chose these four methods when we were involved in a project to evaluate a new professional identity in nurse education and make it more explicit and replicable. This role was the clinical facilitator (CF) who supervised nursing students on placement coordinated their learning in the hospital and acted as a link between university and hospital. The CFs had a professional identity that was primarily as a nurse but with, latterly, increasing elements of nurse teacher. The project thus gave us an opportunity to explore a new hybrid professional identity where experienced nurses were developing a new approach to the organization and supervision of learning in the hospital setting and shifting from a nursing to a teaching identity. Our assumption was that the way in which they supervised student's clinical learning would be a key aspect of their changing professional identity. Their professional identity was as usual a combination of values, knowledge and competence. Our consultative study focused particularly on their competence and their distinctive approach to teaching and clinical learning and this is described in the case study that concludes this chapter.

This chapter begins with a discussion of the nature of professional expertise. The chapter advocates an approach termed the consultative approach as a means of bridging the gap between research and practice. Four methods of implementing a consultative approach are then described. Finally, a case study in consultative research is presented, which is an investigation of the role and professional identity of the Clinical Facilitator in Nurse Education, based on consultation with practitioners using all of the methods discussed in the chapter.

Exploring professional identity

There is very little organized scientific knowledge about the professional identity and expertise of caring professionals and how they learn to be more proficient practitioners. In his recurrent reviews calling for more collaboration between institutions of higher education and professional communities, Eraut (1985, 2000) draws attention to the lack of research on three aspects of professional learning:

1 What is learned during the period of initial qualification apart from the content of formal examinations? In other words: how is a professional identity developed?
2 How professionals learn to apply their initial training in the immediate post-qualification period.
3 How continuing education contributes to professional development.

In simple terms, Eraut (1985, 2000) is saying we do not know enough about the professional identity of, in his case, teachers. His criticism applies across the caring professions as noted by Ellis in 1988.

Ellis (2019) similarly points out that the professionalization of university lecturing is held back by an absence of researched knowledge about effective university teaching and learning. Within this context, I was asked to evaluate the role, practices and expertise of a new category of nurse educator. I was given the opportunity to explore their professional identity through researched knowledge.

One factor inhibiting such research is the implicit nature of professional knowhow. Professional competencies have proved extremely resistant to explicit definition. To what extent this is a problem of method is debatable. It may be more their inherent nature that poses the problem. Eraut (2000) argues that the 'unscripted' and 'intuitive' nature of professional action makes attempts to describe it difficult, although he does not say impossible. I started with the assumption that the implicit could be made more explicit through a consultative approach.

It could be assumed a priori that a key element in the professional identity of the CF was their interaction with the students and colleagues in the hospital and the university. The project therefore had to take account of the debate in the literature on social skills and social skills training.

Interpersonal skills are a key element of professional competence and hence professional identity in the caring professions. There are numerous ways in which interpersonal skills can be described, analyzed and developed (Hargie 2016). One issue is the grain of analysis. Should interaction be described using typical atomistic measures such as eye gaze, level of voice and talk time or should the emphasis be on the social meaning, intention and context of the behavior? For example, in the case of eye gaze, Hargie (2016) points out that the exact same gaze behavior may be dominant, submissive, friendly, a greeting, a signal to start a meeting and so on, depending on what else is going on, including the gazer's other behavior – especially facial expression, the situation, the relationship between participants etc. People do not perceive such events in isolation but in context. Social behavior also occurs in a temporal sequence in which the meaning of one element depends on the preceding and succeeding elements. The process of consultation, including focusing on critical incidents, should establish a functional language for description and analysis of what the professional believes is happening.

Consulting professionals about their identity

There are various methods for the study of interpersonal competence (Hargie 2016). These are reflected in methods to explicate professional competence and identity. In relation to the measurement of professional identity, a theme of this book, there are three basic approaches: measurement, observation and consultation, that is, the use of a psychometric tool, the observation of relevant behavior as naturalistically as possible and asking those concerned, i.e., consulting.

In this book, there are several chapters that look at a particular psychometric approach to the measurement of identity known as Identity Structure Analysis and Ipseus (Weinreich & Saunderson 2005). Instruments are described that have been developed to measure identity and values in nursing, teaching, social work and, prospectively, medicine. These instruments all have the prefix 'match' since they allow the values held by respondents to be matched with an ideal profile.

The observation of professionals in their practice has high face validity but is beset with problems. The main technical problem for naturalistic observation is to determine and obtain a reliable and valid sample of a professional's and client's typical behavior. Both participants have to agree. Once having obtained a sample, the problems are how should it be described, categorized and analyzed. In addition to these practical and theoretical problems, there are ethical and privacy issues to be negotiated. Nevertheless, interesting work has been done which throws a light on professional behavior, self-awareness and identity. An excellent example of this is given by McHale and Cecil in Chapter 20.

As an alternative to the direct observation of professional interaction, and to the psychometric measurement of professional attributes, the researcher can investigate the professionals' own personal beliefs of effective practice. This was the approach we adopted in the CF study described in the case study part of this chapter with the researcher and professional working together to explicate their practice and professional identity. Eraut (2000) supports the same strategy. He presents a case for reconceptualizing the relationship between higher education and the professions. He argues that practice and knowledge of its nature is best explicated through collaborative modes of enquiry linking the academic expertise of researchers with the insights of practitioners (Eraut 2000).

Constituting an ethnography of professional identity

Having advocated consultation with the professionals themselves as a potent method for exploring professional identity, the remainder of this chapter outlines four possible techniques available to the researcher adopting a consultative mode of research and exemplifies their use in a case study. The options considered are as follows:

1   Reconstitutive ethnography
2   CIT
3   The expert system approach
4   The Delphi technique

Only one of these methods is inherently based on consultation, that is, the Delphi technique, and the other three can be employed with various forms of data capture but work particularly well through consultation. Thus, it is possible to construct an expert system through analysis of observational data, and similarly critical incidents can be identified through the analysis of behavior and outcomes. Classically, an ethnography is constructed through participant observation. However, I would argue that each method is enriched through collaborative consultation.

I selected the methods after several literature searches. I chose the methods to provide a structure to what started as a broad intention to have individual interviews and focus groups with the CFs whose work was the object of the research. I was keen to have a collaboration with them from the start. The methods are described later, and some guidance is offered to the prospective consultative researcher through their use in the case study.

My idea of constituting and reconstituting the process of interaction between the CF and the students and other colleagues was the overall organizer for my approach. In this process of questioning and reconstitution, I employed both critical incident and expert system perspectives. Finally, I used a form of Delphi to verify the ethnographic picture which emerged. This ethnography was in the form of a model of CF behavior and consequent student learning (Ellis & Hogard 2001).

Reconstitutive ethnography

Ethnography is the study and description of complex social systems to capture their essential nature. It is a primary technique in social anthropology typically conducted largely through participant observation. Constitutive ethnography is the description of a social system which makes sense to the participants who thus contributive to its constitution. We are suggesting a development of constitutive ethnography where the involvement of the participants is an aim from the start, where their involvement is structured using various approaches and where the construction of the ethnography is iterative. This we call reconstitutive ethnography, the 're' intended to capture its iterative nature. My reconstitutive ethnography involves both CIT and an expert system approach in generating the ethnographic description of social events and structure and the Delphi Technique in returning the participants to the description to reach consensus about it. This approach places the onus on researcher and researched to construct the ethnographic description and to validate it iteratively. The case study in this chapter exemplifies the reconstitutive approach in the process section of the evaluation.

Constituting an ethnography through a critical incident technique

The basic idea in CIT is that a comprehensive set of competencies for a given role can be constructed from identifying a number of critical incidents in the conduct of that role. The researcher's job is to accumulate a number of descriptions of critical incidents both successful and unsuccessful for a given role and from these constructs a competency-based model of the role. At this point role, job, profession and professional identity can be used interchangeably as discussed in the introductory chapter of this book.

These incidents may be gathered in a number of ways but for this chapter, the focus is on how incident descriptions may be garnered from consultation with holders of a role. This approach with the holders of the role of 'clinical facilitator' will be described in the case study next.

The technique itself was first described by Flanagan (1954). His first use of the method was in a study of pilots' competencies during World War II. He was dissatisfied with what he felt were the vague criteria used to evaluate pilots' performances on training programs. These criteria reflected an imprecise and partial description of competencies. This led him to devise the CIT as a way to construct a better model of competencies which would in their turn improve the validity and reliability of assessment.

He worked with pilot instructors who were the experts with whom he consulted. In order to identify critical incidents, the procedure he described (Flanagan 1954) required instructors to complete a short questionnaire answering the following questions: Think of the last time you saw a trainee pilot do something that was effective/ineffective. What led up to this situation? Exactly what did the man do? Why was it effective/ineffective? (Flanagan 1954).

The technique was used as a consultative method requiring, in this case, professional trainers to reflect on the practice they were teaching and identify critical incidents in it which were considered a representative sample of pilot behaviors. These could then be used to produce a comprehensive model of competencies.

Various cues can be used to focus on the generation of incidents. When sufficient critical incidents have been described, these incidents are used through some form of factor analysis to generate a description of the competencies that underpin the critical incidents of good practice. The competencies themselves can then be analyzed to produce a model of good practice. This was the process I used with the CFs to construct a model of their practice and this is described in the case study.

This approach has been used widely since Flanagan's pioneering study. Recent work includes Friedland *et al.* (2017) who elucidated the development and current status of the CIT and focuses on fundamental definitions, guidelines and pros and cons when applied in nursing and healthcare sciences. Steven *et al.* (2020) undertook a review of the technique over the last decade to map and describe existing approaches to recording or using critical incident analysis in nursing and other health professions.

In a useful 'How to' information sheet, Tombs (2019) demonstrates how CIT can be used as a method of data collection in medical education research and indicates how CIT data is analyzed. In an example of a practical application of CIT to professional's perceptions of clinical practice, Wikström *et al.* (2016) report a study which through critical incident analysis described care experiences and actions taken by healthcare professionals when assessing postoperative pain.

Viergever (2019) in an analytical piece considers CIT as more than simply a technique. He presents it as genuine methodology with a clear overall focus that generates a range of studies that apply the technique using various methods for data collection and analysis. The paper describes and justifies the use of a specific format for those methods and unpacks philosophical and practical assumptions. Viergever (2019) warns that due to these assumptions, studies that use the CIT cannot easily make use of additional methodologies simultaneously.

Constituting an ethnography through an expert system approach

An expert system is a system that emulates the decision-making processes of an expert in such a way that this process might be represented as a computerized program. Thus, a complex decision-making process might be analyzed in such a way as to identify its component parts and their sequential dependencies. While such a model might benefit from consultation with the expert whose decisions are being modeled, this is not a necessary condition. The essence of the expert system approach is distinguishing and highlighting the specific elements of a process and their resultant dependencies. Identifying these dependencies and the conditions necessary for the system to work makes clear the stages and the decision-making within the system.

Expert systems are largely computer-based stores of expert knowledge that are used to aid decision-making in applied fields of knowledge. Early examples of expert systems dealt with relatively well-defined though complex problems, such as engineering design, oil technology and citizen's advice. More recently, the expert system approach has been extended to highly technical and semantic areas such as the quality of online health advice (Hu *et al.* 2017) or medical diagnoses (Hossain *et al.* 2017) or in this case study professional interaction between students and facilitator in a hospital ward.

Later in this chapter, we describe a study where we used the idea of an expert system, which is a sequential decision-making process, as a way of eliciting information from CFs about their role in supporting students on placement. This expert system went from the student's first admission through stages of developing and monitoring their activities to the conclusion when the placement was deemed satisfactorily completed. We were also interested in the process involved in coordinating the work of all those who supported the student in the hospital. And, as an overall aim, we wanted to investigate how the initially problematic relationships between the hospital and the university might be studied and improved.

Reconstructing an ethnography using the Delphi technique

This technique is a method of facilitating experts to reach a consensus on a particular issue or problem. Inherent in the method is the idea of iterative presentations of the issue with each successive iteration based on the views expressed and, ideally, the approximation to a consensus. A full treatment of the Delphi technique is given in Chapter 19 by Reid and Hogard which includes a case study of its use in Nurse Education. I used this approach to verify and refine the models of Clinical Facilitation which are described in the case study.

Case study: the use of consultative methods to establish an ethnography of the process of Clinical Facilitation

Introduction

This case study derives from an evaluation of a form of university teaching known as Clinical Facilitation. Clinical Facilitation takes place at the interface of higher education and clinical practice in nursing and involves the supervision of student nurses on their clinical placement. The CF not only provided direct supervision but also organized the inputs of other specialist colleagues. Also, the CF was expected to improve the coordination and communication between the hospital and the university.

In order to undertake the role, CFs had to be experienced and respected nurses with, presumably, a strong professional identity as a nurse. By taking up this new role, they were taking a significant step from providing care to teaching others to provide it. They were therefore adopting a nurse teacher identity or even to some extent an academic professional identity. This hybrid professional identity is therefore an interesting case study in itself.

The evaluation is relevant methodologically to the elucidation of professional identity in two ways. First, the evaluation model employed uses a three-pronged approach to investigate the process of Clinical Facilitation in relation to learning outcomes and the views of the various stakeholders involved. Second, the facilitation itself was investigated and categorized using an innovative form of reconstitutive ethnography. Both the trident evaluation method and reconstitutive ethnography have potential for the identification of professional identity and quality in the caring professions.

Background

A number of problems and issues led to the establishment of the Pilot Clinical Facilitation Project. These included concerns about

- the availability of clinical placements for student nurses,
- the supervision available on these placements (Jacka & Lewin 1986; Polifroni *et al.* 1995),
- the relevance of the competencies and skills that students were developing as a consequence of the placements and
- the collaboration and communication – or lack of it – between service and higher education.

Although student nurses in the United Kingdom now spend half of their time on placements in hospitals and the community, supervisory support for them has weakened as a result of the abolition of the 'clinical tutor' role and the increased load on practitioners (Jowett *et al.* 1994; Twinn & Davies 1996; May *et al.* 1997). Ward staff are so busy caring for patients that they do not have time to supervise students (Bligh 1995; Wilson & Jennett 1997), and research evidence suggests that students are not learning all the skills they need (Luker *et al.* 1996).

In addition, or perhaps because of, many students and newly qualified staff are leaving nursing.

The 18-month pilot scheme, an evaluation of which is presented in this case study, introduced a category of staff called Clinical Facilitators (CFs) into the acute medical and surgical wards of the hospital trusts of an education and training consortium to work with preregistration nursing students. This was in effect a new hybrid of nurse and teacher: a new professional identity.

The CFs were experienced, skilled and up-to-date nurses who were able to work directly with students and with ward and education staff to improve supervision and placement learning (Rowan & Barber 2000). Twelve CFs were appointed to the medical and surgical wards of six NHS Trust sites. The term Clinical Facilitator appears to be of recent origin (Rowan & Barber 2000). However, the job of supervising the learning of nursing students on placement is as old as nurse training itself and has been (and is) undertaken by various persons, including clinical tutors, mentors, assessors/mentors, university link tutors, as well as staff nurses, ward sisters and ward managers (Campbell *et al.* 1994). Nevertheless, the use of a new title for this project encouraged an innovative approach to practice and also allowed for the evaluation that is described here.

The CFs were intended primarily to enhance the competence of preregistration nursing students on clinical placement. On appointment, they were asked to review their objectives and they proposed five key objectives, which were accepted by the education and training consortium. These objectives were

- to work alongside staff to enhance the preregistration students' experience within the clinical settings of acute medicine and surgery, complementing the clinical setting by use of workshops and group settings;
- to improve the clinical competence of preregistration student nurses within the clinical settings of acute medicine and surgery;
- to facilitate broader external/internal communication links;
- to maintain their own clinical professional credibility as a clinical practitioner and
- to monitor the effectiveness of the role.

These problems have been characterized (Ellis & Hogard 2001) as two deficits needing a solution: a deficit in placements and their supervision and a deficit in competence on qualification. The CFs were intended to address these deficits through enhanced supervision of placements.

The evaluation strategy

Following an earlier attempt to evaluate the pilot scheme internally with a single but complex questionnaire, the evaluation proper commenced in Year Two (a year after the pilot began) and ended when the pilot ended in Year Three. Thus, no pre-testing of competence was possible. However, a novel multi-method approach was developed with three main components: (1) outcomes measurement, (2) process analysis and (3) multiple stakeholder perspectives. For this case study, the focus is on the process of Clinical Facilitation and the use of consultative methods to throw a light on these. From the start, this process analysis was conceived as a partnership between the researcher and the CFs. This partnership was thought to be an excellent basis for the use of consultative methods.

A general profile of the CFs shows that there were 14 women and 2 men participating in the scheme (including returning and maternity posts), but no more than 12 in post at any one time. The CFs were all first-level nurses registered on parts 1 and 2 of the UKCC register – that is, the adult branch. They all had at least 5 years of post-registration experience and most had reached senior staff nurse levels of grade F and G, with some coming from ward management positions. The CFs had varying educational qualifications. Most had completed the English National Board 998 course, 'Teaching and assessing in clinical practice'. Some were enrolled on or had completed the City and Guilds 7307: Further and Adult Teaching Certificate or its higher education equivalent, the Postgraduate Certificate in Education. A few CFs already held Bachelor's degrees, while some were studying for that level of qualification. One CF had completed their Master's degree while working as a CF. All were participating in staff development of some kind, for which support had been provided by the consortium.

The project director took a positive and proactive position regarding staff development from the start of the project. Ten percent of the overall budget was set aside for this purpose. The CFs were encouraged to produce personal development objectives, and they were supported to attend courses and study days consistent with those objectives.

While the evaluation addressed outcomes, process and stakeholder perspectives, this case study focuses on the process section where the consultative methods were employed.

Process analysis

Along with outcome measurement and stakeholder perspectives, the second major aspect of the evaluation was the process analysis of what the CFs actually did in practice. This process analysis would elucidate the competency part of professional identity in the threefold model of knowledge; competency and values outlined in Chapter 1. This is the part of the case study which exemplifies the use of the four consultative methods introduced in this chapter. Thus, the identification of the teaching approaches adopted by the CFs was a key objective. This was approached through consultation with the CFs themselves, involving in-depth interviews, focus groups and questionnaires. The objective was to produce a comprehensive description and modeling of Clinical Facilitation that would come from consultation with the participants and would be verified by them as authentic.

It was here that the evaluation was most innovative technically and substantively. There is a dearth of studies that actually describe and analyze the practice of nursing and nurse education. Insufficient use has been made of consultation with professionals themselves. In principle, three approaches could be adopted to elucidate professional practice. One would be based on detailed observation of practice. The second, used extensively, would be determining and codifying practice and procedures from first principles. The third approach would be to arrive at descriptions through consultation with the professionals themselves. These three approaches could be termed the empirical, the analytical and the consultative (Ellis 1988).

The first approach, involving naturalistic observation of the CFs at work, was impractical in the timescale and circumstances of the research; the second would also have been too time-consuming and raised fundamental questions of validity. Hence, it was decided to follow a consultative approach based on in-depth individual interviews and focus groups with the 12 CFs themselves. Models of Clinical Facilitation emerging from the first interviews would then be verified by the CFs themselves in the second round of individual interviews, thus following the iterative approach described by Mehan (1979) as a 'constitutive ethnography' but developed through the use of a Delphi technique as described by Reid and Hogard in Chapter 19.

During the first round of interviews, the CFs were asked, 'what motivated you to become a Clinical Facilitator?' The CFs' responses fell into four broad categories, which tended to overlap. First, there were statements about their commitment to nursing as a profession, to the practice of nursing, to nurse education and to the nursing students. They indicated the ways in which the post would allow them to put this commitment into practice. Second, there were statements about their own competence and suitability for the post, including reference to their practical nursing skills, teaching skills, capacity to motivate and ability to meet challenges. They also saw the post as a logical development of their career from practitioner to educator of novice practitioners. Third, there were references to the potential of the post to improve the learning experience of students and hence the quality of nursing. Finally, there were references to the post bridging the gap between theory and practice, and between higher education and service.

The CFs were then asked, 'what skills should a Clinical Facilitator possess to be successful in the post?' The CFs described an individual who would need to be extremely deft in communication skills, diplomacy and tact in order to work productively between stakeholders in education and service. Not surprisingly, comprehensive nursing experience and clinical credibility were also considered imperative for work as a CF.

In the main part of the interview, the CFs were then encouraged to describe their activities through a form of critical incident analysis (Flanagan 1954). This was approached in several ways. The CFs were asked to describe a typical day's or part day's activities: to recall incidents when their practice was successful and, conversely, when it was less successful. In describing their work, CFs were encouraged to relate accounts of their own activities to those of their students, to students' learning and to aspects of the competent nurse's role. Generally, CFs were able to describe their own activities but found it difficult to relate those activities to specific student learning outcomes.

A detailed list of activities was distilled from the transcripts of the first interviews; these provided the starting point for the second set of interviews, in which CFs were asked to verify, expand or modify the list and, again, to relate their activities to student learning outcomes. They were also invited to comment on a four-level model of Clinical Facilitation and, at the first level, the six aspects of supervision and/or teaching that had emerged from analyzing the transcripts of the first interview. While CFs were able to provide more examples of instances, these did not affect the model, which was verified by the CFs as appropriate. They were keen to emphasize that they supported students in their learning but felt that this commitment to support informed each supervisory behavior rather than being a category itself.

Following these second interviews with the CFs, the four-level model of Clinical Facilitation was confirmed. This model was based primarily on the material from the interviews but also took account of descriptions of possible roles given by managers in higher education in their individual interviews. While recognizing the value of face-to-face supervision and the management of student learning, education managers stressed the potential value of a single coordinator of placement learning for a ward or group of wards who could also contribute to securing and quality-assuring placements in the following ways: direct face-to-face supervision of students; the management of student learning through arranging learning experiences and supervision/instruction of students by others; maintaining an overview of student placement and learning at an organizational level, for example, a group of wards in a hospital; and undertaking a strategic planning role for a higher education institution in securing and quality-assuring clinical placements. The work of these CFs, based on their descriptions, appeared to be primarily at the supervisory and managerial levels, with some contributions at the organizational level. They had no opportunity to fulfill a strategic role. This analysis was based broadly on the expert system approach.

This examination of the CF's role in its organizational context involved an expert system approach describing the path followed by a student from induction to their placement through all the activities and support necessary and culminating in their final report. This support required the harmonization of hospital and university processes and the organization of staff in the hospital.

The responses given by the CFs mainly concerned their work at the supervisory level of direct face-to-face teaching of students, and that is the focus of this chapter. On the basis of the detailed list of activities generated by their responses, the supervisory role was categorized provisionally into six main types of activity or teaching methods as follows:

- Demonstrating a skill to a student
- Pointing out good practice to a student (denotation)
- Giving the student a chance to practice a skill
- Discussing the student's work with them
- Giving the student a chance to practice in a skills laboratory or workshop
- Giving the student a lecture about a skill

Following the second round of interviews, the models were circulated to the CFs, who discussed them at their regular meeting and finally confirmed them as appropriate at a focus group with the researchers.

This process analysis is a good example of the reconstitutive ethnography method that can be a useful tool for the investigation and elucidation of professional client interaction (Hogard 2007) and specifically of teacher–student interaction. It is grounded in the perceptions and reflections of the teachers. It is iterative and progressively focused. It is captured and categorized in a form that can be verified by the teachers. The results of the process analysis can also be considered and validated by the students and other stakeholders. Critically, it can be related to the concurrent or subsequent outcomes of the process.

Conclusion

This case study of consultative methods used to investigate the process of Clinical Facilitation has been drawn from a comprehensive evaluation of a pilot scheme to introduce CFs into the medical and surgical wards of six general hospitals to facilitate the placement learning of student nurses. These facilitators, a new category of staff, were introduced to address two problems: the shortage of adequately supervised placements and the deficit in clinical skills of newly qualified nurses. The context for these problems was national difficulties in recruiting and retaining nurses. The facilitators were distinctive in that, unlike other ward staff and university staff, they were dedicated full time to the supervision and facilitation of student learning in the wards. Clearly, they made a quantitative contribution to supervision and increased the amount that students received. Students, ward staff and university staff were unanimous in agreeing that the CFs had met four of the key objectives, including the central one regarding the enhancement of clinical competence in students. The only doubts were expressed regarding the communication objective, and this might well reflect the imprecise but potentially wide-ranging nature of the objective itself. The use of a critical incident method elucidated the effective practices of CF and enabled these to be summarized in an innovative model. An expert system approach clarified the managerial and interorganizational aspects of the role.

The CFs in this pilot were given a broad brief to enhance the clinical competence of students. How they should work was left largely to the CFs themselves. It was therefore important to capture the details of their working methods. The investigation of the process of Clinical Facilitation used a consultative method involving in-depth interviews with the CFs themselves. This produced a model of Clinical Facilitation that included four possible levels of operation and a six-fold characterization of direct face-to-face supervision. While these six aspects of supervision, including observation of good practice, practice and receiving feedback on practice, are predictable, they are authentic reflections of the views of the facilitators and are indicative of the kind of information that can be adduced regarding professional practice through the use of consultative methods as distinct from direct observation. The six activities were subsequently rated for utility by students, ward staff and university staff. There was a consensus that the most useful methods involved demonstration and observation of good practice, practice and receiving feedback on practice. University staff placed a relatively higher value on lectures and discussion than the other stakeholders, which probably reflects their different perspective on the curriculum as a whole. Further research would be necessary to authenticate these methods and to study their relationship with outcomes. It would also be necessary to identify and evaluate the extent to which others involved in practice education employ such methods and to identify the optimal skills mix between, for example, assessor/mentors, other ward staff, university staff and CFs.

The evaluation of a particular form of teaching described in this case study used two relatively novel approaches which can make a contribution to the elucidation of professional identity and quality in teaching and in other caring professions. The first was the three-pronged approach to the evaluation of a new professional identity focusing on outcomes, process and multiple stakeholder perspectives (Ellis & Hogard 2006). This proved its utility by highlighting the lacuna in outcome measures for the key objective of the teaching and by giving the process of teaching in the form of Clinical Facilitation more attention than is often the case. The second was the use of reconstitutive ethnography, a form of consultation, as an approach to data-gathering regarding the practice of Clinical Facilitation itself (Hogard 2007).

In this chapter, we have advocated consultative methods for the investigation of professional identity. We have described four particular consultative methods and exemplified their use in the investigation of a new hybrid professional role, that of the Clinical Facilitator in Nurse Education.

We would suggest that consultative methods might be used to establish meanings for a professional identity; serve as a qualitative measure of professional knowledge, competence and values and be employed for learning and assessment in the development of a professional identity. They can, in a study, complement psychometric and observational approaches.

While our case study is in Nurse Education, it is our hope that research into the professional identity of the range of caring professions covered in this book might benefit from these consultative approaches.

References

Bligh, J. (1995). The clinical skills unit. *Postgraduate Medical Journal, 71*(842), 730–732.

Campbell, I. E., Larrivee, L., Field, P. A., Day, R. A., & Reutter, L. (1994). Learning to nurse in the clinical setting. *Journal of Advanced Nursing, 20*(6), 1125–1131.

Ellis, R. (1988). *Professional competence and quality assurance in the caring professions.* London: Croom Helm.

Ellis, R., & Hogard, E. (2001). *Evaluation of the pilot project for clinical placement facilitation.* Chester UK: Chester College of Higher Education, School of Nursing and Midwifery.

Ellis, R., & Hogard, E. (2006). The trident: A three-pronged method for evaluating clinical, social and educational innovations. *Evaluation, 12*(3), 372–383.

Ellis, R. (2019). Quality assurance for university teaching; approaches and issues. In: Ellis, R., & Hogard, E. (Eds.), *Handbook of quality assurance for University teaching.* London and New York: Routledge.

Eraut, M. (1985). Knowledge creation and knowledge use in professional contexts. *Studies in Higher Education, 10*(2), 117–133.

Eraut, M. (2000). Non-formal learning and tacit knowledge in professional work. *British Journal of Educational Psychology, 70*(1), 113–136.

Flanagan, J. C. (1954). The critical incident technique. *Psychological Bulletin, 51*(4), 327.

Friedland, B., Henricson, M., & Mårtensson, J. (2017). Critical incident technique applied in nursing and healthcare sciences. *SOJ Nursing & Health Care, 3*(1), 1–5.

Hargie, O. (2016). *Skilled interpersonal communication: Research, theory and practice.* London and New York: Routledge.

Hogard, E. (2007). Using consultative methods to investigate professional client interaction as an aspect of process evaluation. *American Journal of Evaluation, 28*(3), 304–317.

Hossain, M. S., Ahmed, F., & Andersson, K. (2017). A belief rule based expert system to assess tuberculosis under uncertainty. *Journal of Medical Systems, 41*(3), 43.

Hu, Z., Zhang, Z., Yang, H., Chen, Q., & Zuo, D. (2017). A deep learning approach for predicting the quality of online health expert question-answering services. *Journal of Biomedical Informatics, 71*, 241–253.

Jacka, K., & Lewin, D. (1986). Elucidation and measurement of clinical learning opportunity. *Journal of Advanced Nursing, 11*(5), 573–582.

Jowett, S., Walton, I., & Payne, S. (1994). *Challenges and change in nurse education: A study of the implementation of project 2000: Executive summary.* London: NFER.

Luker, K., Carlisle, C., Riley, E., Stilwell, J., Davies, C., & Wilson, R. (1996). Project 2000: Fitness for purpose. *Report to the department of health*. UK: Universities of Liverpool and Warwick.

May, N., Veitch, L., & McIntosh, J. B. (1997). *Preparation for practice: Evaluation of nurse and midwife education in Scotland: 1992 programmes*.

Mehan, H. (1979). *Learning lessons*. Cambridge, MA: Harvard University Press.

Polifroni, E. C., Packard, S. A., Shah, H. S., & MacAvoy, S. (1995). Activities and interactions of baccalaureate nursing students in clinical practice. *Journal of Professional Nursing, 11*(3), 161–169.

Rowan, P., & Barber, P. (2000). Clinical facilitators: A new way of working. *Nursing Standard, 14*(52), 35.

Steven, A., Wilson, G., Turunen, H., Vizcaya-Moreno, M. F., Azimirad, M., Khakurel, J., Porras, J., Tella, S., Pérez-Cañaveras, R., Sasso, L., Aleo, G., Myhre, K., Ringstad, Ø., Sara-Aho, A., Scott, M., & Pearson, P. (2020). Critical incident techniques and reflection in nursing and health professions education: A systematic narrative review. *Nurse Educator*. https://doi.org/10.1097/nne.0000000000000796.

Tombs, M. (2019). Use the Critical Incident Technique (CIT) in Medical Education Research. *How to series*, 1–2.

Twinn, S., & Davies, S. (1996). The supervision of project 2000 students in the clinical setting: Issues and implications for practitioners. *Journal of Clinical Nursing, 5*(3), 177–183.

Viergever, R. F. (2019). The critical incident technique: Method or methodology? *Qualitative Health Research, 29*(7), 1065–1079.

Weinreich, P., & Saunderson, W. (Eds.). (2005). *Analysing identity: Cross-cultural, societal and clinical contexts*. Routledge. London and New York

Wikström, L., Eriksson, K., Fridlund, B., Årestedt, K., & Broström, A. (2016). Healthcare professionals' descriptions of care experiences and actions when assessing postoperative pain – A critical incident technique analysis. *Scandinavian Journal of Caring Sciences, 30*(4), 802–812.

Wilson, D. B., & Jennett, P. A. (1997). The Medical Skills Centre at the University of Calgary Medical School. *Medical Education, 31*(1), 45–48.

World Health Organization. (1999). *The world health report: 1999: Making a difference*. World Health Organization. Geneva

19 The potential contribution of the Delphi technique to the study of professional identity

Norma Reid Birley and Elaine Hogard

Introduction

The Delphi technique is a research tool which can incorporate qualitative, quantitative and mixed methodologies to obtain a professional consensus on complex concepts and constructs such as professional identity. Having originated in structured consensual forecasting, it has since been used widely in medicine, nursing, social work and teaching research to reach expert consensus on topics related to professional identity. We argue that it still has considerable potential to explore meaning, measurement and pedagogy in the caring professions.

In this chapter the concept of professional identity is briefly explored in relation to its meaning, measurement and mastery, so as to define and clarify these, in the context of consideration of the use of the Delphi technique. This methodology is then described, with suggestions about its optimal use, employing the richness of qualitative methods alongside the rigour of quantitative methods. The use of the Delphi as a flexible and potentially powerful method is then explored in relation to professional identity. Finally, a nursing education case study of the use of the Delphi Technique is provided for potential new users and to illustrate its power in the context of professional identity.

Professional identity

Meaning

Professional identity is a concept which permeates the culture, ethos, practice and delivery of the caring professions. The term is widely used both formally and informally, generally with an implicit assumption that its meaning is clear and understood. But, in fact, as Ellis and Hogard (2020) point out in the context of the medical profession, professional identity is often understood interchangeably with such terms as 'profession', 'professional' and 'professionalism'. This undoubtedly is also the case across the spectrum of caring professions, albeit that each profession will have distinctive views and perspectives, informed by such factors as its history, evolution, culture and perceived role in the delivery of the caring services.

Professional identity covers arguably every aspect of the work of the caring professions and their practitioners including self-concept, concepts of peers, knowledge, skills and competencies, and professional and educational standards in both initial and subsequent education. Different caring professions are likely to deconstruct professional identity in distinctive ways, whilst also having much in common.

Crucially, there is general agreement that professional identity depends critically on the values, held by the individual professionals, peers and externally validated professional bodies, who strongly influence accepted wisdom on these often broadly stated values, whilst by no means always defining them precisely. However, several caring professions have made extensive, and sometimes, explicit statements of core values and attributes, which could be further developed into measurable entities and thus contribute to the mastery of professional identity in the caring professions. See, for example, Webb (2017) on professional identity and social work.

The definition of 'values' used by Ellis and Hogard (2020) and adopted in this chapter is 'Values are principles or standards of behaviour. They are not directly observable but are inferred from behaviour'. Professional identity can be viewed from both internal and external perspectives. It may cover the self-concept of the individual professional. This may encompass a wide range of personal and interpersonal factors, besides a multiplicity of experiences, positive and negative, of professional practice of the individual, peers, seniors and subordinates, and the external world.

External perceptions are important and can be either positive or negative from the viewpoint of the practitioner. For example, the impact of the various powerful and esteemed professional bodies of the caring professions can never be underestimated. But some caring professions, notably social work in recent years, have been subject to sustained negative external comment in the context of deaths of children in care, and child sex abuse investigations. Such external influences may well be to the detriment of positive professional identity. So professional identity is a multifaceted concept as indeed are values, which are so central to professional identity. Neither concept is directly observable but must be deduced from behaviours which can be observed. Ellis and Hogard (2020) define values as fundamental beliefs that determine behaviour in a range of situations. But they point out that values themselves being constructs are not directly observable and must be inferred from consistencies in observable behaviour. Values are sometimes called 'attributes' when they clearly align with a set of observable behaviours or a behavioural disposition.

In understanding the meaning of professional identity through the identification of values or attributes, it is often helpful to be more specific about the meaning of each value, and through a process of increasing specification, to reach statements of observable and thus measurable behaviour. This process is central to consideration of the measurement of professional identity, and its mastery in the curriculum and in teaching, learning and assessment to which we turn later in this chapter.

In the caring professions, the concept of 'values' is inextricably linked with codes of professional ethics. Most medical schools in the world still use some form of the Hippocratic Oath, which is, in essence, an attempt to state fundamental values/ethical standards to which graduating medical students publicly swear. In its various versions through the ages, it has remained surprisingly succinct, ranging originally from some five short statements to some eleven (Lasagna, 1964). But it has often been simply characterised as the following.

Primum non nocere – first, do no harm

However, as a statement of the meaning of professional identity, medical ethics or values, arguably no version of the Hippocratic Oath moves one forward in understanding its practical meaning and significance for modern clinical and educational practice, until it is subdivided into a longer list of more specific values. Such subdivision and specification would need to be carried out many times, in order, for example, to describe even some of the values that should underpin the medical curriculum in order to provide graduates who can abide by the Hippocratic Oath. To promote the teaching, learning and assessment of the Oath as the seminal principle of medical education would require a great deal of translation of these more specific values into observable and measurable behaviours. The iterative consensual nature of the Delphi technique is well placed to facilitate this translation.

Measurement

In the context of professional identity, or almost any other conceivable construct, the concept of measurement does not always excite the imagination of many care professionals. Only mathematicians' and psychologists' blood pressures rise to that apparently idiosyncratic challenge. But it matters hugely.

It is a fundamental issue in matters of professional hegemony, credibility and status in the caring professions; it underlies sustained tensions in the status of research and pedagogy within these professions and defines the seminal relationships that determine the care of patients and clients. It is thus a central tenet of professional identity.

These time-worn tensions among the caring professions map very neatly, and not by accident, into the philosophical battle between the relative virtues and shortcomings of qualitative and quantitative research and pedagogical methods of inquiry.

All of this is about 'levels of measurement'. This is a technical term, which has profound implications for research and pedagogy in the caring professions. The classical view of the following four levels of measurement was produced by Stanley Smith Stevens in 1946 and is still widely used and accepted (Stevens, 1946).

Nominal

The nominal level of measurement is usually considered the 'lowest' of the four ways to characterise data. Nominal data deals with names, categories or labels.

The most essential thing about nominal scales is that they do not imply any ordering among the responses. Responses are simply categorised.

Data at the nominal level is qualitative. For example, colour of eyes, nationality, apples or oranges.

Ordinal

Data at the ordinal level of measurement can be ordered, but no meaningful differences can be drawn between the data. Ordinal scales are typically measures of non-numeric, but hierarchical concepts like satisfaction, social class or professional rank.

One of the major drawbacks of an ordinal level of measurement is that it often lacks the capability required to capture important information. In particular, the difference between any two levels of an ordinal scale cannot be assumed to be the same as the difference between any two other levels. For example, hierarchies of professional ranks in any of the caring professions, or any of the taxonomies of social class.

Interval

The interval level of measurement, the next level, deals with data that can be ordered and bears exact comparison. It is to be noted that differences between the data are rigorous, but there is no meaningful baseline. Interval scales are hierarchical numerical scales in which intervals have the same interpretation throughout. However, data at this level does not have a definite starting point. For example, temperature as measured by a thermometer. There is no such thing as 'no' temperature.

Ratio

In the ratio level of measurement, an absolute zero exists that is meaningful. This means that you can construct a meaningful fraction (or ratio) with a ratio variable.

A classic example of a ratio level of measurement is the amount of money you have in your wallet right now (could be £5, etc.). Money is measured on a ratio scale, more than anything else because, in addition to having the properties of an interval scale, it has a true zero point: if you have zero money, this implies the absence of money. Since money has a true zero point, it makes sense to say that someone with 50 pounds has twice as much money as someone with 25 pounds.

So, we have four levels of measurement. For professionals seeking, or nurturing a sense of professional identity, this may seem esoteric and irrelevant, but it actually impacts on every aspect of their daily lives.

There is a hierarchy explicit in the level of measurement concept, which dominates research, development, delivery and pedagogy in the caring professions, and, crucially, inter-professional relationships and interactions. At so-called lower levels of measurement, assumptions tend to be qualitative and open to criticisms of imprecision and idiosyncratic subjectivity. At the so-called higher end of the data spectrum, of which clinical trials would be the gold standard, the reductionism of such research is criticised for its unrealistic and rigid prior conditions, in setting quantifiable and controllable conditions as the epitome of scientific inquiry.

The qualitative advocates in the caring professions argue that they better represent the realities, whilst their antagonists claim their approach lacks scientific rigour and applies only to the limited environment of their immediate work. In contrast, many qualitative champions in the caring professions argue that the reductionism of reality, necessary often for more quantitative work, misses the essence of the caring professions. However, at each level up the widely accepted hierarchy of levels of measurement, any given level includes all of the qualities of the one below it and adds additional analytic potential.

Only the 'lowest' level of measurement – nominal – is characterised by the scientific and medical academic networks as a technique of qualitative methodology in research – and not generally with approbation. The rest tend to be regarded with increasing respect, according to how quantifiable they are. However, it is interesting that the oldest versions of the Hippocratic Oath describe medicine as both an art and a science.

This hierarchy of levels of measurement is inextricably an assumption of research and pedagogy in the caring professions. It has been and continues to be a rationale for hegemony within the caring professions. So, levels of measurement, and associated methods of inquiry matter, and their use, rationale and effectiveness are an essential element of professional identity.

The Delphi technique is well placed to encourage consideration by research experts and others in the professions of appropriate units of analysis and relationships relevant to professional identity and practice. The iterative consideration of options and alternatives can arrive at a functional consensus regarding the nature of, acquisition and analysis of relevant data.

Mastery

If professional identity is, as has been argued, a seminal factor in the beliefs, tenets, values, culture and practice of the caring professions, it must then be mastered in the processes of education, the recruitment of students, the design of the curriculum, the methods of teaching and learning, and crucially assessment of the effectiveness of all of these to deliver the professionals who will exemplify and promote that professional identity.

Starting with the recruitment and selection of students wishing to study in the caring professions, this has historically been a process primarily predicated on credible, nationally and internationally recognised qualifications, such as degrees and baccalaureates. In the caring professions, these have in recent times been supplemented with various types of interviews, structured and unstructured, psychometric testing and profession-specific practical and clinical testing, e.g. the

Objective Structured Clinical Examinations (Harden et al., 2015) used in many medical schools. Accounts of such external more subjectively reported experiences as volunteering, paid work, placements and social and community engagement are also often invited.

All of these more demanding and time-consuming approaches have come under increasing pressure from the huge expansion in higher education in the United Kingdom, and the over-subscription in applications for almost all courses in the caring professions.

Further, as Ellis and Hogard (2020) note, 'Assessing the values held by applicants and their potential for developing the values central to a professional identity is particularly difficult. This approach to selection is called Values Based Recruitment (VBR). VBR is an approach which attracts and selects students, trainees or employees on the basis that their individual values and behaviours align with the values of the selecting organisation'.

In a relatively cost-effective, pioneering initiative to address this, they have devised a web-based psychometric test, Medi-Match, which is being developed at medical schools in Canada and Northern Ireland. Whilst some form of value-based recruitment may be the prerequisite for attracting students with a strong sense of professional identity, in maximising this benefit, it must also inform and permeate curriculum design, teaching, learning and assessment, if mastery of professional identity is to be achieved. The challenges of doing so centrally involve issues of meaning and measurement.

In all of these, it is argued that the Delphi technique has the potential to make a significant contribution.

The Delphi technique

Description

The classical Delphi technique, named after Apollo's Delphic oracle, is a method for the systematic collection and aggregation of informed judgements from a group of experts on specific questions or issues. It is based on a structured or unstructured presentation of relevant information. This information is sent individually, and confidentially, to each expert who then responds to the researcher. The consensus of opinion is collated, and information on the consensus or lack of consensus is sent again to each expert, including the anonymous views of other experts. Each expert is asked to reconsider and respond again in confidence. Again, consensus is collated. Repeat rounds of this process can be carried out until full consensus is reached. It is more usual, however, to halt the process when sufficient consensus is deemed to have been achieved.

A major attribute and advantage of the method is that it removes the interpersonal factors that so often heavily influence emergence of a consensus in face-to-face groups or committees. The method further provides a systematic approach in exploring the judgements of experts. Such judgements are very important in securing high face validity in research and pedagogical inquiry in the caring professions.

In the design of the research materials, it also has arguably an underutilised capacity for flexibility, in enabling optimal selection of qualitative or quantitative or, indeed, mixed-methodologies, which can be exceptionally powerful as a way to deconstruct and study complex concepts in the caring professions, such as professional identity. See the case study in Section 5.

It has generally been recognised that there are three main types of Delphi technique, the numeric, the policy and the historic. These are often aligned with particular levels of measurement and thus provide one of the great strengths of the Delphi technique in utilising quantitative research methods, qualitative research methods or a mix of both.

The classic and still widely cited paper of Strauss and Zeigler (1975) stated that the goal of the numeric Delphi is to specify a single or minimum range of numeric estimates or forecasts on a problem; the goal of the policy Delphi is to define a range of answers or alternatives to a current or anticipated policy problem, and the goal of the historic Delphi is to explain the range of issues that fostered a specific decision or to identify the range of possible alternatives that could have been poised against a specified past decision.

History and development

In the historical development of the Delphi technique, the Delphi concept may be viewed as one of the spin-offs of defence research. The method was developed in the United States in the early 1950s in a study by the Rand Corporation of the likely targets and impact of a Russian bombing campaign. The reason for the development of this new method was that accurate information was unavailable or too expensive to obtain in an area where, in any case, subjective evaluation would also be required. It was believed that consensual forecasts arrived at by a group of experts would be more powerful than individual experts forecasting alone.

Interest in the Delphi method was confined to the defence community until another RAND paper was published by Gordon and Helmer (1964) on the use of the method in technological forecasting. In contrast to its use as a qualitative method in the cold war context, the use of the Delphi in forecasting generally used quantitative levels of measurement which were thus amenable to statistical techniques of analysis.

By the 1960s, use of the method had spread both geographically and in the areas of application. Academics discovered the method relatively late, but in the 1980s, there was increasing use of the method by education researchers and by researchers from a range of social science disciplines including psychology, sociology and social policy. Of the caring professions addressed in this book, the early use of the Delphi in education spread to social work, nursing and medicine.

In the early 1980s, a computer search of the ERIC database of published research (Educational Resources Information Center) to identify Delphi use in Education revealed 368 papers using the Delphi method published since 1966. An updated ERIC search in 2020 revealed nearly 2000 papers. These covered a wide range of applications from education management to personnel management, indices of quality and the identification of physical and mental problems of children. Searches in social work revealed a similar growth in the use of the technique ranging from studies of the needs of client groups through aspects of practice and technique to national policies.

There has been widespread use of the Delphi technique in nursing research where its focus on qualitative data with a potential for quantification has proved popular. It is beyond the remit of this chapter to provide a full up-to-date literature review of the use of the Delphi technique in nursing research, but its markedly increased use since the 1980s has been described by, for example, McKenna (1994) and again by Keeney et al., (2011) which remains a popular handbook not only for nursing but health applications more broadly.

There has been a comparable growth in medicine and medical education and health care generally. Useful review articles include Trevelyan and Robinson (2015) who introduce the Delphi through two studies from which they identify possible pitfalls and recommend best practice. Rowe and Wright (2011) review the use of the Delphi technique over half a century and, in advocating further empirical studies, summarise the lessons that have been learned to date. Humphrey-Murto et al. (2017) review the use of the Delphi and other consensus group methods in Medicine and Medical Education and conclude that such methods including the Delphi are poorly standardised and inconsistently used in medical education research, and improved criteria for reporting are needed.

The impressive number of research citations meanwhile in such sources as Google Scholar testifies to the methodology's sustained popularity and credibility as a research instrument for use with the caring professions. But clearly the method still needs to be standardised with generally accepted procedures. The term Delphi indicates only that a study will be based on some form of iterative sequential consultation with experts to reach a consensus. However, various approaches are adopted to the presentation of options and to the analysis and quantification of results.

Strengths

In the context of the caring professions, seeking consensus through a panel of experts through anonymous and private communications between the researcher and the expert panel has particular advantages. This is because, in general, the face validity of the Delphi is highly valued in the caring professions, reflecting the essential personal and interpersonal essence of these.

It is also the case that expert opinion on clinical and client issues often resides across a wide range of middle and very senior grades. The strictly hierarchical grade structures of the caring professions can open up the possibility of authoritarianism, even when in some caring professions the professional expertise at the middle-grade front-line interface with the public can be seminal. It can be very inhibiting, and it can even be damaging, to challenge the professional view of a senior in the presence of others. The Delphi method enables more junior practitioners to make an equally valued and anonymous contribution.

The method also removes the difficulty that many people have in yielding ground on opinions they have publicly stated. The Delphi allows for second thoughts in privacy. By the same token, it enables a more thoughtful response. Many people feel pressurised into making perhaps over-hasty responses when in a public arena. The Delphi method is most useful in dealing with problems that do not initially lend themselves to highly quantitative and reductive analytical techniques but can be illuminated from subjective judgements on a collective basis. It allows a range of people with possibly diverse backgrounds and expertise to contribute and remove the communication problems that such diverse contributors might experience in a conference or committee process.

The method is, therefore, particularly useful in exploring interdisciplinary issues, a critical element of current good practice in both research and pedagogy in the caring professions. Taking into account the relatively low communication costs, the Delphi method allows the involvement of more professionals in large panels – in fact, it is one of the cheapest research methods available (Reid, 1985).

Weaknesses

There have been, however, criticisms of the Delphi method, many relating to the claim of scientific respectability that is often made for the method. The classical analysts of the method, e.g. Linstone and Turoff (1975), in fact assert that the Delphi method is more of an art than a science. This is interesting in the light of the original Hippocratic Oath – which asserted that medicine was both an art and a science within its historic collection of statements of fundamental medical values – and, by inference, professional identity.

But there is no doubt that many users of the method have presented it as having the properties of a scientific approach. Taking the classical scientific criteria of validity and reliability, does the Delphi method meet these? In professional identity, for example, would it elicit material affirming its designers' and panels' beliefs? If the same structured material were sent to two comparable Delphi panels, would the same consensus emerge? These issues hang on the subjectivity of the Delphi panel, and the possible ephemeral nature of opinions. Uhl (1975) gave a structured questionnaire to a panel of 26 members and reached consensus in three rounds. To test the reliability of that consensus, he gave the same questionnaire to the same panel a year later. The results were more like the initial Delphi round than the final round on the first Delphi process. The consensus did not appear to have been lasting. This still rare and possibly unique investigation of the reliability of the Delphi thus raises concerns about both its validity and reliability.

We, therefore, recommend that where scientific values are important, the Delphi is not necessarily the optimal technique – on these grounds, it fares badly by comparison with such established methodologies as clinical randomised controlled trials, rigorously designed psychometric scale construction or any research design based on the principles of statistical inference.

The latter, however, has particular significance in the size, selection criteria and designation of Delphi panels of experts. It is here that we would argue that the methodological value of the Delphi can in many cases be considerably enhanced by the application of statistical inference, involving sampling in the selection of the expert panel. The size of panels varies to an extraordinary degree in published research. Mostly, the panel is implicitly claimed to be a total population of experts, selected on unevaluated researcher-generated criteria. This rarely bears scrutiny, although neatly swerves the question of generalisability of the research.

Large panels, on the other hand, rarely claim to be a population, but, in many published examples, have produced extremely low response rates, whether sampled representatively or not. Follow-up exhortations to non-response have not become embedded in use of the Delphi, raising serious concerns of response bias, which would rightly be castigated in postal surveys, the nearest methodological neighbour of the Delphi.

One more historical criticism of the Delphi was that its dependence on successive rounds of then postal communications made it relatively time-consuming as a methodology. The potential to address this by electronic communication has been surprisingly under-utilised to date. However, the term 'e-Delphi' has now appeared in the literature, and there are several products cited in studies, including commercial products called e-Delphi, MESYDEL, WELPHI and EDELPHI. See, for example, Meshkat et al (2014), Msibi et al (2018) and Toronto (2017).

In particular, the e-Delphi offers unparalleled convenience, time and cost savings, and data management options, including electronic transfer into statistical analysis packages such as SPSS. Although the e-Delphi technique is a creative and efficient method for facilitating research, there are limitations associated with the Delphi study in this relatively new virtual landscape. (See, for example Helms et al. (2017), or Donohoe and Needham(2009).) They cite reported problems of internet access, connectivity, technological support, management and concerns about anonymity. While many of the issues can be considered to be a reflection of the nature of technology and the internet, some limitations associated with the traditional Delphi can be intensified and new issues can present when the internet is used to facilitate the technique. (See, for example, Donohoe and Needham (2009), Donohoe et al (2012), Cole et al (2013).) It must also be acknowledged that the e-Delphi and other internet-based approaches are simply tools to be used and applied, when appropriate.

The use of e-communication can certainly speed up the iterative rounds of the Delphi, and by using instantly interactive electronic platforms – albeit somehow anonymised – could discard the notion of 'rounds' altogether, allowing consensus to emerge organically with maximum flexibility of personal and interpersonal interaction.

This leads to what is known as Real Time Delphi or RTD. This is a more recent development in the Delphi technique which, due to the electronic platform, allows participants to respond whenever they so choose so that it could be multiple times and thereby moving away from the classic one-point iteration with structured deadlines for single input. Aengenheyster et al (2017) test four Real Time tools and assess them using a system of evaluation categories they have devised. They conclude that further development is required if such instruments are to be widely used.

In principle, the burgeoning social media could be employed in devising new methods of Delphi data capture. For example, crowdsourcing techniques might be employed (Flostrand, 2017). However, whilst possible in theory, experience of social media in producing consensus is discouraging. And it is interesting that quite a number of contemporary writers claim that good old-fashioned e-mail is the best tool for the development of the Delphi in the electronic age (see, for example, Kent and Saffer (2014).)

The Delphi technique is, like all research and pedagogical methods, exemplary when used appropriately, and we would argue to the maximum potential of scientific rigour in its application. We now address this in the context of the meaning, measurement and mastery of professional identity.

Professional identity and the Delphi technique

Meaning

The elaboration and deconstruction of the meaning of professional identity, as an agglomeration of values, professional ethics, and much else besides, must surely be a qualitatively based investigation. Qualitative Delphi materials are well-placed to address this, albeit with quantitative adaptations in panel selection to enable a generalisable inquiry.

The concept of professional identity is widely recognised to adapt over time – our example of the Hippocratic Oath illustrated this – but also is likely to vary, even within a caring profession, depending on the status, seniority, professional role, external or internal viewpoint and self-concept of the individuals. So, for example, in most caring professions, the following constituencies could be seen as in some sense 'owning' a sense of the meaning of professional identity:

- Professional bodies and associations and trades' unions
- Front-line practitioners in face-to-face delivery
- Senior managers with largely administrative roles
- Educationalists who determine admissions, the curriculum, teaching, learning and assessments
- Students who are attracted to the profession as a vocation

It is important in carrying out a Delphi, to be clear which of these, or whether several of these are the relevant constituency for the selection of the expert panel to seek a context-specific consensus on professional identity. This then provides defensible criteria for panel selection, and, we would argue, then allows a more rigorous approach to be taken to panel selection, which will support wider generalisability, applicability and scientific credibility of the study.

If a case can be made for the panel constituency to be a total monopolistic population of relevant experts, in the physical, professional and political environment of the study (and its consequent size is manageable for the study), the panel is self-selected. If not, an appropriate sampling method will improve the study design and the generalisability of its results.

However, if the constituency is, for example, external stakeholders on professional identity such as Professional Bodies and Trade Unions, sampling techniques, preferably random or stratified sampling, should provide a representative panel external perspectives on professional identity, with inferential qualities of generalisation beyond the immediate study.

Many published studies alternatively use selection criteria chosen by the researcher, but this, of course, is open to criticisms of researcher bias.

This use of sampling methods sits easily with an entirely qualitative approach to the study materials, the selection or design of which are the next stage in a Delphi, and in seeking to elaborate on or clarify the meaning of professional identity, the use of a qualitative approach to materials design and analysis is, in the first instance, self-evident.

Either an unstructured approach or a structured approach could be taken. The panel could simply be asked to provide a narrative of their perception of professional identity. Such qualitative methods of analysis as item analysis – for which commercial and academic software are widely available – could then be used to identify coherent themes in the responses. These themes could then provide the materials for an iterative Delphi process of as many rounds as considered necessary in seeking consensus. The usual process of feeding back consensus at each stage and inviting reconsideration where there is no consensus would likely be done electronically by email or some more bespoke or self-designed template (see, for example, Toronto, 2017).

An alternative approach would be to use an extensive relevant literature review to provide a menu of published facets of professional identity, (for example, Webb, 2017) which could then be subjected to item analysis, if necessary, and then, the above process could be followed.

The Delphi, thus, provides a flexible and rigorous approach, encompassing the best methodological approaches, in exploring the meaning of professional identity, for either research or pedagogical purposes.

For an illustrative example of this use of the Delphi Method, see the case study in Section 5.

Measurement

The previous section describes how the Delphi method can elucidate and clarify the meaning of professional identity. If successful, it is likely to result in a nominal taxonomy of consensual values – but in understanding the meaning of professional identity, it can only be a first stage. Because professional identity must be amenable to the realities of its undeniable importance in the practice and delivery of services of the caring professions, their professional interactions with their patients, clients and learners, and the design, teaching, learning and assessment of the curriculum produce the caring professions of the future.

This often means that more quantifiable levels of measurement in research and pedagogical development – 'higher' levels of measure as we described earlier – are needed. Why? Because these are generally more valid and reliable in scientific terms, and they are generally seen as more fair, transparent and defensible in internal, external and public scrutiny – and, most certainly, more externally valued.

This is critical in the modern litigious world in which practitioners, managers, educators and advocates in the caring professions must be able to defend their actions.

Such attributes are also a welcome and necessary element of academic peer review and constructive critique.

Especially as, in the now academic world of quality indicators, permeating the existence of academics and practitioners alike, quantitative indices are paramount. They define the relentless quality league tables that influence recruitment and retention for both students and staff. (See, for example, Hindmarsh and Kingston (2019) or World University Rankings (2020).) And, thus, they matter in every aspect of the work of the caring professions.

The flexibility of the Delphi technique in accommodating both high face-validity qualitative methods and rigorous scientific method has huge unrealised potential in addressing these challenges for the caring professions. We have already addressed how the choice of Delphi panel can be made more scientifically rigorous. But it is in the design of materials that the full potential of the Delphi can be realised.

This is done by formulating the Delphi materials to provide both qualitative and, crucially, quantitative responses, amenable to the spectrum of statistical analysis, and with all of the benefits of statistical inference and generalisability, if rigorous sampling has been applied to the selection of the panel. This is easily applicable to the concept of professional identity.

Techniques for obtaining quantitative measures in a Delphi questionnaire to a panel include, where appropriate:

- construct questions to elicit 'closed' responses, e.g. degrees of agreement (ordinal)
- construct questions/behaviours with binary (yes/no) responses – ordinal – but can be transcribed to 1/0 (ratio),
- construct questions to determine strength of opinion by asking for weightings attached to opinions (interval or ratio) or degrees of agreement (ordinal)

A case study of the potential of the Delphi technique to accommodate all levels of measurement is provided in the context of nursing education in Section 5 and illustrates its potential use in studying professional identity.

Mastery

The mastery of professional identity in its curriculum, teaching, learning and assessment is much more intrinsic to some caring professions than others. Arguably, professionals in school and higher education, and social work are formally through their regulatory and educational systems, less explicitly imbued with the responsibility to train their successors as professionals with the quality of professional identity, than are their colleagues in medicine and nursing. But all caring professions support the placement of learners to varying degrees.

The UK Medical Schools Council Assessment Alliance produced a list of core values and attributes needed to study medicine (MSC Selection Alliance, 2018). These included:

- Motivation to study medicine and genuine interest in the medical profession
- Insight into your own strengths and weaknesses
- The ability to reflect on your own work
- Personal organisation
- Academic ability
- Problem solving
- Dealing with uncertainty
- Manage risk and deal effectively with problems
- Ability to take responsibility for your own actions
- Conscientiousness
- Insight into your own health
- Effective communication, including reading, writing, listening and speaking
- Teamwork
- Ability to treat people with respect
- Resilience and the ability to deal with difficult situations
- Empathy and the ability to care for others
- Honesty

Such an explicit statement of core values and attributes, if generalised from medicine to all the caring professions, provides not only an excellent starting point for incorporation of professional identity into the recruitment of suitable learners but also an agenda for the curriculum. (And some caring professions may well have their own equivalent statements of core values and attributes.) Nonetheless, most educators in the caring professions could easily incorporate these statements into content in curriculum and translate this into appropriate methods of teaching and learning.

Assessment of these qualities, either in recruitment or in the curriculum, could, however, prove more of a challenge. The Delphi technique could provide a valuable contribution to this, as illustrated by an elaboration of the challenges of assessment in the recruitment context, of some of the previously states core values and attributes.

Of this list, very few are readily measurable for assessment, in a way that would enable professional and public confidence. But these probably include academic ability, through recognised national and international qualifications; problem-solving, the setting and assessment of which, in quantifiable, valid; and reliable terms, which is a routine skill of most caring profession recruiters/educators.

In contrast, some of the items require subjective and indirect evidence from applicants – for example honesty and the ability to treat people with respect. The assessment of these is especially challenging and would require direct and sustained observation.

But with some other items, the Delphi offers a method of assessment. As an example:

- Motivation to study medicine and genuine interest in the medical profession.

In assessing this, the first question is: who judges? This is far from uncontroversial – candidates could include professional bodies and registration bodies regulating practice, professional educators, front-line clinicians and their seniors, and learners and applicants themselves. In fact, this attribute may be best illuminated by several Delphi panels of experts in their own constituencies of power and interest, all initially providing statements of the observable behaviours they associate with such motivation to join the profession. However, even if every single constituency of experts were separately and confidentially asked, it is likely that there would be considerable commonality of responses which would be amenable to such techniques as item analysis (Moser and Kalton, 2017), which would reduce the numbers of stated desirable and observable behaviours.

But this use of the Delphi would give equal weight to the constituent panels, even if standardised for sampling methods and size. This might not be professionally or politically acceptable, in which case fewer panels, and those strictly relevant to the study objectives, should be used at the first stage, to whose professional consensus the researcher or pedagogist wishes to give equal weight in the emergence of the observable behaviours, through analysis of the total observable behaviours they specify.

Through the reduction of all thus stated observable behaviours, a taxonomy will emerge, which can be recorded as a quantifiable, binary measure of being observed to be present or absent. To combine these into a total score, a technique such as factor analysis (Moser and Kalton, 2017) could be used to give appropriate weightings to each behaviour. Alternatively, the assignment of weightings of a Delphi panel of professional experts could be used (see case study in Section 5).

Then the question arises as to who should assess potential recruits in these behaviours. This could be done by school teachers, mentors in relevant work placements or by medical academics within psychometric testing laboratories often used in recruitment in the caring professions.

Thus, the Delphi technique can provide a method for the curriculum, in the quantitative, valid and reliable assessment of a stated core value in the recruitment of medical professionals.

We stress that we do not offer the above as an optimal design and method to address the motivation of medical or other caring professional applicants, especially as it could be impracticably time-consuming. But rather, we offer it to illustrate the potential role of the Delphi technique in the mastery of assessment of professional identity in student recruitment.

A further such application is now illustrated in the case study in Section 5, in the context of nurse education in the clinical setting.

A case study of the Delphi technique and its applicability to professional identity

This case study involves the use of the Delphi method in the evaluation of clinical settings as environments for nursing education. The terms of reference of the study (Reid, 1983) were 'to examine the factors which determine the suitability of a clinical area for nurse training and to determine the number of learners who can then be effectively supported'. During the first phase of the work, which was a feasibility study, hundreds of nurses were informally interviewed and asked which criteria they considered to be important in determining the suitability of a ward for nurse training. There was no shortage of suggestions, ranging from resource and manpower factors to attitudinal and motivational factors. It became clear, however, that all the factors put forward were assumed rather than proven determinants of good ward-based education. A trawl of the research literature revealed that there was no instance of any factor having been shown to directly affect the efficacy of a clinical-learning setting. On the contrary, published studies tended to concentrate on one or two relevant factors, e.g. communication among ward staff, and to study such factors on the implicit assumption that they were determinants of good, ward-based education. No researcher had ever attempted to assess the ward as a learning environment and then investigate the reasons or factors which explained this.

It was decided to design a study that would both evaluate the wards as clinical-learning environments and collect information on factors that might explain variations.

The collection of empirical data on explanatory factors was relatively straightforward: data on staffing levels and skill mix obtained from off-duty rotas, data on bed occupancy and turnover obtained from bed-state forms, data on the organisation and daily work of the ward obtained from activity analysis, data on patient-dependency obtained using the Barr dependency method (Barr et al., 1973) and data on attitudes and motivation and opinions obtained from a variety of questionnaires administered to staff and students.

The evaluation of wards as clinical-learning environments was a good deal more difficult. It was not just a question of how to measure or assess, but what should be measured and assessed. After consultation with the nursing profession and colleagues with experience in educational evaluation, some principles were generally agreed: that wards should be evaluated against explicit educational criteria, in terms of both the quantity and quality of education provided in a ward placement.

There was a readily available means of obtaining the desired educational criteria, since every school of nursing had in the previous months been required to produce educational objectives for each clinical placement in the basic nurse training programmes. Perusal of these objectives for each of the six schools of nursing in Northern Ireland revealed a common core for any given placement, with only small local variations. This common core was extracted and used as a baseline. For each clinical placement, this comprised a list of educational objectives.

Evaluation using an objectives model is controversial and has been the topic of many books and articles by educationalists. Even those most critical of the objectives model, however, concede its validity in contexts such as nurse training. For a defence of the objectives model in this context, see Reid (1983).

These lists of educational objectives now provided a baseline from which to evaluate the quantity of nurse training provided by the wards. The assessment of quantity was relatively straightforward for each objective the number of exposures to practice during the placement. It was recognised that an exact estimate of exposures would be difficult to obtain retrospectively but that an ordinal variable indicating frequency of exposure could be used, i.e. How often have you performed this activity during this placement? Answers were on the scale: 'frequently', 'fairly often', 'a few times', 'once only' or 'never'.

The evaluation of the quality of the ward as a learning environment was considerably more complex. Since the overall objective of a clinical placement is to produce a safe and competent practitioner, it was clear that one focus of an evaluation of quality must be the learner.

Four possible approaches were considered: the learners' or trained staff's perceptions of the quality of the ward as a learning environment, formal examination or test results of the learners.

Using learner or staff perception involved all of the usual problems in basing an evaluation on the perceptions of parties with vested interests. Even if reliable and valid instruments could be designed, no more would be achieved than an accurate account of perceptions. While it was felt that such perceptions were relevant and valuable, it was not thought appropriate that they should be the sole basis of a ward evaluation. In the event, some material of this kind was incorporated within the questionnaires, but it was not used directly in the evaluation of wards.

The use of examination results from formal tests within nurse training was considered. Results from final examinations in the form of written papers were immediately ruled out as these could not be linked to any particular ward placement (some eight clinical placements to different wards occurred during RGN training). There were, however, formal ward-based assessments that contributed to the final mark obtained. These assessments were designed by educators in the schools of nursing and were administered by clinical teachers or tutors at the end of selected clinical allocations. It was reluctantly decided that these marks could not be used for three reasons:

- The independence of the research study was important, and the researchers did not wish to be perceived as having a particular link with any branch of the nursing profession, e.g. school or service, or to be seen as management-sponsored. The cooperation of learners was vital to the study, and it was felt that to use the results of ward-based assessments could compromise the integrity of the research team, in which the team would become identified in the students' minds as part of the hierarchy within the nursing profession. This could have jeopardised or weakened the students' contribution to other aspects of the study.
- The stress caused to learners by ward-based assessments had been noted, and while this is a flaw in any examination situation, it was felt that many learners suffered from nervousness to the point that the results of ward-based examinations were not a good indicator of the quality of the learning environment.
- The instruments used to assess learners included marking systems that depended on value judgements made by the test administrator. It was felt that there was an unnecessarily high degree of subjectivity in these instruments.

Surprisingly an international literature search revealed nothing suitable for use in assessing learner competence. The task was, therefore, to design new test schedules. Criteria in the design of these schedules were that they should reduce value judgement to a minimum and that they should be acceptable and credible within the nursing profession.

It was the latter criterion that led to the selection of the Delphi technique in the design of the test schedules. It was considered important that nurse educators be involved in their design, both to draw on their expertise and to enhance the credibility of the research. Each of the six schools of nursing was asked to nominate two nurse educators to participate in the Delphi panel. There was no randomness in the selection of the educators, since the schools were asked to select educators with experience in the development of ward-based assessments. In practice, two educators had been responsible for this in each of the schools. The Delphi panel, thus, constituted a population in the environment of the study.

The research team then designed the materials for the Delphi technique, based on investigation of competence of all learners relative to all educational objectives.

It was decided to select three activity-related objectives for each of three cohorts of learners who would be present onwards. To minimise individual variance, it was desirable to include as many learners as possible in this exercise, so medical wards were selected because of the high density of learners on these wards. Three cohorts of learners were allocated to medical wards: introductory module (first year), medical module (second year) and preparation-for-responsibility module (third year). For these three modules, the selected activity-related objectives were as follows:

- Introductory module: Bed-bathing; taking and recording temperature, pulse and respiration; and giving a verbal report
- Medical module: Administration of medicines to four patients; testing the urine of a diabetic patient and admission of a patient
- Preparation-for-responsibility module: Taking charge of a ward; written report and communication

These activities were selected because they represented the spirit of the modules and because they covered psychomotor, interpersonal and caring aspects of performance within each module. Guidelines were developed for the selection of patients to ensure as far as possible that the tests were being carried out in comparable circumstances. These guidelines also affected the design of the Delphi materials in which the dependency levels and emotional states of patients were specified, allowing exclusion of particularly ill or difficult patients. A full list of guidelines is provided in Reid (1985). The research team then designed, for each activity, a list of nursing behaviours that should be observed. As far as possible, each behaviour was observable as either present or absent.

The total lists of behaviours for each activity were surprisingly long. The first draft for a bed-bath of a single patient included 90 behaviours! The final number of items was 87! The nine test schedules thus devised were sent to the Delphi panel who were asked:

- To suggest any additional behaviours that had been omitted from the draft
- To suggest any deletions of unnecessary behaviours
- To suggest any subdivision of behaviours that would aid clarity
- To suggest any change in the sequencing of behaviours
- To provide a weight for each behaviour indicating its relative importance

A structured form for the recording of these responses was sent to each panel member (Reid, 1983).

The provision of weights for each behaviour within an activity was a crucial stage in the process, which resulted in a scoring system. It is clear that not all behaviours within an activity are of equal importance. Some are crucial to safety, some are relatively unimportant. The Delphi panel were free to select their own range of weights and interpretation but were asked to specify this. Some chose weights between one and five, others between one and three and others between one and ten. After the first-round returns were received, these weights were all translated to a scale between one and three and the average weight for each item, correct to one decimal place and rounded up or down to the nearest half score, was fed back to respondents, alongside their own first-round weight, translated, where necessary, on to the 1–3 scale.

Feedback was also provided on additions, deletions and re-sequencing, in the form of redrafted schedules incorporating the consensus of first-round opinion as judged by the researchers. Comment was invited in the same way as for round one, and the returns at this stage revealed a high level of consensus on the second draft, including the average weights. The Delphi technique could have been used to attempt to gain consensus on a handful of remaining items, but it was decided that this would be too time-consuming. (The previous rounds took some 4 months.) This would not be a problem with contemporary electronic communication.

It was, therefore, decided to convene the group for a meeting on the remaining items. At this meeting, solutions were sought to which all panel members could accede, and to which no panel member strongly dissented. Full consensus on this basis was achieved in a 3-hour meeting.

These completed assessment schedules enabled a total quantitative score to be calculated for each learner for each selected activity. A full set of test schedules for all nine competence tests is provided in Reid (1985).

This was a modified Delphi exercise in which a committee forum followed two rounds of the process. This reflects the comment made by a number of writers about the then time-consuming nature of the Delphi technique, prior to the electronic age.

The technique was, however, very successful in providing consensus. There was full cooperation from the panel, which may have been attributable to the fact that the researchers knew personally, or came to know personally, each individual in the panel. There was regular telephone contact with the panel, not on the substance of the exercise, but in clarifying any queries and encouraging panel members to continue to cooperate in this then time-consuming exercise. The final level of consensus was very high.

The results of this study were very widely disseminated. Two thousand booklets were distributed amongst ward and school nursing staff in Northern Ireland. A detailed report went out of print at 300 copies, which were sent out by request throughout the United Kingdom. Over a thousand letters concerning the study were received. A variety of journal articles and a book (Reid, 1985) were published.

This degree of interest reflected the radical conclusions of the research, which were highly critical of the then apprenticeship system of nurse training. Since the findings were uncomfortable for some within the nursing profession (although widely accepted and welcomed by the vast majority), it would not have been surprising if the research instruments had been challenged. There has not been a single criticism of which the authors are aware of the methods of assessment, either in the written communications or during any of some 30 public presentations of the work across the United Kingdom to hundreds of nurses. It is suggested that the credibility of the research instruments on assessment owes much to the Delphi technique, through which they were produced.

All of this bodes well for the use of the Delphi technique to translate the concept of professional identity in the caring professions, for both research and pedagogy. In its meaning, the Delphi offers the essential professional endorsement in a qualitative form, with high face validity, and, if the expert panel is scientifically chosen, with generalisability to the entire profession. In the measurement of professional identity, the Delphi offers every possible flexibility and sophistication of analysis, which will contribute to its credible integration in the education of the caring professionals of the future, and, thus, its mastery.

Acknowledgements

The author thanks Miss Pam Compton, former Sub-Librarian, University of Ulster, who undertook many of the computer-literature searches required for this work. The contribution of Mrs. Laurie Gilbert to some of the ideas in this chapter was most valuable, and it was Mrs Gilbert who first proposed the use of the Delphi method in the case study described.

The contribution of Mr Charles Reid, former IT Manager of Stranmillis University College, was invaluable in unravelling formatting problems within original sources used.

References

Aengenheyster, S., Cuhls, K., Gerhold, L., Heiskanen-Schüttler, M., Huck, J., & Muszynska, M. (2017). Real-Time Delphi in practice—A comparative analysis of existing software-based tools. *Technological Forecasting and Social Change, 118*, 15–27.

Barr, A., Moores, B., & Rhys-Hearn, C. (1973). A review of the various methods of measuring the dependency of patients on nursing staff. *International Journal of Nursing Studies, 10*(3), 195–208.

Cole, Z. D., Donohoe, H. M., & Stellefson, M. L. (2013). Internet-based Delphi research: Case based discussion. *Environmental Management, 51*(3), 511–523.

Donohoe, H., Stellefson, M., & Tennant, B. (2012). Advantages and limitations of the e-Delphi technique: Implications for health education researchers. *American Journal of Health Education, 43*(1), 38–46.

Donohoe, H. M., & Needham, R. D. (2009). Moving best practice forward: Delphi characteristics, advantages, potential problems, and solutions. *International Journal of Tourism Research, 11*(5), 415–437.

Ellis, R. and Hogard, E. (2020 in press). Professional Identity: Values, Selection and Career Choice In Dent, J., Harden, R. M., & Hunt, D. Eds. *A Practical Guide for Medical Teachers*. Elsevier Health Sciences.

Flostrand, A. (2017). Finding the future: Crowdsourcing versus the Delphi technique. *Business Horizons, 60*(2), 229–236.

Gordon, T. J., & Helmer, O. (1964). *Report on a Long-Range Forecasting Study* (No. P-2982). RAND CORP SANTA MONICA CALIF.

Harden, R. M., Lilley, P., & Patricio, M. (2015). *The Definitive Guide to the OSCE: The Objective Structured Clinical Examination as a Performance Assessment*. Elsevier Health Sciences.

Hindmarsh, A., & Kingston, B. (2019). *Times Good University Guide 2020*. J. O'Leary (Ed.). Harper Collins.

Helms, C., Gardner, A., & McInnes, E. (2017). The use of advanced web-based survey design in Delphi research. *Journal of Advanced Nursing, 73*(12), 3168–3177.

Humphrey-Murto, S., Varpio, L., Wood, T. J., Gonsalves, C., Ufholz, L. A., Mascioli, K., ... & Foth, T. (2017). The use of the Delphi and other consensus group methods in medical education research: A review. *Academic Medicine*, *92*(10), 1491–1498

Keeney, S., McKenna, H., & Hasson, F. (2011). *The Delphi Technique in Nursing and Health Research*. John Wiley & Sons.

Kent, M. L., & Saffer, A. J. (2014). A Delphi study of the future of new technology research in public relations. *Public Relations Review*, *40*(3), 568–576.

Lasagna, L. (1964). *Hippocratic Oath–Modern Version*. *WGBH Educational Foundation*.

Linstone, H. A., & Turoff, M. (Eds.). (1975). *The Delphi Method*. Reading, MA: Addison-Wesley.

McKenna, H. P. (1994). The Delphi technique: A worthwhile research approach for nursing?. *Journal of Advanced Nursing*, *19*(6), 1221–1225.

Meshkat, B., Gethin, G., Cowman, S., Ryan, K. (2014) *Using an e-Delphi technique for developing best practice in day surgery in Ireland*. Department of Health, Ireland.

Moser, C. A., & Kalton, G. (2017). *Survey Methods in Social Investigation*. Routledge.

MSC Selection Alliance (2018) *Statement On The Core Values And Attributes Needed To Study Medicine*. Medical Schools Council, London.

Msibi, P. N., Mogale, R., De Waal, M., & Ngcobo, N. (2018). Using e-Delphi to formulate and appraise the guidelines for women's health concerns at a coal mine: A case study. *Curationis*, *41*(1), 1–6.

Reid, N. G. (1983). *A multivariate statistical investigation of the factors affecting nurse training in the clinical area* (Doctoral dissertation, University of Ulster).

Reid, N. G. (1985). *Wards in Chancery?: Nurse Training in the Clinical Area*. Royal College of Nursing of the United Kingdom. Research Series.

Rowe, G., & Wright, G. (2011). The Delphi technique: Past, present, and future prospects—Introduction to the special issue. *Technological Forecasting and Social Change*, *78*(9), 1487–1490.

Stevens, S. S. (1946). On the theory of scales of measurement. *Science 103*(2864) 677–680.

Strauss, H. J., & Zeigler, L. H. (1975). The Delphi technique and its uses in social science research. *The Journal of Creative Behavior*, *9*(4), 253–259.

Toronto, C. (2017). Considerations when conducting e-Delphi research: A case study. *Nurse Researcher*, *25*(1). 10–15.

Trevelyan, E. G., & Robinson, N. (2015). Delphi methodology in health research: how to do it?. *European Journal of Integrative Medicine*, *7*(4), 423–428.

Uhl, N.P. (1975) 'Consensus and the Delphi process.' Paper presented at the Annual Meeting of the American Educational Research Association, Washington, D.C., (ERIC Document ED 104 201

Webb, S.A. (2017) (ed) *Professional Identity in Social Work*, Routledge.

World University Rankings (2020) *Times Higher Education*, Elsevier.

20 Observing identity

Measuring professional identity empirically in the healthcare professions

Calum T. McHale and Joanne E. Cecil

Professional identity in the healthcare professions

Professional identity, specifically how it is formulated, develops and manifests, has been the focus of increasing academic interest over the past decade (Cruess et al., 2015). The concept of professional identity is complex, with multiple constituent components broadly defined as the internalisation of knowledge, values, attitudes and beliefs that are shared within a professional group and define that particular profession and the development of interpersonal skills (Adams et al., 2006; Matthews et al., 2019; Wilkinson et al., 2009). Within the health professions, professional identity has become an important construct. Previous research has associated the specific constituent components of professional identity with numerous practitioner and patient-related outcomes, including greater career satisfaction (Afonso et al., 2014), a desire to actively engage with improvements in quality of care and the reduction of medical errors (Campbell et al., 2007) and improved patient perceptions of practitioners' professionalism and communication skills (Abadel & Hattab, 2014). Conversely, a lack of professional identity may reduce practitioners' perceived professional values, confidence and willingness to advocate for their profession (Turner & Knight, 2015).

Professional identity has been shown to facilitate more efficient working within the health service. Healthcare professionals who have a clear concept of their professional identity understand where they fit into healthcare teams, as well as transition and adapt within the workplace. For example, having a more clearly defined professional identity allows practitioners to better understand practice boundaries and distinguish their professional role from other healthcare professions, which is important for working efficiently within a modern multidisciplinary approach to healthcare (Brown et al., 2000). Furthermore, a focus on professional identity formation (i.e. the 'process' of becoming a healthcare professional) during education may contribute to a more successful transition from study to the workplace (Ashby et al., 2016) and to enabling a strong group identity, the latter of which has been shown to play a protective role in healthcare students well-being (Mavor et al., 2014). Thus, professional identity is central to shaping healthcare professionals' practice and has implications for safe and effective clinical practice and patient care. As such, understanding the formulation of professional identity is a focal point of healthcare research, and the development of clear professional identities has become a core component in medical education and continual professional development.

Understanding the concept of professional identity

Professional identity is a self-representation, formed over time by the internalisation of characteristics, values, norms, beliefs and attitudes associated with the healthcare professions, resulting in an individual "*thinking, acting and feeling*" like a healthcare professional (Cruess et al., 2014). The concept of healthcare or medicine as a distinct profession, with specific values and ethical practices, dates back to classical Greece and Hippocrates (Chadwick & Mann, 1950). In the modern day, most healthcare organisations and professional healthcare registration bodies have comprehensive publications, which describe what they expect of their affiliates in terms of values and practices, in other words, what it means to be a professional. For example, the National Health Service (NHS) has a constitution that established the core principles and values of the NHS, the rights of patients and the responsibilities that professionals have to ensure that these values and principles are upheld (UK Government, 2015). Similarly, the General Medical Council (GMC) has thorough guidance on "professionalism in action", in which they highlight, not only the core values and beliefs that doctors should hold, but also how they should translate these into behaviours and practices for the benefit of the profession and for their patients (General Medical Council, 2013).

Much of the academic research on professional identity has focussed on the complex concept of how professional identity develops in healthcare professionals by providing a greater understanding of what precisely constitutes professional identity. At its core, professional identity comprises internal and external aspects and is understood to be the degree to which an individual internalises and relates with humanistic values and professional qualities associated with the healthcare profession (Branch, 2015; Cruess et al., 2014; Ellis & Hogard, 2020; Swick, 2000). These values and qualities may include, but are not limited to, altruism, respect, honesty, integrity and empathy (Ong et al., 2020). Clinical competency, such as knowledge, situational awareness, decision-making and communication skills, as well as a reflective capacity, are also identified as key components of professional identity (Ong et al., 2020; Swick, 2000; Wilkinson et al., 2009).

Professional identity is understood to develop in a similar way to personal identity, through socialisation and experience (Cruess et al., 2015; Willetts & Clarke, 2014). Research into the formation and development of professional identity in healthcare professionals propose that identity is continually being influenced, challenged and modified by experiences in practice and professional socialisation (Ashby et al., 2016; de Lasson et al., 2016; Trede et al., 2012).

Dr Clare Gerada, former Chair of the Council of the Royal College of General Practitioners, has proposed that professional identity is closely intertwined with personal identity (Gerada, 2016). In essence, professional identity is the result of a complex consolidation of one's own personal values and beliefs with taught or observed professional values and beliefs and is therefore unique to the individual.

The theory of psychosocial development proposes that personal identity develops in stages and that each stage is heavily influenced by social interaction and experiences (Sokol, 2009). Professional identity is a group identity and scholars have drawn on social identity theory to understand professional identity formation in healthcare professionals (Willetts & Clarke, 2014). Social learning and identity theories emphasise that knowledge acquisition takes place within a social context and that belonging to a group, self-categorisation within groups and in-group behaviour are important for personal identity formation (Bandura & Walters, 1977; Turner & Oakes, 1986). Within professional organisations, social norms develop as a means to express the central values of that organisation or a particular organisational identity and reinforce behaviours that express these values (Furnham, 2012).

Although professional identity is itself an individuals' cognitive internalisation of values and beliefs, it is expressed through actions, behaviours and practices that exhibit these values and beliefs. This manifestation of the values and beliefs of professional identity through action has been called professionalism (Cruess et al., 2014; Royal College of Physicians, 2005). Professionalism in healthcare has been interpreted as integrity and adherence to ethical and practice principles (Hilton & Slotnick, 2005; Jha et al., 2006; Lane, 2018; Swick, 2000), effectively communicating with patients and colleagues (Hilton & Slotnick, 2005; Swick, 2000; Wagner et al., 2007), being consistent and reliable (Ainsworth & Szauter, 2006; Frohna & Stern, 2005; Van De Camp et al., 2004) and having autonomy and a commitment to continuous self-improvement (Cohen, 2006; Royal College of Physicians, 2005; Swick, 2000). For healthcare professionals, professional identity may be more closely related to professionalism (i.e. behaviours and practices, interacting with patients and colleagues) than the internalised concept of individual membership to the healthcare professions (Barbour & Lammers, 2015; Vough, 2012). The GMC and Royal College of Physicians emphasise that professionalism is a partnership between medical professionals and their patients and that every interaction with patients is an opportunity to enact the principles and values of the medical profession (General Medical Council, 2013; Royal College of Physicians, 2018).

Measurement of professional identity

A number of researchers have examined comprehensive approaches to assess professional identity within healthcare as a single concept (Ellis et al., 2015; Kalet et al., 2017; Tan et al., 2017); however, because professional identity is a complex, abstract, even philosophical concept, quantifying and measuring it is challenging. Recent work by Buck et al. (2019), investigating self-report assessment of professional identity formation in medical students, concluded that current approaches to assessing professional identity as a single concept are lacking and that attempting to assess the broad concept of professional identity with a single approach may not be possible (Buck et al., 2019). As such, professional identity is typically assessed through more specific cognitive and behavioural factors (i.e. professionalism) because they can be more consistently defined, observed and measured.

Systematic reviews by Wilkinson et al. (2009) and Matthews et al. (2019) have highlighted the breadth of approaches taken by researchers to measure and assess professional identity and professionalism. These approaches have included psychometric evaluation (Matthews et al., 2019), self-reported reflections via surveys and interviews, structured feedback from mentors, colleagues and patients and assessment through directly observed behaviours and practices (Wilkinson et al., 2009). Psychometric evaluation focuses on the assessment of the internalised cognitive aspects of professional identity, including strength of professional identity (Adams et al., 2006), professional self-concepts (Cowin, 2001) and professional values and ethics (Ellis et al., 2015; Weis & Schank, 2009). Self-report approaches, via surveys and interviews, assess individuals opinions and perceptions about aspects of professionalism and professional identity, such as attitudes towards professionalism (Blackall et al., 2007), the ability to reflect on experiences (Aukes et al., 2007) and cultural competence (Godkin & Savageau, 2001). Feedback from others can include assessment of knowledge through exams, ratings of professional behaviour completed by mentors (van de Camp et al., 2006), simulated patient rating scales (van Zanten et al., 2005) for trainees and students, or peer-review and appraisals from colleagues or supervisors (Evans et al., 2004) and patient satisfaction questionnaires (General Medical Council, 2020) for working health professionals. Directly observed behaviours and practices have used the model whereby a mentor or examiner will observe and assess clinical competency, professional behaviour and communication practices in students and trainees via predetermined simulated consultations (Norcini et al., 2003; Singer et al., 1996). This model is useful for a consistent approach to examination or appraisal, where an examiner is assessing the presence of individual specific professional practices, such as whether someone followed a particular practice protocol, said an empathic statement or did not exceed their allotted time. However, each observable behaviour is cognitively complex and occurs within a unique context. Looking beyond the behaviours and communication produced by healthcare professionals, and interrogating their function, meaning and context, can provide an insight into the more complex internalised aspects of professionalism and professional identity. This research-driven approach to the direct observation of healthcare consultations is most usefully conducted by video or audio recordings of these interactions, as it allows for repeated observation and a more objective and comprehensive analysis of the communications and behaviours (Coleman, 2000; McHale et al., 2016).

Direct observation of clinical interactions

Direct observation of clinical interactions is an established research approach within healthcare education and communication and can take the form of live observations of the interaction or audio-visually recording the interaction for subsequent review (Fromme et al., 2009; McHale et al., 2016). Observation of healthcare students interacting with patients is used to assess clinical and communication skills (Kogan et al., 2009) and has been associated with improved student outcomes, such as self-reflection and task performance (Hammoud et al., 2012). Additionally, direct observation is a commonly used approach in healthcare communication research to investigate topics such as patient-centred communication and emotional expression (Epstein et al., 2005; McHale et al., 2019; Zhou et al., 2013). The primary advantage of direct observation when researching behaviours and communication practices is that it negates the subjectivity and risk of bias introduced by relying solely on self-report from the individuals engaging in the interaction. The Hawthorne effect, or observation bias, whereby the knowledge of being observed will result in changes to behaviour, has the potential to introduce bias into this research approach (McCambridge et al., 2014). However, review evidence suggest that direct observation methodologies have minimal impact on healthcare professionals' behaviour and practices (Themessl-Huber et al., 2008).

Direct observation for use in the assessment of professionalism and professional identity is crucial because it captures many aspects of professional identity in a reliable, valid and feasible way (Wilkinson et al., 2009). Recent review evidence has suggested that integrating direct observation into research approaches is important for understanding the more complex aspects of professional identity that are specific to particular professions (Barbour & Lammers, 2015). Research assessing professionalism in medical students apply observation and rating scales to actual or simulated interactions with patients and focus on clarity of communication, demeanour, approachability and involving patients in discussions (Abadel & Hattab, 2014). Thus, direct observation for the assessment of professional identity has a key place in medical education. We propose that many of the values and attitudes associated with professional identity in the healthcare professions can be meaningfully studied through the detailed analysis of communication and behavioural practices, observed directly from interactions with patient during clinical consultations.

Direct observation of communication during primary care consultations: a case study

Direct observation can be used within healthcare to provide a unique insight into the subtle nuances of clinical communication and can provide a greater understanding of the factors that influence these communication processes. Clinical communication practices are a core component of professionalism and professional identity (General Medical Council, 2020; Royal College of Physicians,

2005, 2018), as established earlier in this chapter. Thus, here we present a case study on healthcare communication to illustrate how direct observation methodologies can be practically employed to provide a comprehensive analysis of communication and identify and quantify communication practices consistent with professionalism and professional identity.

Introduction

Communication is key to healthcare. Patient-centred communication aims to establish a partnership with the patient by building rapport and acknowledging patient concerns and emotions, facilitating patient understanding and enabling patients to express their thoughts and opinions and, ultimately, to help patients take control of their health and healthcare decisions (King & Hoppe, 2013). Patient-centred communication has become the gold standard of healthcare communication and is considered by various healthcare organisations and professional bodies as a core component of healthcare professionalism (General Medical Council, 2013; Royal College of Physicians, 2018). This widespread advocacy of patient-centred communication is a result of its robust associations with improvements in practitioner–patient relations (Pinto et al., 2012) and numerous patient outcomes, including improved therapeutic alliance between practitioners and patients (Pinto et al., 2012), and increased patient satisfaction and adherence to treatment (Finset, 2011; Zolnierek & Dimatteo, 2009). Patient-centred communication has also been related to improved patient health outcomes (Stewart, 1995), including improvements in patient weight management and patient weight loss (Cox et al., 2011; Pollak et al., 2007, 2010), which is the focus of this case study. Direct observation has become an established research methodology for investigating communication-related processes in primary care; however, directly observed communication processes around patient weight and weight management in primary care are understudied and poorly understood (McHale et al., 2016).

Excessive body weight is a worldwide public health crisis. Globally, almost 2 billion adults are now considered to have overweight and 650 million have obesity (World Health Organisation, 2020). Critically, obesity is associated with mortality and multiple chronic health conditions (Carmienke et al., 2013; Guh et al., 2009; Kramer et al., 2013). Primary healthcare is the first point of access to the health service and is responsible for the management of most chronic health conditions. Primary care is well placed to discuss weight-related issues with patients and provide access to weight management services. Research has shown that primary care can successfully implement weight management interventions to patients with overweight and obesity in practice (Aveyard et al., 2016; Tsai et al., 2013). Despite this potential, weight issues are rarely discussed with patients with overweight and obesity and weight management is inconsistently offered (Booth et al., 2015; Kraschnewski et al., 2013; Laidlaw et al., 2015; McHale et al., 2016).

The aim of the research, showcased in this case study, was to directly observe and analyse weight-related discussion between patients with overweight and obesity and their practitioners in routine primary care consultations. Specifically this research sought to (i) identify the prevalence of weight-related discussion within primary care consultations in Scotland; (ii) provide a comprehensive understanding of the content and context of weight-related discussion; (iii) associate communication processes with outcomes, including whether weight was discussed in a consultation and whether there was a tangible weight-related outcome for the patient.

Methodology

The analysis presented in this case study formed part of a larger programme of doctoral research to investigate weight-related discussion in routine primary care consultations and the patient and practitioner factors that may influence communication interactions between primary care practitioners and their patients with overweight and obesity, using direct observation (McHale et al., 2016, 2019, 2020). This research was cross-sectional and employed multiple methods, including questionnaires, semi-structured interviews and video recording to address the research aims. Routine consultations between primary care practitioners and patients were video recorded in seven NHS primary care practices across Scotland. Following the consultation, patients met with a researcher who measured their height (centimetres) and weight (kilograms) using a calibrated set of scales and a stadiometer so that body mass index (BMI) could be calculated. To avoid biasing consultation discussions towards weight issues, all participants were informed that the study was observing general clinical communication processes. The study focus on weight discussion was disclosed to participants after all video recording was completed in each practice (McHale et al., 2019).

As this research targeted weight discussion, communication was coded only in those consultations where the patient was assessed to have an overweight or obese BMI (≥ 25 kg/m^2). Communication was systematically coded directly from the video recordings using the Roter interaction analysis system (RIAS) (Ong et al., 1998; Roter & Larson, 2002). This system comprehensively attributes a code to every utterance, spoken by both the healthcare professional and patient. Utterances are defined as the smallest possible discernible communication segment to which a code can be meaningfully attributed. Codes within RIAS are organised into five functional communication groupings (Table 20.1).

Codes within three of these functional groupings (information provision, data gathering and procedural statements) focus on practical or technical communication that function to gather and provide information about health-related issues or move discussion forwards. Codes within the remaining two function groups (partnership building and activating, and emotional expression and responsiveness) focus on socio-emotional and patient-centred communications that function to build rapport, are affective (e.g. empathy, laughing, worry/concern etc.) or seek to involve patients actively in the discussions and decisions made about their health and care.

Table 20.1 The Roter interaction analysis system (RIAS)

Communication functional group	RIAS codes
Information provision	• Gives information (medical condition, therapeutic regimen, lifestyle, psychosocial, other) • Counsels or directs behaviour (medical condition/ therapeutic regimen/lifestyle/psychosocial)[a]
Data gathering	• Asks closed-ended questions (medical condition, therapeutic regimen, lifestyle, psychosocial, other) • Asks open-ended questions (medical condition, therapeutic regimen, lifestyle, psychosocial, other)
Partnership building and activating	• Asks for understanding • Asks for opinion[a] • Asks for permission[a] • Back-channel (e.g. uh-huh, mm hm, go on)[a] • Paraphrases, checks for understanding • Transitions[b] • Requests for service or medication[b] • Bids for repetition
Emotional expression and responsiveness	• Personal remarks, social conversation • Laughs, tells joke • Shows approval • Gives compliment • Shows agreement or understanding • Empathy • Shows concern or worry • Reassures, encourages or shows optimism • Legitimises • Partnership[a] • Self-disclosure[a] • Shows disapproval • Shows criticism • Asks for reassurance
Procedural statements	• Transitions[a] • Gives orientation, instruction[a]

[a] Practitioner only.

[b] Patient only.

Communication coding was facilitated by using The Observer XT (Noldus Information Technology, 2020), a dedicated behavioural analysis software, which allows for real-time coding of audio-visual data (i.e. timestamping of codes). Codes were consistently applied after having observed each communication utterance. Any part of the observed communication that was dedicated to weight discussion was separated from the rest of the communication using a binary code that was active for the duration of the video (i.e. weight discussion vs. not weight discussion). Weight discussion was defined as any explicit mention of, or clear inference to, patient weight by either the patient or primary care practitioner, regardless of whether it resulted in subsequent weight discussion (McHale et al., 2019).

RIAS code frequencies were calculated by exporting coded data from The Observer XT into Microsoft Excel and using the pivot table function. Codes were organised into their functional groups then divided according to whether or not there was weight discussion within the consultation and according to who they were attributed to (practitioner or patient). Codes during consultation that contained weight discussion were also divided into those during weight discussion and those during all other consultation discussion. Differences in code counts were examined for statistical differences using chi-square (χ^2) analysis.

Results: analysis of communication and practices in the context of patient weight issues

The results of these analyses have been published elsewhere (McHale et al., 2019). A total of 14 primary care practitioners, 12 general practitioners and 2 practice nurses participated in the research. In total, 305 patients participated in the study, 218 of these patients (71.4%) were measured to have an overweight or obese BMI. The mean BMI of the patient sample was 28.74 kg/m^2. Only 54 patients with overweight or obesity (24.7%) discussed weight with their practitioner during their consultation. Of the 54 consultations that contained weight discussion, only 14 (26%) had any weight-related outcomes for the patient.

Our findings identified clear communication patterns, in that practitioners exhibited less patient education and counselling communications [χ^2 = 19.336 (1), $p < 0.001$] and more partnership building and activating communications [χ^2 = 37.348 (1), $p < 0.001$] during consultations that contained weight discussion when compared with consultations that did not contain weight discussion (Table 20.2).

Table 20.2 Primary care practitioner and patient communication, coded with the RIAS, according to whether weight discussion occurred during the consultation

	n RIAS codes (% of all RIAS codes)	
RIAS communication functional group	*Consultations containing no weight discussion (n = 164)*	*Consultations containing weight discussion (n = 54)*
Practitioner communication		
Patient education and counselling	10,515 (41.5%)	4125 (39%)**
Emotional expression and responsiveness	6724 (26.54%)	2843 (26.88%)
Partnership building and activating	3451 (13.62%)	1703 (16.1%)**
Procedural talk	2352 (9.28%)	939 (8.88%)
Question asking	2297 (9.07%)	968 (9.15%)
Patient communication		
Information provision	10,944 (52.39%)	4921 (54%)*
Emotional expression and responsiveness	8333 (39.89%)	3504 (38.45%)*
Activation	919 (4.40%)	416 (4.56%)
Question asking	692 (3.31%)	272 (2.98%)

Chi-square $p < 0.05$*, $p < 0.01$**.

Table 20.3 Primary care practitioner and patient communication during weight discussion compared with all other consultation discussion

RIAS communication functional group	n RIAS codes during all other discussion (% of all other discussion)	n RIAS codes during weight discussion (% of all weight discussion)
Practitioner communication		
Patient education and counselling	3778 (39.23)	347 (36.60)
Emotional expression and responsiveness	2594 (26.94)	249 (26.27)
Partnership building and activating	1528 (15.87)	175 (18.46)*
Question asking	889 (9.23)	98 (10.34)
Procedural talk	841 (8.73)	79 (8.33)
Patient communication		
Information provision	4413 (53.44)	508 (59.42)**
Emotional expression and responsiveness	3215 (38.93)	289 (33.80)***
Activation	374 (4.53)	42 (4.91)
Question asking	256 (3.10)	16 (1.87)

Chi-square $p < 0.05$*, $p < 0.01$**, $p < 0.001$***

Additionally, patients whose consultations contained weight discussion exhibited significantly more information provision communication [$\chi^2 = 6.568$ (1), $p = 0.01$] and less emotional expression and responsiveness communications [$\chi^2 = 5.532$ (1), $p = 0.019$] compared with patients whose consultations did not contain weight discussion (Table 20.2).

Practitioners were found to use significantly more partnership and activating communications during weight discussion than they did during all other consultation discussion [$\chi^2 = 4.295$ (1), $p = 0.04$] (Table 20.3). Despite a relative reduction of 3% in practitioner use of patient education and counselling communications during weight discussion when compared with other consultation discussion, this difference was not statistically significant ($p > 0.05$). Patients used significantly more information provision communications [$\chi^2 = 11.139$ (1), $p = 0.001$] and significantly less emotional expression and responsiveness communication [$\chi^2 = 15.075$ (1), $p < 0.001$] during weight discussion than they did during all other consultation discussion (Table 20.3).

Discussion of case study results within the context of professional identity

A key finding of our research presented in this case study was that weight discussion between primary care practitioners and patients with overweight and obesity was scarce and seldom resulted in any tangible weight-related outcome (McHale et al., 2019). This finding, that weight discussion occurs seldom in primary care consultations, supports our previous direct observation work (Laidlaw et al., 2015) and contributes robust evidence to this area of research, where weight discussion prevalence is inconsistently defined and reported (McHale et al., 2016). Notably, this finding is inconsistent with the perceptions of primary care practitioners, who self-report to regularly discuss weight issues with patients with overweight and obesity (Laidlaw et al., 2019; McHale et al., 2020). These data highlight the limitations of relying on self-report evidence when studying clinical practices and illustrate the value of directly observing clinical interactions in order to obtain a more accurate and objective understanding of clinical practices.

When directly observed at consultation level, the professional identity and professionalism of these primary care practitioners could reasonably be called into question. Through not routinely discussing weight issues with patients with clinical overweight and obesity, their practices were not consistent with the UK clinical guidelines (Health Improvement Scotland, 2010; National Institute for Health and Care Excellence, 2014). Furthermore, most patients were not offered a solution to a potentially serious health issue (weight) that was made explicit during the consultation. However, through the use of video observation and an intricate analysis of the content, function and context of clinical communication processes, behaviours and practices were observed that were consistent with professionalism and the values and beliefs associated with professional identity.

We found that primary care practitioners altered their communication approach, using significantly less directive patient education and counselling communications and significantly more patient-centred partnership building and activating communication, when discussing weight-related issues compared with all other types of consultation discussion. Effective patient-centred communication such as shared-decision-making (partnership building) and active patient participation in clinical discussions (activating) are core components of professionalism in healthcare (Royal College of Physicians, 2018). This shift in practitioner communication style highlights that practitioners perceive a difference in how patient weight issues should be discussed compared with other issues during their consultations with patients. Transitioning to a more patient-centred approach when discussing weight issues is consistent with recommended weight management guidelines (Health Improvement Scotland, 2010; National Institute for Health and Care Excellence, 2014) and behaviour change counselling approaches, such as assessing readiness to change and motivational interviewing (Lane et al., 2005; Ogunleye et al., 2015). Thus, identifying this subtle change in communication approach during weight discussion is significant because it provides an insight into primary care practitioners' professional identity, in terms of their knowledge and understanding of clinical guidelines, and how they professionally demonstrate this identity through flexible and adaptive communication practices.

A significant advantage of the research-driven approach of direct observation of clinical communication is that patient communication can be investigated in the same level of detail as practitioner communication. Patient communication is known to be understudied in existing research that has used direct observation to examine weight discussion in primary care (McHale et al., 2016). Our analysis found that when primary care practitioners increased their use of partnership building and activating communication, patients appeared to respond to this change by significantly increasing their information provision communications during weight discussions. Through this comprehensive and descriptive analysis of communication code frequencies, we are provided with detailed information relevant to professional practice, including whether primary care practitioners' attempts to implement a patient-centred communication approaches are producing the desired impact on patient communication responses. In our case, patients responded to practitioners' patient-centred communication by talking more and providing more health-related information (McHale et al., 2019). Other clinical communication coding schemes exist that examine a more sequential relationship between brief and consecutive sections of practitioner and patient communication. One such scheme is the Verona coding definitions of emotional sequences (VR-CoDES), which codes patients' implicit and explicit expressions of emotion (i.e. cues and concerns) and how practitioners respond to these expressions (Del Piccolo et al., 2011; Del Piccolo et al., 2017). Practitioner responses can 'provide space' for subsequent discussion about the emotional expression (e.g. acknowledgement, exploration or empathy) or 'reduce space' for subsequent discussion (e.g. ignore, explanation or changing the subject). The VR-CoDES system is often implemented as an effective way to measure patient-centred communication, specifically active listening and empathy (Del Piccolo, 2017; Epstein et al., 2017). Consideration and analysis of patient communication is equally valuable when examining clinical communication practices and can provide an insight into aspects of professional identity and professionalism, such as compassion, empathy, reflective listening and patient centredness. As such, it should be considered as a key component in healthcare education.

Importantly, directly observed communication practices should be analysed and interpreted with consideration of the wider contextual factors. Research exploring primary care practitioners' beliefs about obesity and weight management emphasises how complicated weight issues can be for primary care practitioners and highlight various internal and external barriers to effective weight discussion. For example, there are differing opinions among primary care practitioners about whether it is truly their role and responsibility to manage non-symptomatic weight issues, or whether it is a lifestyle issue and primarily the responsibility of the patient (Al-Ghawi & Uauy, 2009; Dewhurst et al., 2017; Laidlaw et al., 2019; McHale et al., 2020). Thus, for some practitioners, the management of weight issues clearly conflicts with how they perceive their role (i.e. professional identity) as a primary care practitioner. Further, primary care practitioners perceive weight issues as more complex than other (medical) health issues, in that they are heavily influenced by psychological and social factors, over which practitioners have limited (perceived) ability to change (McHale et al., 2020). There is apprehension among practitioners about discussing weight issues for fear of upsetting or offending patients and damaging their relationship with their patients (Blackburn et al., 2015; McHale et al., 2020; Michie, 2007). Beneficence and avoidance of maleficence in patient care are core values of professional identity in the healthcare professions (Ellis & Hogard, 2020); therefore, primary care practitioners' apprehension about patients negative reaction to discussing weight issues fit closely with these core values and may explain why weight discussion occurs so seldom in primary care.

Together, these data highlight the significance of employing a direct observation approach to examine clinical communication interactions. We propose therefore that direct observation, particularly video observation, has the potential to provide a comprehensive understanding of aspects of practitioner professional identity and professionalism. This systematic analysis of clinical communication allows an examination of the nuanced, more transient, aspects of communication in additional to content, context and function of communication. Through this methodology, we can interrogate professional behaviours and gain a comprehensive insight into the professional values and beliefs behind these behaviours. This research-driven approach provides a more robust and objective assessment of internalised aspects of professional identity because the communication can be examined repeatedly, more objectively and with varied evidence-based coding tools.

Implications and recommendations

There is increasing emphasis, within the healthcare professions, on developing professional identity through social learning, mentoring and role modelling (Royal College of Physicians, 2018). As such, future research to assess, measure and monitor professional identity in healthcare professional should focus more directly on observable professional behaviours and practices, in addition to written appraisals or self-reported perceptions. In this chapter, we report a research-driven approach for interrogating clinical communication practices, which are core components of professionalism and manifestations of professional identity. By comprehensively examining clinical communication (both patient and practitioner communication), as well as the content, function and context of the communication, a unique and more objective insight into healthcare practitioners' professional identity can be achieved. By observing trainees and practitioners as they work, we believe that this model of direct observation for the assessment of professional identity can be integrated into both medical education and the workplace for the purposes of quality assessment or continued professional development.

References

Abadel, F. T., & Hattab, A. S. (2014). Patients' assessment of professionalism and communication skills of medical graduates. BMC Medical Education, 14, 28–28.

Adams, K., Hean, S., Sturgis, P., & Clark, J. M. (2006). Investigating the factors influencing professional identity of first-year health and social care students. Learning in Health and Social Care, 5(2), 55–68.

Afonso, P., Ramos, M. R., Saraiva, S., Moreira, C. A., & Figueira, M. L. (2014). Assessing the relation between career satisfaction in psychiatry with lifelong learning and scientific activity. Psychiatry Research, 217(3), 210–214.

Ainsworth, M. A., & Szauter, K. M. (2006). Medical student professionalism: are we measuring the right behaviors? A comparison of professional lapses by students and physicians. *Academic Medicine, 81*(10).

Al-Ghawi, A., & Uauy, R. (2009). Study of the knowledge, attitudes and practices of physicians towards obesity management in primary health care in Bahrain. *Public Health Nutrition, 12*(10), 1791–1798.

Ashby, S. E., Adler, J., & Herbert, L. (2016). An exploratory international study into occupational therapy students' perceptions of professional identity. *Australian Occupational Therapy Journal, 63*(4), 233–243.

Aukes, L. C., Geertsma, J., Cohen-Schotanus, J., Zwierstra, R. P., & Slaets, J. P. (2007). The development of a scale to measure personal reflection in medical practice and education. *Medical Teacher, 29*(2–3), 177–182.

Aveyard, P., Lewis, A., Tearne, S., Hood, K., Christian-Brown, A., Adab, P., Begh, R., Jolly, K., Daley, A., Farley, A., Lycett, D., Nickless, A., Yu, L.-M., Retat, L., Webber, L., Pimpin, L., & Jebb, S. A. (2016). Screening and brief intervention for obesity in primary care: a parallel, two-arm, randomised trial. *The Lancet, 388*(10059), 2492–2500.

Bandura, A., & Walters, R. H. (1977). *Social learning theory* (Vol. 1). Englewood Cliffs, NJ: Prentice-Hall.

Barbour, J. B., & Lammers, J. C. (2015). Measuring professional identity: a review of the literature and a multilevel confirmatory factor analysis of professional identity constructs. *Journal of Professions and Organization, 2*(1), 38–60.

Blackall, G. F., Melnick, S. A., Shoop, G. H., George, J., Lerner, S. M., Wilson, P. K., Pees, R. C., & Kreher, M. (2007). Professionalism in medical education: the development and validation of a survey instrument to assess attitudes toward professionalism. *Medical Teacher, 29*(2–3), e58–e62.

Blackburn, M., Stathi, A., Keogh, E., & Eccleston, C. (2015). Raising the topic of weight in general practice: perspectives of GPs and primary care nurses. *BMJ Open, 5*(8), e008546.

Booth, H. P., Prevost, A. T., & Gulliford, M. C. (2015). Access to weight reduction interventions for overweight and obese patients in UK primary care: population-based cohort study. *BMJ Open, 5*(1), e006642.

Branch, W. T. (2015). Teaching professional and humanistic values: suggestion for a practical and theoretical model. *Patient Education and Counseling, 98*(2), 162–167.

Brown, B., Crawford, P., & Darongkamas, J. (2000). Blurred roles and permeable boundaries: the experience of multidisciplinary working in community mental health. *Health & Social Care in the Community, 8*(6), 425–435.

Buck, E., West, C., Graham, L., Frye, A. W., & Teal, C. R. (2019). Challenges to assessing professional identity in medical students: a tale of two measures. *Medical Education Online, 24*(1), 1649571.

Campbell, E. G., Regan, S., Gruen, R. L., Ferris, T. G., Rao, S. R., Cleary, P. D., & Blumenthal, D. (2007). Professionalism in medicine: results of a national survey of physicians. *Annals of Internal Medicine, 147*(11), 795–802.

Carmienke, S., Freitag, M. H., Pischon, T., Schlattmann, P., Fankhaenel, T., Goebel, H., & Gensichen, J. (2013). General and abdominal obesity parameters and their combination in relation to mortality: a systematic review and meta-regression analysis. *European Journal of Clinical Nutrition, 67*(6), 573–585.

Chadwick, J., & Mann, W. N. (1950). *The medical works of Hippocrates.* Oxford: Blackwell Scientific Publications.

Cohen, J. J. (2006). Professionalism in medical education, an American perspective: from evidence to accountability. *Medical Education, 40*(7), 607–617.

Coleman, T. (2000). Using video-recorded consultations for research in primary care: advantages and limitations. *Family Practice, 17*(5), 422–427.

Cowin, L. (2001). Measuring nurses' self-concept. *Western Journal of Nursing Research, 23*(3), 313–325.

Cox, M. E., Yancy, W. S., Jr., Coffman, C. J., Østbye, T., Tulsky, J. A., Alexander, S. C., Brouwer, R. J. N., Dolor, R. J., & Pollak, K. I. (2011). Effects of counseling techniques on patients' weight-related attitudes and behaviors in a primary care clinic. *Patient Education and Counseling, 85*(3), 363–368.

Cruess, R. L., Cruess, S. R., Boudreau, J. D., Snell, L., & Steinert, Y. (2014). Reframing medical education to support professional identity formation. *Academic Medicine, 89*(11), 1446–1451.

Cruess, R. L., Cruess, S. R., Boudreau, J. D., Snell, L., & Steinert, Y. (2015). A schematic representation of the professional identity formation and socialization of medical students and residents: a guide for medical educators. *Academic Medicine, 90*(6), 718–725.

de Lasson, L., Just, E., Stegeager, N., & Malling, B. (2016). Professional identity formation in the transition from medical school to working life: a qualitative study of group-coaching courses for junior doctors. BMC *Medical Education, 16,* 165.

Del Piccolo, L. (2017). VR-CoDES and patient-centeredness. The intersection points between a measure and a concept. *Patient Education and Counseling, 100*(11), 2135–2137.

Del Piccolo, L., de Haes, H., Heaven, C., Jansen, J., Verheul, W., Bensing, J., Bergvik, S., Deveugele, M., Eide, H., Fletcher, I., Goss, C., Humphris, G., Kim, Y. M., Langewitz, W., Mazzi, M. A., Mjaaland, T., Moretti, F., Nübling, M., Rimondini, M., Salmon, P., Sibbern, T., Skre, I., van Dulmen, S., Wissow, L., Young, B., Zandbelt, L., Zimmermann, C., & Finset, A. (2011). Development of the Verona coding definitions of emotional sequences to code health providers' responses (VR-CoDES-P) to patient cues and concerns. *Patient Education and Counseling, 82*(2), 149–155.

Del Piccolo, L., Finset, A., Mellblom, A. V., Figueiredo-Braga, M., Korsvold, L., Zhou, Y., Zimmermann, C., & Humphris, G. (2017). Verona coding definitions of emotional sequences (VR-CoDES): conceptual framework and future directions. *Patient Education and Counseling, 100*(12), 2303–2311.

Dewhurst, A., Peters, S., Devereux-Fitzgerald, A., & Hart, J. (2017). Physicians' views and experiences of discussing weight management within routine clinical consultations: a thematic synthesis. *Patient Education and Counseling, 100*(5), 897–908.

Ellis, R., Griffiths, L., & Hogard, E. (2015). Constructing the nurse match instrument to measure professional identity and values in nursing. *Journal of Nursing & Care, 4*(245), 1–10.

Ellis, R., & Hogard, E. (2020). Professional identity: values, selection and career choice. In J. Dent, R. Harden, & D. Hart (Eds.), *A practical guide for medical teachers* (6th ed.). Amsterdam, London, and Oxford: Elsevier.

Epstein, R. M., Duberstein, P. R., Fenton, J. J., Fiscella, K., Hoerger, M., Tancredi, D. J., Xing, G., Gramling, R., Mohile, S., Franks, P., Kaesberg, P., Plumb, S., Cipri, C. S., Street, R. L., Jr., Shields, C. G., Back, A. L., Butow, P., Walczak, A., Tattersall, M., Venuti, A., Sullivan, P., Robinson, M., Hoh, B., Lewis, L., & Kravitz, R. L. (2017). Effect of a patient-centered communication intervention on oncologist-patient communication, quality of life, and health care utilization in advanced cancer: the VOICE randomized clinical trial. *JAMA Oncology, 3*(1), 92–100.

Epstein, R. M., Franks, P., Fiscella, K., Shields, C. G., Meldrum, S. C., Kravitz, R. L., & Duberstein, P. R. (2005). Measuring patient-centered communication in patient–physician consultations: theoretical and practical issues. *Social Science & Medicine, 61*(7), 1516–1528.

Evans, R., Elwyn, G., & Edwards, A. (2004). Review of instruments for peer assessment of physicians. *BMJ*, *328*(7450), 1240.

Finset, A. (2011). Research on person-centred clinical care. *Journal of Evaluation in Clinical Practice*, *17*(2), 384–386.

Frohna, A., & Stern, D. (2005). The nature of qualitative comments in evaluating professionalism. *Medical Education*, *39*(8), 763–768.

Fromme, H. B., Karani, R., & Downing, S. M. (2009). Direct observation in medical education: a review of the literature and evidence for validity. *Mount Sinai Journal of Medicine*, *76*(4), 365–371.

Furnham, A. (2012). *The psychology of behaviour at work: the individual in the organization*. London: Psychology Press.

General Medical Council. (2013). *Good medical practice*. Retrieved 30th May 2020 from https://www.gmc-uk.org/ethical-guidance/ethical-guidance-for-doctors/good-medical-practice.

General Medical Council. (2020). *Collecting colleague and patient feedback for revalidation*. Retrieved 9th June 2020 from https://www.gmc-uk.org/registration-and-licensing/managing-your-registration/revalidation/revalidation-resources/collecting-colleague-and-patient-feedback-for-revalidation.

Gerada, C. (2016). Physician, heal thyself? *The Hippocratic Post*. Retrieved 29th May 2020 from https://www.hippocraticpost.com/mental-health/physician-heal-thyself/.

Godkin, M. A., & Savageau, J. A. (2001). The effect of a global multiculturalism track on cultural competence of preclinical medical students. *Family Medicine*, *33*(3), 178–186.

Guh, D. P., Zhang, W., Bansback, N., Amarsi, Z., Birmingham, C. L., & Anis, A. H. (2009). The incidence of co-morbidities related to obesity and overweight: a systematic review and meta-analysis. *BMC Public Health*, *9*(1), 88.

Hammoud, M. M., Morgan, H. K., Edwards, M. E., Lyon, J. A., & White, C. (2012). Is video review of patient encounters an effective tool for medical student learning? A review of the literature. *Advances in Medical Education and Practice*, *3*, 19–30.

Health Improvement Scotland. (2010). *SIGN guideline: management of obesity*. Retrieved 11th June 2020 from https://www.sign.ac.uk/sign-115-management-of-obesity

Hilton, S. R., & Slotnick, H. B. (2005). Proto-professionalism: how professionalisation occurs across the continuum of medical education. *Medical Education*, *39*(1), 58–65.

Jha, V., Bekker, H. L., Duffy, S. R., & Roberts, T. E. (2006). Perceptions of professionalism in medicine: a qualitative study. *Medical Education*, *40*(10), 1027–1036.

Kalet, A., Buckvar-Keltz, L., Harnik, V., Monson, V., Hubbard, S., Crowe, R., Song, H. S., & Yingling, S. (2017). Measuring professional identity formation early in medical school. *Medical Teacher*, *39*(3), 255–261.

King, A., & Hoppe, R. B. (2013). "Best practice" for patient-centered communication: a narrative review. *Journal of Graduate Medical Education*, *5*(3), 385–393.

Kogan, J. R., Holmboe, E. S., & Hauer, K. E. (2009). Tools for direct observation and assessment of clinical skills of medical trainees: a systematic review. *JAMA*, *302*(12), 1316–1326.

Kramer, C. K., Zinman, B., & Retnakaran, R. (2013). Are metabolically healthy overweight and obesity benign conditions? *Annals of Internal Medicine*, *159*(11), 758–769.

Kraschnewski, J. L., Sciamanna, C. N., Stuckey, H. L., Chuang, C. H., Lehman, E. B., Hwang, K. O., Sherwood, L. L., & Nembhard, H. B. (2013). A silent response to the obesity epidemic: decline in US physician weight counseling. *Medical Care*, *51*(2), 186–192.

Laidlaw, A., McHale, C., Locke, H., & Cecil, J. (2015). Talk weight: an observational study of communication about patient weight in primary care consultations. *Primary Health Care Research & Development*, 16(3), 309–315.

Laidlaw, A., Napier, C., Neville, F., Collinson, A., & Cecil, J. E. (2019). Talking about weight talk: primary care practitioner knowledge, attitudes and practice. *Journal of Communication in Healthcare*, 12(3–4), 145–153.

Lane, C., Huws-Thomas, M., Hood, K., Rollnick, S., Edwards, K., & Robling, M. (2005). Measuring adaptations of motivational interviewing: the development and validation of the behavior change counseling index (BECCI). *Patient Education and Counseling*, 56(2), 166–173.

Lane, S. (2018). Professionalism and professional identity: what are they, and what are they to you? *Australian Medical Student Journal*, 8(2), 10–15.

Matthews, J., Bialocerkowski, A., & Molineux, M. (2019). Professional identity measures for student health professionals – a systematic review of psychometric properties. *BMC Medical Education*, 19(1), 308.

Mavor, K. I., McNeill, K. G., Anderson, K., Kerr, A., O'Reilly, E., & Platow, M. J. (2014). Beyond prevalence to process: the role of self and identity in medical student well-being. *Medical Education*, 48(4), 351–360.

McCambridge, J., Witton, J., & Elbourne, D. R. (2014). Systematic review of the Hawthorne effect: new concepts are needed to study research participation effects. *Journal of Clinical Epidemiology*, 67(3), 267–277.

McHale, C. T., Cecil, J. E., & Laidlaw, A. H. (2019). An analysis of directly observed weight communication processes between primary care practitioners and overweight patients. *Patient Education and Counseling*, 102(12), 2214–2222.

McHale, C. T., Laidlaw, A. H., & Cecil, J. E. (2016). Direct observation of weight-related communication in primary care: a systematic review. *Family Practice*, 33(4), 327–345.

McHale, C. T., Laidlaw, A. H., & Cecil, J. E. (2020). Primary care patient and practitioner views of weight and weight-related discussion: a mixed-methods study. *BMJ Open*, 10(3), e034023.

Michie, S. (2007). Talking to primary care patients about weight: a study of GPs and practice nurses in the UK. *Psychology, Health & Medicine*, 12(5), 521–525.

National Institute for Health and Care Excellence. (2014). *Weight management: lifestyle services for overweight or obese adults – Public health guideline [PH53]*. Retrieved 11th June 2020 from https://www.nice.org.uk/guidance/ph53

Noldus Information Technology. (2020). *The Observer XT Version 12*. https://www.noldus.com/observer-xt.

Norcini, J. J., Blank, L. L., Duffy, F. D., & Fortna, G. S. (2003). The mini-CEX: a method for assessing clinical skills. *Annals of Internal Medicine*, 138(6), 476–481.

Ogunleye, A. A., Osunlana, A., Asselin, J., Cave, A., Sharma, A. M., & Campbell-Scherer, D. L. (2015). The 5As team intervention: bridging the knowledge gap in obesity management among primary care practitioners. *BMC Research Notes*, 8(1), 810.

Ong, L. M., Visser, M. R., Kruyver, I., Bensing, J. M., Van Den Brink-Muinen, A., Stouthard, J., Lammes, F. B., & De Haes, J. C. (1998). The Roter interaction analysis system (RIAS) in oncological consultations: psychometric properties. *Psycho-Oncology*, 7(5), 387–401.

Ong, Y. T., Kow, C. S., Teo, Y. H., Tan, L. H. E., Abdurrahman, A., Quek, N. W. S., Prakash, K., Cheong, C. W. S., Tan, X. H., Lim, W. Q., Wu, J., Tan, L. H. S., Tay, K. T., Chin, A., Toh, Y. P., Mason, S., & Radha Krishna, L. K. (2020). Nurturing professionalism in medical schools. A systematic scoping review of training curricula between 1990-2019. *Medical Teacher*, 1–14.

Pinto, R. Z., Ferreira, M. L., Oliveira, V. C., Franco, M. R., Adams, R., Maher, C. G., & Ferreira, P. H. (2012). Patient-centred communication is associated with positive therapeutic alliance: a systematic review. *Journal of Physiotherapy*, 58(2), 77–87.

Pollak, K. I., Alexander, S. C., Coffman, C. J., Tulsky, J. A., Lyna, P., Dolor, R. J., James, I. E., Brouwer, R. J. N., Manusov, J. R., & Østbye, T. (2010). Physician communication techniques and weight loss in adults: project CHAT. *American Journal of Preventive Medicine*, 39(4), 321–328.

Pollak, K. I., Ostbye, T., Alexander, S. C., Gradison, M., Bastian, L. A., Brouwer, R. J. N., & Lyna, P. (2007). Empathy goes a long way in weight loss discussions: female patients are more likely to step up weight loss efforts when a physician shows empathy and offers support. *Journal of Family Practice*, 56(12), 1031–1037.

Roter, D., & Larson, S. (2002). The Roter interaction analysis system (RIAS): utility and flexibility for analysis of medical interactions. *Patient Education and Counseling*, 46(4), 243–251.

Royal College of Physicians. (2005). *Doctors in society: medical professionalism in a changing world*. https://shop.rcplondon.ac.uk/products/doctors-in-society-medical-professionalism-in-a-changing-world?variant=6337443013

Royal College of Physicians. (2018). *Advancing medical professionalism*. Retrieved 30th May 2020 from https://www.rcplondon.ac.uk/projects/outputs/advancing-medical-professionalism

Singer, P. A., Robb, A., Cohen, R., Norman, G., & Turnbull, J. (1996). Performance-based assessment of clinical ethics using an objective structured clinical examination. *Academic Medicine*, 71(5).

Sokol, J. T. (2009). Identity development throughout the lifetime: an examination of Eriksonian theory. *Graduate Journal of Counseling Psychology*, 1(2), 14.

Stewart, M. A. (1995). Effective physician-patient communication and health outcomes: a review. *CMAJ*, 152(9), 1423.

Swick, H. M. (2000). Toward a normative definition of medical professionalism. *Academic Medicine*, 75(6).

Tan, C. P., Van der Molen, H. T., & Schmidt, H. G. (2017). A measure of professional identity development for professional education. *Studies in Higher Education*, 42(8), 1504–1519.

Themessl-Huber, M., Humphris, G., Dowell, J., Macgillivray, S., Rushmer, R., & Williams, B. (2008). Audio-visual recording of patient–GP consultations for research purposes: a literature review on recruiting rates and strategies. *Patient Education and Counseling*, 71(2), 157–168.

Trede, F., Macklin, R., & Bridges, D. (2012). Professional identity development: a review of the higher education literature. *Studies in Higher Education*, 37(3), 365–384.

Tsai, A. G., Wadden, T. A., Volger, S., Sarwer, D. B., Vetter, M., Kumanyika, S., Berkowitz, R. I., Diewald, L. K., Perez, J., Lavenberg, J., Panigrahi, E. R., & Glick, H. A. (2013). Cost-effectiveness of a primary care intervention to treat obesity. *International Journal of Obesity*, 37(1), S31–S37.

Turner, A., & Knight, J. (2015. A debate on the professional identity of occupational therapists. *British Journal of Occupational Therapy*, 78(11), 664–673.

Turner, J. C., & Oakes, P. J. (1986). The significance of the social identity concept for social psychology with reference to individualism, interactionism and social influence. *British Journal of Social Psychology*, 25(3), 237–252.

UK Government. (2015). *The NHS Constitution: the NHS belongs to all of us*. Retrieved 30th May 2020 from https://www.gov.uk/government/publications/the-nhs-constitution-for-england.

van de Camp, K., Vernooij-Dassen, M., Grol, R., & Bottema, B. (2006). Professionalism in general practice: development of an instrument to assess professional behaviour in general practitioner trainees. *Medical Education, 40*(1), 43–50.

Van De Camp, K., Vernooij-Dassen, M. J., Grol, R. P., & Bottema, B. J. (2004). How to conceptualize professionalism: a qualitative study. *Medical Teacher, 26*(8), 696–702.

van Zanten, M., Boulet, J. R., Norcini, J. J., & McKinley, D. (2005). Using a standardised patient assessment to measure professional attributes. *Medical Education, 39*(1), 20–29.

Vough, H. (2012). Not all identifications are created equal: exploring employee accounts for workgroup, organizational, and professional identification. *Organization Science, 23*(3), 778–800.

Wagner, P., Hendrich, J., Moseley, G., & Hudson, V. (2007). Defining medical professionalism: a qualitative study. *Medical Education, 41*(3), 288–294.

Weis, D., & Schank, M. J. (2009). Development and psychometric evaluation of the nurses professional values scale—revised. *Journal of Nursing Measurement*, (3), 221–231.

Wilkinson, T. J., Wade, W. B., & Knock, L. D. (2009). A blueprint to assess professionalism: results of a systematic review. *Academic Medicine, 84*(5).

Willetts, G., & Clarke, D. (2014). Constructing nurses' professional identity through social identity theory. *International Journal of Nursing Practice, 20*(2), 164–169.

World Health Organisation. (2020). *Overweight and obesity*. Retrieved 8th June 2020 from https://www.who.int/en/news-room/fact-sheets/detail/obesity-and-overweight

Zhou, Y., Collinson, A., Laidlaw, A., & Humphris, G. (2013). How do medical students respond to emotional cues and concerns expressed by simulated patients during OSCE consultations? – a multilevel study. *PLoS One, 8*(10).

Zolnierek, K. B. H., & Dimatteo, M. R. (2009). Physician communication and patient adherence to treatment: a meta-analysis. *Medical Care, 47*(8), 826–834.

21 Conclusion

Professional identity and the curriculum

Roger Ellis and Elaine Hogard

One of our aims in producing this book was to offer ideas for the professional training curriculum in the caring professions. We invited all contributors, whatever their topic, to reflect on the three themes of the book of which Mastery is one. In principle, therefore, all of the chapters in this book should have some implications for the initial training curriculum, some more obviously than others.

A consensus has emerged in the book that a comprehensive model of Professional Identity (PI) should be the overall organising idea in the curriculum. If such an approach was adopted, this would have implications for selection; aims and objectives, teaching and learning methods, assessment and careers guidance. In the remainder of this chapter, we will look at ideas for a curriculum with PI as its overarching theme and organiser. The curriculum could be called the 'Curriculum for Professional Identity Development' or CuPID which may be a useful acronym to keep the curriculum aim on the PI target!

We will now consider the implications of CuPID for aspects of the professional training curriculum in relation to:

- Overall design and aims and objectives
- Selection
- Content
- Teaching and learning methods
- Assessment
- Careers guidance

Overall design and aims and objectives

The idea of CuPID is that PI, broadly defined, as encompassing knowledge, competence and values, would be the organising concept for the curriculum as a whole. Obviously, the prerequisite for this is that curriculum developers should first produce their model of PI. It would then be a touchstone for all parts of the curriculum.

Developing a model of PI would have several advantages. It would both give a wholistic justification for the curriculum and also determine its component parts.

The model should determine the aims and objectives for the curriculum as a whole and for all its elements. It should be possible to justify any curricular elements with regards to its content, teaching and learning and assessment through its contribution to the development the desired PI in students. This identity should be articulated and communicated at all points in the programme from selection onwards to give a direction and coherence to all parts of the programme. In this sense, CuPID is both integrative regarding the unity of the curriculum as a whole and reductionist in validating its component parts.

Our model for PI has three main components. These are in brief knowledge, competence and values. Thus, a PI is made up of what the professional knows, what the professional can do and the values that should underpin these cognitions and actions. This trichotomy is easily identified in training curricula. There are of course strong traditions of theoretical knowledge playing a key role in the curriculum. One conventional model is to include modules in foundation sciences, whatever these might be thought to be, followed by more applied modules that culminate in modules that address particular specialisms. This knowledge can be taught through a well-established pattern of lectures and seminars and assessed through course work and written exams, including Multiple Response Papers or MCQ's, which simplify marking.

The teaching and learning of the second element, competencies, has seen the most development over the last 20 years with competency-based curricula emerging in all the caring professions. This necessitates an analysis of the professional role to identify those skills or competencies that are required, the construction of practical training programmes to develop these and then the devising of appropriate forms of performance-based assessment. Typically, this part of the curriculum is taught through practical placements in the field of professional activity, linked with some form of practicum in the university. There are problems in devising and implementing reliable and valid assessment methods for such placement activities. In some cases, this is made more manageable, whilst still demanding through such testing methods as Objective Structured Clinical Examinations (OSCEs) (Harden et al., 2015) and multiple mini interviews (MMIs) (Pau et al, 2013).

The third element, values, remains the most problematic to identify, teach, learn and assess. In addressing the measurement part of the book's title, we have introduced a particular approach to measuring PI: ISA/Ipseus. There could, of course, be others, but the important thing is to have some way of measuring the value orientation of applicants, students and graduates. Given such a measure, it can be used to aid selection and as a check at points in the programme to measure progress towards an appropriate values base. It can be used to track the development of an important part of PI.

As explained in Chapter 17, the development of such a measure requires the identification of appropriate values, from the literature, from professional codifications and from ethnographic work with key stakeholders in the profession and the community. A list of values then becomes part of the PI model and can inform teaching, learning and assessment in the same way as knowledge and competency listings.

In constructing the PI model for a programme, planners will obviously draw on current curriculum documents and reviews. The importance of identifying these knowledge and competency components lies in their inclusion in the PI model that will be the touchstone for the relevance curriculum and its components.

Once constructed, the model should then translate into overall aims and objectives and aims and objectives for its individual parts. Every part must be justified for its contribution to the development of each student's PI. This must be a conscious decision by faculty members and apparent to students at every stage of their programme. While students will, of course, question the relevance of parts of their programme, the answer should always be in relation to the PI model of which they should be well aware.

Selection

Selection is the culmination of the Application Process when decisions are made as to who should be admitted to a programme. Selection should be based on valid and reliable evidence about a candidate. This evidence is evaluated against standards in comparison with other candidates and in the context of the number of places available. This process should be transparent, fair and defensible.

Selection should be predictive of success on the programme and ultimately as a professional practitioner. Programmes will consist of academic and practical learning components together with the development of a PI and its values.

Selection for the academic component is the most straightforward since it can be based on national examination results and also, when available, on dedicated standardised tests for prospective students. Using these results in selection helps meet the requirement for transparency, fairness and defensibility.

Gauging potential for practical learning and professional development is more problematic. The applicant may be required to produce evidence of relevant practical activities. Evidence may be drawn from a wide range of experiences including:

- Work experience placements
- Experience of paid employment
- Volunteer work
- Participation in social activities
- Educational experience

However, the availability, acceptability and evaluation of this evidence are relatively unreliable and dubiously valid.

Practical assessments may be built into selection through simulations or even preliminary OSCEs. Use can be made of MMIs where each interview requires a practical response. Face-to-face interviews may include an assessment of communication skills and also the inference from responses that applicants hold the right values.

Assessing the values held by applicants and their potential for developing the values central to a PI is particularly difficult. This approach to selection is called values-based recruitment (VBR). VBR is a method that draws upon and chooses individuals whose values are in keeping with the respective institution (NHS Employers, 2014).

Professional values are of course not directly observable but have to be inferred from behaviour in the professional role. Clearly this is not feasible for applicants. Methods that are used to assess values prior to selection can include:

- Structured interviews;
- Multiple mini interviews;
- Selection centres; and
- Situational Judgement Tests (for screening).

Scoring these activities depends on valid and reliable inference from behaviour to values by trained observers. The candidate's response to questions or in a personal statement depends on their ability to reflect on their own values. This self-report evidence is of doubtful validity since it assumes that applicants are able to reflect on their values and that they will report them honestly rather than saying what they believe is required. A more cost-effective approach may be to require applicants to complete an appropriate psychometric test assuming a suitable one is available.

We have developed such a VBR test for selection in Nursing programmes, Nurse Match, and are working on something similar for medicine and social work as described in Chapter 18. The idea is to build into selection procedures psychometrically sound evidence of the professionally related values held by applicants and the extent to which these match those which an ideal professional should hold. The test may be tailored in part to the particular values that would be consistent with the distinctive regional mission of the school.

In summary, selection should be driven by judgements on the applicant's potential to develop the PI specified for the programme. Thus, selection should be the first place where the CuPID approach is apparent.

Content

It is not our intention in this chapter to suggest specific content that should be included in the professional curriculum. Our main point is that all content should meet the requirements of the CuPID approach; that is, it should demonstrate its relevance to the PI model identified for the programme. The question should be asked: how does this content contribute to the development of a PI? Of course, the danger here might be a kind of circularity where particular knowledge is specified for the knowledge component of the PI model; coverage of this knowledge then leads to content in a particular module that is then justified in relation to the PI model.

This brings into play another assumption of the PI model which is that its component parts should be integrated into a wholistic identity. Thus, specific knowledge should relate, where possible, to specific actions that are underpinned by values. For example, in a medical programme, courses in anatomy and physiology underpin the medical sciences that inform the diagnostic practices of a physician which should be carried out in a manner that is technically competent and informed by a respect for persons. We expressed an early form of this approach in what we called the Action Focus Curriculum where all the content in a programme was justified by its contribution to professional action (Ellis, 1992). Our current approach develops that by integrating the values component of the PI model adopted.

Teaching and learning

There is a substantial literature in all the caring professions regarding teaching and learning, although as we pointed out recently (Ellis and Hogard, 2019) this lacks a systematic and organised empirical and theoretical base. Within this literature the development and teaching of values receives relatively less attention. There is a general belief evident in several chapters in this book that professional values are best developed through some form of personal mentoring by an experienced professional, particularly in the workplace. Such mentoring would we would suggest be enhanced by a shared focus on the kind of PI model we are advocating.

Supervising and mentoring in the workplace is undertaken by people with a kind of hybrid PI combining expertise in the profession with expertise as a teacher. The Clinical Facilitators we described in Chapter 18 were examples of this kind of hybrid being qualified as both Nurses and Educationalists and required to bridge the gap between the hospital and the university to maximise professional development for students on placement.

The question we posed was how do they do it? What teaching and learning methods do they employ and what could be learned from this for placement supervision not just in Nursing but caring professions more broadly. The evaluation is described in detail in Chapter 18, but it is worth extracting their characterisation of their methods that were elicited through consultation with them. This is the coal face of PI development.

The responses given by the Clinical Facilitators to the researcher mainly concerned their work at the supervisory level of direct face-to-face teaching of students. On the basis of the detailed list of activities generated by their responses, the supervisory role was categorised provisionally into six main types of activity or teaching methods:

- demonstrating a skill to a student;
- pointing out good practice to a student (denotation);
- giving the student a chance to practise a skill;
- discussing the student's work with them;
- giving the student a chance to practise in a skills laboratory or workshop; and giving the student a lecture about a skill.

This process is a good example of how teaching and learning activities can integrate theory and practice in relation to the PI development of student nurses. It has to be assumed that the practise denotated and encouraged was informed by appropriate values, but this was not explored in the study. The main point is that it could have been addressed if the supervision was in relation to a PI model.

Assessment

Assessment is a vital part of any programme. It is intended to demonstrate that the objectives of the programme have been met and that, in a professional programme, graduating students are fit to practise. Assessment stages throughout the programme are referred to as formative and those at the end as summative. Assessment provides feedback to students on whether they are meeting objectives and how effective their learning has been. Finally, assessment also provides important data for teachers on how effective their teaching has been. The remainder of this section looks at ways that might optimise this feedback for identity development.

In our CuPID approach, we are suggesting an enhanced and central role for assessment in a student's personal identity development. Assessment should clearly relate to the PI model adopted for the curriculum in respect of knowledge, competence, values and their integration. There are two problems with this aspiration. First, assessment is most established with regard to knowledge, developing with regard to competence, but problematic for values. In this context, values can be relatively neglected or assumed. A CuPID assessment scheme will require creativity in devising assessments that relate to values, as well as, knowledge and competence, but which are also where possible integrated as the PI should be. Assessment and its requirements can take on a separate life of their own being a preoccupation of students and faculty but not central to the development of a PI.

Several contributors have drawn attention to Programmatic Assessment as addressing the problems of assessment and optimising its teaching and learning potential. This approach was developed by Van der Vleuten et al. (2012) in the Netherlands and represents a radical paradigm shift and restructuring of assessment in, in their case, a medical programme. There are certainly features of Programmatic Assessment that would enhance the focus on PI that we are advocating, but this can be done without adopting the whole approach. Readers may be interested in adopting programmatic assessment as a whole but guidance for that is beyond the scope of this chapter. Van der Vleuten et al (2015) set out clearly the steps to follow to implement such an assessment programme. While Programmatic Assessment has been developed for Medical Education, we believe it has the potential to be applied in the curricula of other professions.

There are several features of Programmatic Assessment that could improve any curriculum. First is the idea that assessment should be considered as a learning and teaching programme in itself (Van der Vleuten et al., 2012). This is radical notion since assessment is often seen as no more than a necessary pendant to the main elements in the curriculum rather than a programme in itself. Second, and following on from this, the students should be encouraged to learn from their assessment results and guided to see how these results can enhance the development of their PI. This process of identity development should be supported by an individual mentor who helps the students to learn from assessment results and their experience of them.

In considering assessment as a programme, objectives should be set which clearly point to the development through assessment of an aspect of PI whether this is concerned with knowledge, competence or values.

There should be an overall master plan for assessment that relates clearly to the overarching structure of the curriculum, in this case, the development of a student's PI. The various points when assessment information is recorded should cohere to illuminate aspects of the PI model adopted.

Examination regulations should be concerned not only with pass/fail and remediation but should also specify the kind of feedback that is provided and its function in learning and identity development.

The collection, storage and analysis of assessment data should be underpinned with a robust and secure system that can provide detailed information of each student's profile and their PI development. This profile should be readily available for confidential individual mentoring. The information provided for students should be both qualitative and quantitative. Their responses should be compared with ideal responses. They should be encouraged to consider how their understanding, performance and value position, revealed by their results, might be enhanced to contribute to their PI development.

Throughout their programme each student should have a PI development mentor whose role would include providing constructive analysis of assessment results and deciding steps to enhance professional development.

In summary, then we are suggesting that assessment should be conceived, not only as a necessary series of standards, but as a key learning programme for the development of the student's PI.

Careers choice and guidance

Careers choice is the process whereby students make, ideally, a well-informed, realistic decision about their future career. This choice involves, in principle, a matching of the student's emergent PI with that of the specialism they choose. Careers guidance is the process provided by the school that enables this decision. While some form of choice, possibly less than ideal, will happen inevitably, careers guidance appears to vary widely between schools.

As an example, Medicine is a vocational degree with a large number of postgraduate options. Comparable lists could be produced for each of the caring professions and should be available to all students.

Jobs directly related to a medical degree include:

- Anaesthetist
- Cardiologist
- Clinical radiologist

- General practice doctor/community physician
- Hospital doctor
- Neurologist
- Ophthalmologist
- Pathologist
- Psychiatrist
- Surgeon

Jobs where the degree would be useful include:

- Children's nurse
- Adult nurse
- Clinical scientist, genomics
- Higher education lecturer
- International aid/development worker
- Medical sales representative
- Medical science liaison
- Mental health nurse
- Midwife
- Naturopath
- Paramedic
- Physician associate
- Research scientist (life sciences)
- Science writer

Within medicine and other caring professions, there are routes into research, teaching, administration and management, in addition to the clinical specialisms.

Ideally, for each of these possible careers, there will be a comprehensive identity profile with which the student's developing PI can be matched.

Choice is a function of both personal and external factors and may continue for some throughout the student's undergraduate programme (Pianosi et al, 2016). Factors that are reported as influencing students' career choices range from personality and personal attributes, to gender differences, to issues of prestige and income. Lifestyle issues and role models are identified as prominent factors influencing students (Yang et al, 2019). While all this factors have been demonstrated to have an influence on choice, few studies have addressed career choice on a broad scale integrating factors. We could find no studies where PI was considered in relation to choice. Clearly, identity and PI will have a bearing on choice, but there is an absence of research that follows this line of enquiry.

It is recognised by programme accreditors in, for example, medicine that the school has an important role in supporting and facilitating career choice. However, the standards set by, for example, CACMS are general and lack specific guidance. Somewhat more helpful the GMC requires that all doctors in training must have an educational supervisor who should provide, through constructive and regular dialogue, feedback on performance and assistance in career progression (Hogard et al, 2019). The training programme director should also have career management skills (or be able to provide access to them) and be able to provide career advice to doctors in training within their programme.

There is not a wealth of research studies of the effectiveness of career guidance. However, our impression is that careers guidance, as part of the undergraduate curriculum, is relatively neglected, variable in form and doubtfully effective.

To address this, we would suggest that Careers Guidance should be treated as other parts of the curriculum with learning objectives, a syllabus, teaching and learning methods and assessment. It should also be subject to the programme evaluation process. This part of the curriculum should as all others be clearly related to the central focus on the student's developing PI. When there are a number of possible routes, identity profiles should be constructed for these options and students encouraged to match their developing identity profiles with these options.

Conclusion

In this chapter, we have proposed that the development of a PI should be the focus of the training curriculum. This identity should be characterised through its knowledge, competence and values components. This central focus should be apparent in selection, course structure, aims and objectives, teaching and learning, assessment and careers guidance. We have labelled this approach with the acronym CuPID: Curriculum for Professional Identity Development. We would be interested to work with professional teams looking to develop or review their curriculum in this manner.

References

Ellis, R. (1992). An action-focus curriculum for the interpersonal professions. *Learning to Effect*, 69–86.

Ellis, R., & Hogard, E. (Eds.). (2019). *Handbook of Quality Assurance for University Teaching*. London and Ne York: Routledge.

Harden, R. M., Lilley, P., & Patricio, M. (2015). *The Definitive Guide to the OSCE: The Objective Structured Clinical Examination as a Performance Assessment*. London: Elsevier Health Sciences.

Hogard, E., Hunt, D., Lichtenstein, J., Walters, T., & Ellis, R. (2019). Quality assurance in medical education: accreditation and teaching standards in Australia, the USA, Canada and the UK. In *Handbook of Quality Assurance for University Teaching* (pp. 100–114). Routledge.

NHS Employers (2014). Values-Based Recruitment Interviews: Example Pre-reading Material: Accessible from: http://www.nhsemployers.org/-/media/Employers/Documents/Recruit/VBI%20Training%20Example%20Pre-reading.docx.

Pau, A., Jeevaratnam, K., Chen, Y. S., Fall, A. A., Khoo, C., & Nadarajah, V. D. (2013). The multiple mini-interview (MMI) for student selection in health professions training – a systematic review. *Medical teacher*, 35(12), 1027–1041.

Pianosi, K., Bethune, C., & Hurley, K. F. (2016). Medical student career choice: a qualitative study of fourth-year medical students at Memorial University, Newfoundland. *CMAJ open*, 4(2), E147.

Van der Vleuten, C. P., Schuwirth, L. W., Driessen, E. W., Dijkstra, J., Tigelaar, D., Baartman, L. K., & van Tartwijk, J. (2012). A model for programmatic assessment fit for purpose. *Medical teacher*, 34, 205–214.

Van Der Vleuten, C. P., Schuwirth, L. W. T., Driessen, E. W., Govaerts, M. J. B., & Heeneman, S. (2015). Twelve tips for programmatic assessment. *Medical teacher*, 37(7), 641–646.

Yang, Y., Li, J., Wu, X., Wang, J., Li, W., Zhu, Y., Chen, C., & Lin, H. (2019). Factors influencing subspecialty choice among medical students: a systematic review and meta-analysis. *BMJ open*, 9(3), e022097.

Index

Printed in the United States
By Bookmasters